How to choose?

HOW TO CHOOSE?
A Comparison of the U.S. and Canadian Health Care Systems

Edited by
Robert Chernomas
and
Ardeshir Sepehri

POLICY, POLITICS, HEALTH AND MEDICINE Series
Vicente Navarro, Series Editor

Baywood Publishing Company, Inc.
Amityville, New York

12/98

36900731

Library of Congress Catalog Number: 97-14841
ISBN: 0-89503-180-9 (Cloth)

Library of Congress Cataloging-in-Publication Data

     Main entry under title:

How to choose? : a comparison of the U.S. and Canadian health care
    systems / edited by Robert Chernomas and Ardeshir Sepehri.
        p.   cm. - - (Policy, politics, health and medicine series)
    Includes bibliographical references and index.
    ISBN 0-89503-180-9 (cloth)
     1. Medical care- -United States. 2. Medical care- -Canada.
I. Chernomas, Robert.   II. Sepehri, Ardeshir.   III. Series.
RA395.A3H68   1997
362.1'0971- -dc21   97-14841
                                        CIP

For my brother Fred,
who would have understood, he always did.
R.J.C.

TABLE OF CONTENTS

Introduction

Robert Chernomas and Ardeshir Sepehri

North America has witnessed a quasi-experiment in its health care institutions over the past quarter of a century. As late as the 1960s the U.S. and Canadian health care systems were virtually identical: both spent the same amount of money on health care as a percentage of GNP and delivered their services in a similar way. By 1971 the systems' financing and decision-making processes began to diverge significantly. Canada continued to consolidate its single-payer system while the United States continued its market-oriented system.

As a result, researchers have begun to examine a number of issues related to this "experiment," ranging from economics to medicine to political outcomes. These researchers have focused their lenses on intercountry comparisons of a diversity of issues, including:

- *Costs of health care,* requiring a determination of: (*a*) how to measure intercountry health cost trends and (*b*) what should be included in this measure.
- *Access,* to determine what percentage of the population of each country has access to what level of care: the *quality of outcome,* to determine whether one system does a better job of performing medical services than the other.
- *System satisfaction and acceptability,* to determine whether the population of each country is satisfied with its system and the degree to which it would find the alternative system acceptable.

COMPARATIVE INSTITUTIONAL BACKGROUND

In the two decades preceding 1971, Canada's health care system was evolving from a system in which private insurance dominated the financing side and fee-for-service providers dominated the delivery side. By 1971 the privately funded system had evolved into a publicly funded system based on single insurers—the provincial governments—with costs shared by the federal

1

government in exchange for federal rules. Private insurance is prohibited from covering the same benefits as the public system. The delivery system is composed largely of nonprofit community hospitals and self-employed physicians. Hospitals are funded on the basis of global budgets, and physicians are paid on a fee-for-service basis negotiated with the provincial governments.

By 1971 the federal government had in place a system that funded 50 percent of physician and hospital costs paid by the provincial governments. The Federal Provincial Fiscal Arrangements and Established Programs Act of 1977 replaced this matching grant system. These grants are based on the federal government's national average per capita payments increased annually by the average nominal growth in GDP. The change was introduced as a cost-control measure since the open-ended nature of the matching grant approach was thought to limit the provinces' incentives to control costs.

This change added incentive for the provincial governments to cut costs. The resulting stringent negotiations over hospital budgets and physicians' fees encouraged hospitals to raise user fees and physicians to practice extra-billing so that out-of-pocket expenditures would pay an increasing share of health care costs, thus reducing the share from government revenues. The shift in 1977 to the indexed per capita grant system was followed by an increase in extra-billing and user fees as provinces searched for additional ways to raise revenues.

In January 1984 the Alberta government passed legislation requiring hospitals to levy charges if they wanted to spend beyond their global budgets. Three months later the federal government passed the Canada Health Act, which stipulated that federal payments to the provinces would be reduced by the amount of user charges by hospitals and extra-billings by physicians. The Act is the basis for the Canadian health care system. It describes the five criteria for a provincial plan to be eligible for a federal subsidy.

- *Public administration*—Each provincial plan must be run by a nonprofit, public authority accountable to the provincial government.
- *Comprehensiveness*—Provinces must provide coverage for all necessary physician and hospital services including dental surgical services rendered in hospitals.
- *Universality*—Insured services must be universally available to all residents of the province under uniform terms and conditions. For new residents, the waiting period to entitlement cannot exceed three months.
- *Portability*—Each provincial plan must be portable so that eligible residents are covered while they are temporarily out of the province.
- *Accessibility*—Reasonable access to insured services is not to be impaired by charges or other mechanisms. In addition, reasonable compensation must be made to physicians and dentists for providing insured health services.

These federal criteria ensure that the 12 separate health plans in Canada are largely similar: all provinces provide insurance for medically necessary services to citizens at zero price at the point of delivery.

As a result of economic stagnation and conservative economic policy (e.g., deindexing the per capita grant) the federal contribution, as a percentage of total public spending on health care, has been declining over time, while per capita health expenditures have been growing. The result is increasing pressure on the provinces and private sector to meet the financial needs of the health care system. The provinces in turn have reduced the number of services covered, and the private sector has begun to take on a larger role.

Currently, the federal government retains its considerable influence on the provincial health care plans, and the federal contribution is still sufficient to ensure that provinces uphold the standards outlined in the Canada Health Act. However, if the federal government's share of total public spending on health care continues to decline, the provinces will bear more of the financing responsibility. The provincial Ministries of Health may then become more independent. If continued, this trend would cast doubt on the ability of the federal government to maintain standards for health care in Canada.

The U.S. health care system is the most market-oriented system and the United States is the only major industrialized country without a national health care system, relying on out-of-pocket payments and private insurance for the majority of its health care spending. Health expenditure trends in the 1960s and 1970s were strongly expansionary as public and private funding grew. The subsequent failure of piecemeal cost-containment efforts has led third-party payers in one of two directions. The federal government and many state governments have introduced prospective reimbursements and have often chosen to cut those reimbursements to providers based on sheer monopsony power. Private insurers have moved toward more utilization control and the adoption of other managed care techniques to restructure the incentives of providers and patients. These techniques include control over decisions about health care services provided, either prospectively or retrospectively, limiting or influencing patients' choice of providers, and negotiating different payment terms or levels with certain providers.

Physicians are paid under a variety of arrangements, including fee-for-service, salaries, or, increasingly, capitation and other risk-sharing arrangements. While fee-for-service arrangements may encourage high-cost low-benefit health care, managed care uses risk-sharing primary care physicians as gatekeepers to specialists and hospital sectors in order to control costs. This growing institutional arrangement has also raised issues of quality of care.

Hospitals, like physicians, are paid in several ways with an increased emphasis on prospective pricing. Increasingly, rates are a fixed payment per diagnosis, such as diagnosis-related groups under Medicare, or are per diem or cost-per-case rates. Relatively low payments by Medicare, Medicaid, and managed care entities have led hospitals to shift costs to private insurers and to outpatient services.

One consequence of rising health care costs and cost containment pressures is that a large and growing portion of the U.S. population is without health insurance, while many more are underinsured. In addition, private insurers and HMOs try to avoid insuring high-risk individuals, with the result that those with greatest need for health insurance coverage must pay the highest premiums or go without coverage. In a word, it is a system of rising costs and declining access requiring structural reform if an efficient and equitable health care system is to evolve.

OVERVIEW OF THE BOOK

Comparing the U.S. and Canadian health care systems has been a significant part of the search for a more efficient, efficacious, and equitable health institution. Part I of this book explores the economists' debate over the relative costs of the two health care systems. It examines the different means of measuring health costs used by economists as well as what should and should not be included in these measurements. The authors debate these issues from theoretical, institutional, and empirical vantage points. The first two chapters, by Evans and colleagues and Fuchs and Hahn, describe the Canadian health care system and its cost-control mechanisms, and Chapter 3 by Newhouse, Anderson, and Roos provides a comparative analysis of hospital spending in the United States and Canada. In Chapter 4 Neuschler argues that the Canadian health care system's expenditures, when measured properly, are relatively more expensive in comparison to the U.S. system than previously thought, but Barer, Welch, and Antioch suggest that Neuschler has relied on a flawed measurement methodology and has ignored significant institutional circumstances. Krasny and Ferrier argue in Chapter 5 that with respect to cost, access, quality, and political acceptability the U.S. systems' advantages over the Canadian system are greater than conventionally perceived because researchers tend not to incorporate all the relevant factors. Waldo and Sonnefeld suggest, however, that Krasny and Ferrier are selective in their choice of the relevant factors that need to be incorporated into the comparative analysis. Part I ends with a chapter by Chernomas and Sepehri providing an economist's overview of the debate on cost and what is to be measured with respect to the Canadian and U.S. health care systems.

Part II explores the debate on access and quality in the U.S. and Canadian systems. Critics of the Canadian system argue that its universal system of access is deeply flawed by a rationing problem in the form of waiting lists. Critics of the U.S. system argue that a large and growing percentage of the population has inadequate access to a system that is neither efficient nor relatively efficacious. In addition, Part II includes research that makes intercountry comparisons of medical outcomes for the same interventions on similar patients in both countries. The chapters by Himmelstein, Woolhandler, and Wolfe (Chapter 7), Bodenheimer (Chapter 8), and Morgan (Chapter 11) explore access to health care in the United States. Himmelstein and Woolhandler compare access in the two countries (Chapter 9) while Ramsay and Walker (Chapter 10) measure the waiting time for patients in the Canadian system. Chapters 12–15 provide data on medical interventions in the two countries with respect to appropriateness and outcomes.

Part III incorporates surveys and debate on the U.S. and Canadian health care systems in terms of satisfaction, interest, and willingness to accept either the U.S. market-driven system or the Canadian single-payer system. In Chapter 16 Himmelstein and Woolhandler provide a graphic review of public opinion surveys on the Canadian and U.S. health care systems. The final chapter presents a debate between Blendon and Altman, who provide evidence that Americans are inconsistent about their goals for the U.S. health care system, and Navarro, who suggests that Americans are not schizophrenic with respect to their health care system.

In the Conclusion we present an update of trends in Canada and the United States, and suggest directions for future research.

PART I. THE RELATIVE COSTS OF THE CANADIAN AND U.S. HEALTH CARE SYSTEMS

CHAPTER 1

Controlling Health Expenditures—
The Canadian Reality

Robert G. Evans, Jonathan Lomas, Morris L. Barer,
Roberta J. Labelle, Catherine Fooks, Gregory L. Stoddart,
Geoffrey M. Anderson, David Feeny, Amiram Gafni,
George W. Torrance, and William G. Tholl

American interest in the Canadian health care system appears to be on the rise, as evidenced in a three-part article by Iglehart (1–3) in *The New England Journal of Medicine.* Such interest has been intermittent in the past, depending in part on the position of national health insurance on the U.S. political agenda. In the early 1970s, the most recent period [as of 1989] during which national health insurance seemed imminent, Americans paid considerable attention to the structure, logic, and history of the Canadian system (4). At the time, that system had just been established in its entirety. Although its origins and organization were documented, there had been little experience with universal, public coverage, and data were not yet available on its performance. Universal hospital coverage was a decade or more old (in Saskatchewan, a quarter century), but the extension of insurance to cover physicians' services was very new. Then the moment passed, national health insurance moved off the American agenda, and after a variety of attempts to regulate the health care system at arm's length, competition and the marketplace became the dominant ideas of the 1980s. In this context the Canadian experience was of little relevance.

So far, however, market forces, at least as applied in practice, have been even less successful in containing the growth of health care expenditures than were the regulatory efforts of the 1970s (5, 6). The one major success in this field, prospective payment and diagnosis-related groups, is virtually a pure type of regulatory

Reprinted by permission of *The New England Journal of Medicine* from 320(90), pp. 571–577, 1989. Copyright 1989, *Massachusetts Medical Society.*

intervention, despite its being occasionally clothed in market rhetoric. At the same time, the proportion of the American population with no insurance coverage or grossly inadequate coverage is believed to be both large and growing (7, 8), and there is increasing uneasiness about the effect of market forces in health care on the interests of both patients and providers (9–11). In this context, the radically different Canadian approach to funding may deserve a second look—not as a panacea, but as evidence that perhaps things could be different. By now [1989] that system has generated nearly two decades of experience that can be compared with the American record.

To an American audience, the most striking feature of the Canadian experience may be the association of universal coverage with substantially lower expenditures for health services. Despite (or, as many Canadians would argue, because of) universal access on equal terms and conditions, overall costs in Canada have risen more or less in line with the growth of national income, rather than eating up a steadily increasing share of it, as in the United States.

Before 1971, when the Canadian funding system was more similar to the American one, health care costs consumed a share of national income that was virtually identical in both countries and was rising steadily. In 1971 it reached 7.4 percent in Canada, as compared with 7.6 percent in the United States. After 1971, however, the Canadian share remained stable, whereas in the United States it continued to rise (5,12–14). By 1981 their spending shares were 7.7 and 9.2 percent, respectively. In the 1982 recession, the share of expenditures for health care rose sharply in both countries, to 8.6 and 10.2 percent (12, 14). In both systems, health care escaped the effects of the recession—an interesting and unstudied observation. But the Canadian share stabilized at its new level; preliminary estimates for 1987 show it still at 8.6 percent. In contrast, the United States share continued to rise. Estimates for 1987 are in excess of 11 percent (5, 15).

The large and growing gap between the United States and Canada drives home the point that, for good or ill, the form of funding adopted by Canada does permit a society to control its overall outlays on health care. Furthermore, it is unnecessary to impose financial barriers to access in the process. In this chapter we sketch some of the basic institutional and statistical facts of that process, and their implications for physicians in particular.

Cost control, although successful in general, can be a bruising political process, producing much sound and fury. External observers who rely on newspaper reports may not always get a clear picture, either of the critical issues in dispute or of the distinction between facts and rhetoric. Further confusion arises from casual interpretations of the comparative data, such as that by Feder et al. (16). Looking at the period from 1970 to 1984, they noted that health spending in Canada rose faster than in the United States, but that the gross national product (GNP) rose faster still. They concluded that the apparent success of the Canadian system with cost control was illusory, and that the stability of the share of the GNP applied to health care was simply the result of rapid economic growth. A more detailed look at the data shows this conclusion to be incorrect.

NATIONAL INCOME AND HEALTH EXPENDITURES
IN CANADA AND THE UNITED STATES

Table 1 provides the relevant data for Canada and the United States over the period referred to by Feder et al. The Canadian GNP does in fact outpace the American by 2 percent per year. But after adjustment for the more rapid rate of inflation in Canada, our advantage shrinks to 0.7 percent. When adjusted further for the slightly faster growth of the Canadian population, the difference in real per capita growth rates is less than half a percent per year—respectable enough over the long term, but not enough to account for the divergence in the shares of the GNP spent on health. The oversight of confusing nominal with real rates of GNP growth leads Feder et al. to their erroneous conclusion.

The relevant base year for examining the effect of national health insurance on health spending is not 1970, however, but 1971. Quebec, the second-largest province, with about a quarter of the Canadian population, adopted its health plan in October 1970, and New Brunswick began its plan on January 1, 1971. Correspondingly there was a substantial jump, from 7.1 to 7.4 percent, in the share of the GNP applied to health care for all of Canada.

Table 2 shows the annual rates of increase in total health spending in Canada and the United States since the completion of universal Medicare coverage in Canada. Spending in nominal dollars did rise somewhat faster in Canada, by 0.7 percent per year. But when account is taken of the more rapid rate of general inflation in Canada and the slightly faster rate of population growth, health spending in constant dollars per capita rose more slowly in Canada, by 1.6 percent per year.

Table 1

Average annual percentage increases in gross national product (GNP),
1970 to 1984[a]

Measures of GNP	Canada	United States	Difference[b]
Current dollars	12.1%	9.8%	2.0%
Constant dollars	3.4	2.7	0.7
Constant dollars per capita	2.2	1.7	0.4

Sources: [a]Data for the United States are from the Health Care Financing Administration (5) and the Bureau of Economic Analysis (17); data for Canada are from the Department of Finance (18, 19).
[b]Differences in annual growth rates must be calculated geometrically, not by subtraction $[d = (1 + r_1)/(1 + r_2) - 1]$. Rates have been rounded after calculation.

Table 2

Average annual percentage increases in total expenditures for health care,
1971 to 1985[a]

Measures of health expenditures	Canada	United States	Difference[b]
Current dollars	13.1%	12.3%	0.7%
Constant dollars[c]	4.3	5.8	−1.4
Constant dollars per capita[c]	3.1	4.8	−1.6

Sources: [a]Data for the United States are from the Health Care Financing Administration (5), Gibson et al. (14), and the Department of Commerce (17); data for Canada are from Health and Welfare Canada (12, 13) and the Department of Finance (18, 19).
[b]Differences in annual growth rates must be calculated geometrically, not by subtraction $[d = (1 + r_1)/(1 + r_2) - 1]$. Rates have been rounded after calculation.
[c]These constant-dollar measures are not real output measures for the health sector; they have not been adjusted by price indexes specific to the health sector. Rather, they are adjusted for changes in the general level of prices, economy-wide, as reflected in price indexes based on gross national expenditures, and they therefore reflect the increase in generalized purchasing power that is absorbed by the health care sector, in the form of either increased resource inputs or health sector–specific inflation.

To put this more concretely, in 1985 Americans spent an average of $1,710 each on health care (5). If their rate of cost escalation since 1971, in real terms, had been the same as that in Canada, they would have spent only $1,362, or 20 percent less. Preliminary estimates for 1987 show Americans spending just under $2,000 each for health care. Detailed Canadian data are not [as of 1989] available, but the spending gap is clearly continuing to widen. One may estimate conservatively that if the Canadian rates of escalation in real cost since 1971 had prevailed in the United States, health spending would by 1987 be about $450 less, on average, for every person in the country, or at least $100 billion less in all.

THE PROCESS OF COST CONTROL IN CANADA

How such control has been achieved, and with what effects, continues to form a major part of the agenda for research in health services in Canada (20). As Iglehart pointed out (2), virtually the entire difference between Canada and the United States in the share of GNP that is spent on health is accounted for by three components: insurance overhead, or costs of prepayment and administration; payments to hospitals; and payments for physicians' services. In 1985, these three items took up 0.59, 4.18, and 2.07 percent, respectively, of the U.S. GNP, and 0.11, 3.48, and 1.35 percent of the Canadian GNP.

Relative to the expenditures that might have been generated by a system comparable to Canada's, in 1985 Americans spent about $20 billion more for insurance and prepayment costs, and just under $30 billion more for each of physicians' services and hospital costs.

Administration and Prepayment Expenses

In relative terms, the most extraordinary difference between Canadian and American spending is in the area of administration and prepayment expenses. In 1985 the overhead component of health insurance—the share of premiums that goes not to the reimbursement of physicians, hospitals, and other providers, but to paying for the handling of the flow of paper and dollars—cost Americans $95 each, out of their overall $1,710. Canadians spent $21—and those were Canadian dollars. Indeed, Canadians spent less per capita to administer universal comprehensive coverage than Americans spent to administer Medicare and Medicaid alone (about $26 U.S. per capita (5)).

A universal, tax-financed system can simply be much less costly to administer, at all levels, and the Canadian system is. On the revenue side, once a tax system is in place, as it is in all modern societies—with income tax, sales tax, and everything else—the additional cost of raising more funds is minimal. (Some Canadian provinces continue to collect premiums, which are taxes in all but name. They are related to family size, but not to risk status; they cover only a portion of the total plan outlays; they are compulsory for most of the population; and most important, coverage is not conditional on payment.)

On the expense side, all the costs of determining coverage and eligibility are avoided—everyone is eligible, and for the same benefits. Patients drop out of the payment system entirely, and reimbursement takes place between the public insurer and the provider. There are no marketing expenses, no costs of estimating risk status in order to set differential premiums or decide whom to cover, and no allocations for shareholder profits; the process of claims payment, although not free of costs, is greatly simplified and much cheaper. In this area it is obvious that the public sector is more efficient and less costly than the private sector (21), a fact that was recognized early on in Canada. The 1964 Royal Commission on Health Services, which drew up the blueprint for Canada's universal system, described the private administration of insurance as "an uneconomic use of . . . limited resources" (22). This "uneconomic use" accounts for nearly one-quarter of the difference in cost for health insurance between Canada and the United States.

Nor is that the end of the story. Himmelstein and Woolhandler (23) calculate that in the United States, the provider-borne overheads for hospitals, nursing homes, and doctors' offices (the accounting costs of complying with the requirements for documentation by a multiplicity of insurers, as well as coping with the determination of eligibility, direct billing of patients, and collections) amounted to $62.1 billion in 1983. They estimate that shifting to a national health insurance system could save $21.4 billion in the administrative costs of hospitals and physicians' offices. This would be 6 percent of total health care costs, or 0.63 percent of the GNP in 1983—leading to the startling conclusion that the costs of running the American payment system itself, independent of the costs of patient care, may account for more than half the difference in cost between the Canadian and the U.S. systems.

For the Canadian physician, differences in the costs of insurance administration show up as a lower overhead for practice. The problems of determining insurance status and managing the collections process disappear, along with the problem of uncollectible accounts. The costs of compliance with the requirements of the health care reimbursement system also show up outside the area of health expenditures as it is normally defined, particularly in the budgets of the social welfare services, and to no inconsiderable degree in the monetary and nonmonetary costs borne by individual patients and their families. Furthermore, the considerable research, legal, and regulatory efforts required to put the complex and varied reporting and compliance requirements in place are not without cost, but will be counted as outside the health care system.

There is private insurance for some forms of health care in Canada. But for hospital and medical care, such coverage is prohibited for services that are included in the public plans. The original intent was quite explicit—to prevent private firms from skimming off the good risks, supporting the development of multiclass service, or both. But the restriction also has the very important effect of making provincial governments to all intents and purposes the sole funders of hospital and medical care, and of creating a bilateral bargaining situation as the foundation for cost control in these sectors.

The Effect on Hospitals

In Canada, controlling hospital costs is a two-part process. Operating budgets are approved, and funded almost entirely, by the Ministry of Health in each province, but they include no allowance for capital expenditures. New facilities, equipment, major renovations, and the like are funded from a variety of sources, but they require the approval of the same provincial agency, which generally also contributes the major share of financing. This process of centralized approval prohibits hospitals from accessing private capital markets, and has historically limited their efforts to support expansions of capacity from community sources. So far, it has been relatively successful in limiting such expansion (24), but somewhat less successful in managing the diffusion of major equipment (25, 26).

Centralized control over operating costs is more complete. Annual global budgets are negotiated between ministries and individual hospitals. Although political pressures have often forced governments to pick up the deficits of hospitals that are unable or unwilling to stay within these budgets, this process has resulted in a significantly less rapid rise in hospital expenditures in Canada than in the United States (27, 28).

The more rapid rate of escalation of hospital costs in the United States since 1971 has been shown to result from major differences in the growth in hospital costs per patient day at constant hospital input prices, or intensity of servicing

(27–30). This measure increases in response to increases in the number of nursing hours or drugs, or in the use of operating rooms, magnetic resonance imaging, and other such complex technology, per day of inpatient care. In the case of particular technologies that are embodied in specifically countable items like machines, capacities available per capita have tended to increase less rapidly in Canada. On the other hand, changes in the intensity of servicing in hospitals also include relative increases in internal administrative costs. Therefore, some portion of the apparent relative increase in servicing intensity simply reflects the increasing administrative intensity of the American hospital system.

But the different trends in servicing intensity also reflect quite different patterns in the use of beds in acute care hospitals. In Canada, a growing share of such beds has been occupied by patients over 65 years of age, whose stays exceed 60 days and whose daily care requirements are well below average. These patients prevent physicians from using the beds in question to treat short-term patients (31).

Thus, Canada can have higher rates of hospitalization and greater average lengths of stay than the United States, yet also have lower per capita hospital expenditures (32). Even if such expenditures, in terms of the cost of hospital care, are less different than is usually believed (because so much of the U.S. expenditure is for administrative activity), it does appear that the resulting mix of hospital activities favors intensive, high-technology services in the United States and long-term, chronic care in Canada. Nor should this come as a surprise, given the history of cost and procedural reimbursement in the United States, and of global budget-constrained funding in Canada. Which is preferable, in terms of value for money or benefits to patients, is harder to say. Possibly, each system generates its own forms of overuse and underuse.

One product that is clearly generated by the Canadian system, structured as it is to place the sole responsibility for control of hospital resources on the provincial governments, is intense, continuing public debate. The rhetoric of underfunding, shortages, excessive waiting lists, and so on is an important part of the process by which providers negotiate their share of public resources—including their own incomes (33). Furthermore, there are reasons for the noticeable recent increase in such rhetoric. Increases in the supply of physicians per capita, in the face of a relatively constant supply of beds, have resulted in steady reductions in the number of short-term hospital beds available to each physician since 1971 (27). As bed availability and operating budgets have undergone increasing scrutiny, hospital administrators responded first (in the mid-1970s) by rationalizing administrative operations, and more recently by joining physicians in stepped-up rhetoric and pressure about underfunding (34).

The difficulty for health policy and funding is that, since the boy always cries wolf (and must do so, given the political system of funding), one does not know if the wolf is really there. The political dramatics should not mislead external observers into believing that the wolf is always at hand. What varies most between the two nations in the method of establishing total hospital expenditures is the centralized, overtly political process in Canada, in contrast to the largely decentralized, institution-centered, and only implicitly political process in the United States. The Canadian controls on hospital expenditures impinge on individual physicians by limiting the complementary resources that are available to them. In this way, the environment of medical practice is changed, and practice patterns change in response. But individual physicians are not subject to any substantial direct intervention by hospital management or third parties. In this sense, Canadian physicians are actually much more autonomous than their American counterparts.

The Effect on Physicians

From 1971 to 1985, the share of the American GNP going to physicians rose by over 40 percent. By contrast, Canadian physicians had an increase of only 10 percent. The stories that U.S. physicians hear about disaffected Canadian physicians, outmigration, underfunding, and occasional strikes correspond to an underlying reality of less generous funding. Despite the rhetoric, however, there has been no mass bailout of physicians from Canada. The supply of physicians per capita has risen throughout the period, is currently growing at between 1.5 and 2 percent per year, and is projected to continue its growth for the foreseeable future (35). At the end of 1985 there were about 490 people per physician in Canada—very similar to the U.S. ratio. As in the United States, the policy concern is with surpluses, not shortages (36). There may be some loss of superstars to the United States, but that is hard to document—individual anecdotes do not make a trend. In any case, there is always some leakage of stars in any field from countries with small populations to populous neighbors (the Gretzky effect).

The main explanation for the difference in outlays to physicians is that real fees have increased much faster in the United States than in Canada (27, 37). This difference, in turn, has resulted from the effect of universal public coverage on the process of fee determination. Increases in the general levels of fees and rules of payment are negotiated periodically between provincial medical associations and Ministries of Health. Over the long term, this complex negotiation process has had a major impact on the overall rate of escalation of fees (37). Ironically, for a society that believes in the influence of competitive markets, the increasing supply of physicians in the United States seems to be associated with an acceleration in fee increases. In 1986, the rise in fees relative to the overall Consumer Price Index was one of the largest on record (5).

Two other related issues have been particularly contentious for Canadian physicians—billing at rates above those reimbursed by the provincial plans ("extra billing") and the growth in the use of services per physician. Since 1971 these factors have become increasingly prominent in the political negotiating process, although the first one may at last have been pushed off center stage.

With the passage of the Canada Health Act in 1984 (38), the right to "extra bill" was removed in all provinces in which such billing had previously occurred. This act, passed unanimously by the House of Commons, was a response to public perceptions that extra billing was undermining the fundamental principle of universal access on uniform terms and conditions. The termination of extra billing was met with intense opposition from physicians in some provinces, however, culminating in a lengthy strike in Ontario (2, 39). Physicians argued that the threat of widespread extra billing was a safety valve, protecting them against overly aggressive bargaining by the Ministries of Health and helping to push up public reimbursement rates. Although relatively few physicians engaged in extra billing, the majority strongly supported the option. They were unable to mobilize any sizable public support, however.

The extreme distress among physicians in Ontario appears to have been based largely on symbolic considerations. The right of ultimate access to the patient's economic resources seems to have had a meaning difficult for nonphysicians to understand. In fact, no change has occurred in the prevailing pattern of private, fee-for-service practice with reimbursement at uniform, negotiated rates. But Canadian physicians do have real concerns about the future, which have been linked to the extra-billing issue.

Once governments have achieved control over fee levels by ensuring that the public reimbursement rates represent payment in full, it is feared that the next step in cost control will be to restrict the amount or type of care provided, or at least the number and mix of services for which reimbursement will be made. This is particularly likely if physicians increase their delivery of services to compensate for the loss of extra billing, for a stagnant fee structure, or both.

The latter possibility has been an important consideration in recent American discussions of physicians' reimbursement under Medicare (40, 41). Analyses of the U.S. experience with fee freezes in the early 1970s clearly demonstrated that increased billing occurred as a response (42, 43). Billing activity per physician has risen faster in Canada than in the United States since 1971, in a manner consistent with this concern, although in Canada fee controls have clearly moderated the rate of escalation of expenditures for physicians' services, not just that of fees. Until recently, the provincial governments have been willing to accept an additional rise in expenditures (increases in physicians' productivity or more creative billing, depending on one's point of view) over and above increases in fees and numbers of physicians. Nationally, this has averaged 1 to 2 percent per year since 1971 (37).

This exception was Quebec, where over a four-year period of unchanged fees (1971 to 1975) the increase became so large as to create a fiscal problem (37, 44). Starting in 1976, Quebec introduced modifications to the reimbursement process that limited its liability for increases in services, billings, or both (per practitioner and in the aggregate) that exceeded preset target levels. From a billing standpoint, 26 office-based diagnostic and therapeutic procedures were bundled into the office visit. These procedures had been billable separately, in addition to the basic visit fee, and during the early 1970s their number and cost per office visit had risen rapidly. Their consolidation into the office-visit fee removed one of the principal mechanisms by which Quebec physicians had been able to stem some of the erosion in their real incomes during the period of unchanged fees (37).

In addition, there are ceilings on the quarterly gross billings of individual practitioners, above which physicians are reimbursed at only 25 percent of the allowable fee. For the profession as a whole, negotiated fee increases are implemented in steps, conditional on the rate of increase in use. If the rate of use per physician (i.e., average gross receipts) rises faster than a predetermined percentage, subsequent fee increases are scaled down or eliminated.

None of these measures impinge directly on the autonomy of individual physicians in their practices, however. Specific clinical decisions are not reviewed by the reimbursement agency, nor are therapeutic protocols established. If the aggregated bill for all clinical decisions exceeds the limits, then fees to either the individual or the group as a whole will be scaled down, but physicians remain free to determine their own practice patterns.

Committees to review patterns of practice have existed for years in each province, under various names. But they were established to monitor a very small number of practitioners whose patterns deviated radically from those of their peers, and to look for fraud or incompetence. Such committees have neither the mandate nor the resources to go beyond statistical outliers in their investigations; even in this role, a 1986 commentary suggests that they are not very aggressive or effective (45).

Since 1985, British Columbia, Alberta, Saskatchewan, Manitoba, and Ontario have all negotiated contracts setting limits on aggregate billings. British Columbia attempted to go further, by restricting the numbers of new physicians entitled to reimbursement by the provincial plan and controlling their locations of practice (46). This policy, however, was successfully challenged on constitutional grounds. It was sustained at the provincial court, but overturned on appeal, and leave to appeal further was denied by the Supreme Court of Canada.

The absence of intrusion by any of these measures into the autonomy of individual practice contrasts markedly with the situation in the United States, where managed care systems and prospective payment, designed to alter individual physicians' care of individual patients, have become the principal tools for the control of expenditures for physicians' services. In the absence of a centralized bargaining mechanism between physicians and payers—a single-source payer—there is no way to limit the overall levels of billings. Hence the leap from constraints on capacity (as by a certificate of need) straight to the level of minute scrutiny of the behavior of individual physicians or the treatment of specific diseases.

Thus, many Americans already feel the threats to clinical freedom that Canadian physicians fear for the future. Whether such fears actually materialize will probably depend in large part on whether the provincial governments can continue to contain overall expenditures. What is disturbing, however, is that the current aggregate approaches to control of the use of services leave unexplored the cost-effectiveness, and even the efficacy, of the actual services provided. Such concerns, if left unaddressed by the profession itself, may become the catalysts for more detailed scrutiny of the use of services within the fee-negotiation process in Canada. To date, we see little evidence of this, but a decade ago there was little sign of the now widespread practice of bargaining over aggregate use along with fees. The context of policy decisions changes more slowly in Canada than in the United States, but it does move forward.

Orchestrated Outrage versus Diffuse Distress

Thus, the major difference between the two countries with respect to health expenditures lies in the degree of centralization of the cost-control process. In the United States the battles are fought in a myriad of private struggles between physicians and their employers, or their hospitals (or their competitors). When the struggle becomes public, as in the call by Minnesota physicians for unionization (47), it takes the form of a series of isolated and localized incidents. The general pattern is obscured. In Canada, by contrast, the struggle over shares of income between physicians and the rest of the society is played out as large-scale public theater, with all the rhetorical threats and flourishes that political clashes require (48). Physicians in Canada, and perhaps also in the United States, may perceive the Canadian conflicts as more severe and as arising from the presence of a universal public-payment system. That system serves to focus and channel such conflicts and to bring them into the headlines, but is has also afforded Canadian physicians a greater degree of professional autonomy.

Whatever the liabilities of such an overt and at times rancorous process, the Canadian approach has controlled health care costs more effectively. In the end, this may be the root of the sense of unease among Canadian physicians, who face a problem common to physicians in every country with a rapidly rising supply, including the United States. In such circumstances, every community of physicians must struggle for an ever-increasing share of national income or accept falling personal incomes. In the process, they must urge on the rest of society the benefits of buying the additional services that the additional numbers of physicians make possible (some would say inevitable)—and of doing so at fees that will sustain their own incomes. Whether such benefits are real or illusory is important from the standpoint of health policy, but irrelevant to the needs of the medical community.

The rest of society, or at least a sector of it, attempts to resist this expansion under the banner of cost control. When such resistance is organized collectively through public insurance, it is relatively successful. When it is disorganized and fragmented, an inconsistent and contradictory mix of strategies, as in the United

States, it has so far been unsuccessful. Again, that observation is logically independent of whether the lack of success in the United States reflects waste, or whether the Canadian success leads to "underfunding."

In such an environment the pressure on physicians can only grow. To the extent that they resist such pressures successfully and continue to expand their share of the national income, as in the United States, the public and private responses to cost escalation will become increasingly radical. Major institutional changes are already transforming the American health care system to an extent much greater than has been the case in the more conservative Canadian environment. Fears and anecdotes about the erosion of professional autonomy, and even of incomes, are becoming increasingly widespread. In the United States, corporate competitors or employers may turn out to be more ruthless than public regulators.

Such are the costs of economic success. The Canadian environment is more stable and predictable precisely because its cost-control processes work relatively well. But in Canada, whatever has happened or may happen can be blamed on government and on the evils of "socialized medicine." Anxiety and dissatisfaction are easily, if not always accurately, focused and channeled collectively through the process of public negotiation. In the United States, it is harder for individual practitioners to find the villains, and still harder to identify an effective response. At the same time, it is easier to misinterpret the experience of other countries with more visible bargaining processes.

REFERENCES

1. Iglehart, J. K. Canada's health care system. *N. Engl. J. Med.* 315: 202–208, 1986.
2. Iglehart, J. K. Canada's health care system. *N. Engl. J. Med.* 315: 778–784, 1986.
3. Iglehart, J. K. Canada's health care system: Addressing the problem of physician supply. *N. Engl. J. Med.* 315: 1623–1628, 1986.
4. Andreopoulos, S. (ed.). *National Health Insurance: Can We Learn from Canada?* Wiley, New York, 1975.
5. Division of National Cost Estimates, Health Care Financing Administration. National health expenditures, 1986–2000. *Health Care Financ. Rev.* 8(4): 1–35, 1987.
6. Fein, R. *Medical Care, Medical Costs: The Search for a Health Insurance Policy.* Harvard University Press, Cambridge, Mass., 1986.
7. Wilensky, G. R. Viable strategies for dealing with the uninsured. *Health Aff. (Millwood)* 6(1): 33–46, 1987.
8. Library of Congress, Congressional Research Service. *Health Insurance and the Uninsured: Background Data and Analysis.* Government Printing Office, Washington, D.C., 1988.
9. Fuchs, V. R. The "competition revolution" in health care. *Health Aff. (Millwood)* 7(3): 5–24, 1988.
10. Brook, R. H., and Kosecoff, J. B. Competition and quality. *Health Aff. (Millwood)* 7(3): 150–161, 1988.

11. Gray, B. H. (ed.) for the Institute of Medicine. *For-Profit Enterprise in Health Care.* National Academy Press, Washington, D.C., 1986.
12. Canada, Health and Welfare Canada. *National Health Expenditures in Canada 1975–1987.* Ottawa, 1985.
13. Canada, Health and Welfare Canada. *National Health Expenditures in Canada 1970–1982.* Ottawa, 1985.
14. Gibson, R., et al. National health expenditures, 1983. *Health Care Financ. Rev.* 6(2): 1–29, 1984.
15. Ginzberg, E. A hard look at cost containment. *N. Engl. J. Med.* 316: 1151–1154, 1987.
16. Feder, J., Scanlon, W., and Clark, J. Canada's health care system. *N. Engl. J. Med.* 317: 320, 1987.
17. Department of Commerce, Bureau of Economic Analysis. *Survey of Current Business* 67(9), September 1987.
18. Canada, Department of Finance. *Quarterly Economic Review: Annual Reference Tables, June 1987.* Ottawa, 1987.
19. Canada, Department of Finance. *Economic Review April, 1985.* Ottawa, 1985.
20. Evans, R. G. Finding the levers, finding the courage: Lessons from cost containment in North America. *J. Health Polit. Policy Law* 11: 585–615, 1986.
21. Reinhardt, U. E. On the B-factor in American health care. *Washington Post.* August 9, 1988, p. 20.
22. Canada, Royal Commission on Health Services (Hall Commission). *Report* Vol. 1, p. 745. Ottawa: Queen's Printer, 1964.
23. Himmelstein, D. U., and Woolhandler, S. Cost without benefit: Administrative waste in U.S. health care. *N. Engl. J. Med.* 314: 441–445, 1986.
24. Bellerose, P.-P., and Tholl, W. Capital Spending in the Health Sector. Presented at the Annual Meeting of the Canadian Health Economics Research Association, Halifax, Canada, June 8, 1987.
25. Feeny, D., Guyatt, G., and Tugwell, P. *Health Care Technology: Effectiveness, Efficiency and Public Policy.* Montreal: Institute for Research in Public Policy, 1986.
26. Deber, R. B., and Leatt, P. Technology acquisition in Ontario hospitals: You can lead a hospital to policy, but can you make it stick? In *Proceedings of the Third Canadian Conference on Health Economics,* edited by J. M. Home, pp. 259–277. University of Manitoba, Winnipeg, 1987.
27. Barer, M. L., and Evans, R. G. Riding north on a south-bound horse? Expenditures, prices, utilization and incomes in the Canadian health care system. In *Medicare at Maturity: Achievements, Lessons and Challenges,* edited by R. G. Evans, G. L. Stoddart, pp. 53–163. University of Calgary Press, Calgary, 1986.
28. Detsky, A. S., Stacey, S. R., and Bombardier, C. The effectiveness of a regulatory strategy in containing hospital costs: The Ontario experience, 1967–1981. *N. Engl. J. Med.* 309: 151–159, 1983.
29. Barer, M., and Evans, R. G. Prices, proxies and productivity: An historical analysis of hospital and medical care in Canada. In *Price Level Measurement,* edited by E. Diewert and C. Montmarquette, pp. 705–777. Statistics Canada, Ottawa, 1983.
30. Detsky, A. S., et al. Global budgeting and the teaching hospital in Ontario. *Med. Care* 24: 89–94, 1986.

31. Evans, R. G., et al. The long good-bye: The great transformation of the British Columbia hospital system. *Health Serv. Res.,* 1989.
32. Newhouse, J. P., Anderson, G. M., and Roos, L. L. What accounts for differences in hospital spending between the United States and Canada: A first look. *Health Aff. (Millwood)* 7(5): 6–16, 1988.
33. Reinhardt, U. E. Resource allocation in health care: The allocation of lifestyles to providers. *Milbank Q* 65: 153–176, 1987.
34. Murray, V. V., Jick, T. D., and Bradshaw, P. Hospital funding constraints: strategic and tactical decision responses to sustained moderate levels of crisis in six Canadian hospitals. *Soc. Sci. Med.* 18: 211–219, 1984.
35. Barer, M. L., Gafni, A., and Lomas, J. Accommodating rapid growth in physician supply: Lessons from Israel, warnings for Canada. *Int. J. Health Serv.* 19: 95–115, 1989.
36. Lomas, J., Barer, M. L., and Stoddart, G. L. *Physician Manpower Planning: Lessons from the MacDonald Report.* Ontario Economic Council, Toronto, 1985.
37. Barer, M. L., Evans, R. G., and Labelle, R. J. Fee controls as cost control: Tales from the frozen north. *Milbank Q.* 66: 1–64, 1988.
38. Heiber, S., and Deber, R. Banning extra-billing in Canada: Just what the doctor didn't order. *Can. Public Policy* 13: 62–74, 1987.
39. Barer, M. L., and Antioch, K. *Bill 94 and the Ontario Physicians' Strike: Lobbying as Professional Emasculation.* University of British Columbia, Vancouver, 1987.
40. United States Congress, Office of Technology Assessment. *Payment for Physician Services: Strategies for Medicare.* Government Printing Office, Washington, D.C., 1986: 146–150.
41. United States Congress, Congressional Budget Office. *Physician Reimbursement under Medicare: Options for Change.* Government Printing Office, Washington, D.C., 1986: 10–12.
42. Holahan, J., and Scanlon, W. Price Controls, Physician Fees and Physician Incomes from Medicare and Medicaid. Working paper no. 998-5. Urban Institute, Washington, D.C., 1978.
43. Gabel, J. R., and Rice, T. H. Reducing public expenditures for physician services: The price of paying less. *J. Health Polit. Policy Law* 9: 595–609, 1985.
44. Contandriopoulos, A.-P. Cost containment through payment mechanisms: The Quebec experience. *J. Public Health Policy* 7: 224–238, 1986.
45. Wilson, P. R., Chappell, D., and Lincoln, R. Policing physician abuse in British Columbia: An analysis of current policies. *Can. Public Policy* 12: 236–244, 1986.
46. Barer, M. L. Regulating physician supply: The evolution of British Columbia's Bill 41. *J. Health Polit. Policy Law* 13: 1–25, 1988.
47. Doctors' dilemma: Unionizing. *New York Times.* July 11, 1987, pp. 13, 21.
48. Tuohy, C. J. Conflict and accommodation in the Canadian health care system. In *Medicare at Maturity: Achievements, Lessons and Challenges,* edited by R. G. Evans and G. L. Stoddart, pp. 393–434. University of Calgary Press, Calgary, 1986.

CHAPTER 2

How Does Canada Do It? A Comparison of Expenditures for Physicians' Services in the United States and Canada

Victor R. Fuchs and James S. Hahn

American interest in the Canadian health care system is growing rapidly for two principal reasons (1–3). First, costs have escalated in the United States to such an extent that health care now [1990] accounts for approximately 11.5 percent of the gross national product, whereas in Canada the comparable figure is about 9 percent. Second, one in seven Americans has no health insurance, and tens of millions of others have incomplete coverage; in contrast, Canada provides comprehensive, first-dollar health insurance to all its citizens. If U.S. spending could be held to the Canadian percentage, the savings would amount to more than $100 billion a year.

There have been numerous descriptions of the evolution of national health insurance in Canada and of the current federal-provincial system (4–6). A detailed statistical analysis of trends in Canada and the United States has identified prospective global budgets for hospitals and negotiated fee schedules for physicians' services as major reasons for lower spending in Canada (7). Other studies have focused on hospital costs (8, 9), drug prices (10–12), the use of surgical services (13, 14), and administrative costs (15).

This study concentrates on per capita expenditures for physicians' services because in this important sector the ratio between U.S. and Canadian spending is particularly large (1.72 in 1985). In other words, after adjustment for population size and the overall purchasing power of the Canadian dollar, Americans spend 72 percent more than Canadians for physicians' services. The comparable ratio

Reprinted by permission of *The New England Journal of Medicine* from 323(13), pp. 884–890, 1990. Copyright 1990, *Massachusetts Medical Society*.

for hospital expenditures is 1.34, and for all other health expenditures combined it is 1.30.

How does Canada do it? Do Canadians receive fewer physicians' services? Are the higher U.S. expenditures attributable entirely to higher fees? Do higher fees result from the use of more resources to produce a given quantity of services (more physicians, nurses, equipment, and the like), or do they reflect higher prices for those resources (higher physicians' net incomes, nurses' salaries, and the like)?

Our principal objective was to provide quantitative answers to these questions. Our analysis of the ratio between the United States and Canada was supplemented by a parallel comparison of Iowa and Manitoba. The state and the province have small, relatively homogeneous populations, and we had special access to data for the two regions. Our analysis of the ratio between Iowa and Manitoba in per capita expenditures for physicians' services (1.51) served as a check on the comparison between the United States and Canada and helped to sharpen our understanding of the reasons for the differences between countries in spending, fees, and use. The effect of physicians' services on the health of Americans and Canadians is not addressed in this chapter.

METHODS

Data on health care expenditures, the number of physicians who care for patients, vital statistics, and socioeconomic variables for the United States, Canada, Iowa, and Manitoba for 1985 were gathered from published sources (16–34), and the appropriate ratios were calculated. All data in Canadian dollars were converted to U.S. dollars according to the purchasing-power-parity exchange rate of $1 U.S. equals $1.22 Canadian. This rate, calculated each year by the Organization for Economic Cooperation and Development, is based on the relative prices of the same comprehensive basket of goods and services in the two countries. All dollar amounts mentioned in this study are in U.S. dollars. Total expenditures for physicians' services were allocated to procedures or to evaluation and management according to a formula based on the distribution of specialists in each country (or region). Details of the allocation are available elsewhere.[1]

Fees

The necessary data on physicians' fees were not available—except from Manitoba—in published form. We therefore relied on data made available to us

---

[1] See NAPS document no. 04801 for 20 pages of supplementary material, from NAPS c/o Microfiche Publications, P.O. Box 3513, Grand Central Station, New York, NY 10163-3513.

on a confidential basis by the Health Insurance Association of America, California Blue Shield, Iowa Blue Cross and Blue Shield, and Health and Welfare Canada. Fees in the United States for surgery (33 procedures) and evaluation and management (22 kinds of visits that we combined in five broad categories to achieve comparability with the Canadian data) are based on billed charges reported to the Health Insurance Association of America by its members. The association did not have data for ancillary services; charges for radiology (eight procedures) and anesthesiology (eight procedures) were therefore obtained from California Blue Cross and adjusted to the levels of the association by comparing surgery fees from both sources. Billed charges for Iowa for the same procedures and visits were provided by Iowa Blue Cross and Blue Shield. A list of the procedures and types of visits according to CPT-4 code (Current Procedural Terminology, fourth revision), as well as the precise methods we used to calculate the fee ratios, is available elsewhere (see footnote on p. 24).

All U.S. and Iowa charges were reduced by 20 percent to measure the fees actually received by American physicians more accurately. There are services that are provided but never paid for; there are differences between what is billed and what insurance companies will allow; preferred-provider and health maintenance organizations extract explicit or implicit discounts from billed charges; physicians who accept Medicare assignment may receive less than their usual fee; and Medicaid is frequently the lowest payer of all. A survey of the Medical Group Management Association for 1985 reported that fee-for-service cash collections were 15 percent less than gross fee-for-service billed charges (35). It is widely believed that the collection ratio for such groups is higher than the ratio for physicians in solo practice or small partnerships. A sample of Medicare-approved charges for 30 major services and procedures showed a median difference from Health Insurance Association of America billed charges of –23 percent (36). Reducing U.S. billed charges by 20 percent therefore appeared appropriate. No such adjustment was necessary for Canada because bills are paid fully and promptly by the provincial governments according to predetermined, annually negotiated rates.

Fees in Manitoba were taken from the physicians' manual of the Manitoba Health Services Commission and included an adjustment for services provided in rural areas. Because overall Canadian fees were unavailable, Manitoba fees were adjusted to an all-Canada level according to a ratio of benefit rates between Canada and Manitoba that we calculated using provincial data assembled by Health and Welfare Canada. Because there is considerable interest in the United States in reimbursement for procedures as compared with reimbursement for evaluation and management, we calculated separate fee ratios for the two categories of services.

Quantity of Services per Capita

In principle, the quantity of services per capita is the sum of all the visits, tests, operations, and other services provided by physicians. Because comprehensive data to measure these services directly were not available, we estimated the ratios between the United States and Canada and between Iowa and Manitoba by dividing the ratio of expenditures per capita by the appropriate fee ratio. Because expenditures equal the product of fees and the quantity of services, this method provided an indirect measure of the relative quantity of services provided.

Price of Resources

Physicians' services are produced through the use of resources such as physicians, nurses, equipment, and office supplies. We estimated the ratio of the prices of these resources for the United States and Canada (and for Iowa and Manitoba) from physicians' net incomes, nurses' salaries, and other relevant data. The overall ratio was a weighted average (weighted according to expenditures) of the price ratios for four categories of resources: physicians, other personnel, office, and equipment and supplies. This average was then adjusted to take liability-insurance premiums into account.

Quantity of Resources

Of the four categories of resources listed above, we only had data on quantity for the number of physicians. We therefore estimated the ratio of the quantity of resources per capita for the United States and Canada (and for Iowa and Manitoba) by dividing the ratio of expenditure per capita by the ratio of the price of resources. Because expenditures equal the product of the price of resources and the quantity of resources, this method provided an indirect measure of the quantity of resources.

RESULTS

Table 1 presents selected background statistics for each country and for Iowa and Manitoba in order to put the data on expenditures in context. Most of the populations of the United States, Canada, and Manitoba are urban, whereas more than half of Iowa's population is rural, which helps to explain the low number of physicians per capita in that state. Despite its huge territory, 90 percent of Canada's population lives in a narrow band of land just north of the border with the United States. Manitoba, like Canada in general, has a large area, most of which is thinly populated. More than half of Manitoba's population and more than three-quarters of its physicians live in one city, Winnipeg. The elderly are relatively more numerous in the United States and in Iowa; were all other things

Table 1

Selected background statistics, 1985[a]

Variable	United States	Canada	Iowa	Manitoba	Ratio of United States to Canada	Ratio of Iowa to Manitoba
Population (thousands)	283,739	25,358	2,905	1,070	—	—
Percent rural	26.3	24.3	52.3	28.8	—	—
Percent in cities of						
≥ 100,000	25.4	34.5	10.5	55.5	—	—
Percent over 65 years old	12.0	10.4	14.2	12.5	—	—
Births (per 1000)	15.8	15.1	14.3	16.0	—	—
Gross national (domestic) product per capita[b]	16,703	14,801	14,490	13,791	1.13	1.05
Patient-care physicians (per 1000)[c]	1.81	2.05	1.21	2.02	0.88	0.60
Private-practice general practitioners and family physicians	0.24	0.90	0.29	0.88	0.26	0.33
Other[c]	1.57	1.15	0.92	1.14	1.37	0.81
Short-term general hospitals (per 1000)[d]						
Beds	4.20	4.43	5.22	4.89	0.95	1.07
Admissions	140	136	142	153	1.03	0.93
Days	994	1,293	1,084	1,317	0.77	0.82
Life expectancy at birth (yr)						
Men	71.2	72.9	73.1	72.9	0.98	1.00
Women	78.2	79.7	80.2	79.7	0.98	1.01
Infant mortality (per 1000)	10.6	8.0	9.5	9.9	1.33	0.96

[a]Sources: Data were collected from references 16 through 29. Calculations in this and the subsequent tables were performed with unrounded numbers.

[b]Values are in 1985 U.S. dollars. Canadian figures were adjusted according to the purchasing-power-parity exchange rate. $1.00 U.S. equals $1.22 Canadian.

[c]Values include interns and residents.

[d]Canadian data include rehabilitation units.

equal, this would lead to a slightly higher use of medical services. The higher per capita gross national product in the United States would tend to increase health care expenditures per capita, mostly through higher incomes for physicians, nurses, and other personnel.

The differences in the number of physicians per capita, both in the aggregate and according to the type of physician, are worthy of special note. On a per capita basis there are more physicians who care for patients in Canada than in the United States, and many more in Manitoba than in Iowa. The disparity with respect to general practitioners and family physicians is very large. In most specialties and subspecialties, however, the ratio between the United States and Canada is much greater than 1. Rates of hospital admission are similar in the two countries; the average length of stay is considerably longer in Canada, partly because some of Canada's short-term general hospitals include rehabilitation units.

Canada does better than the United States with respect to life expectancy and infant mortality, but Iowa does slightly better than Manitoba. There is no reason to believe that access to or the quality of medical care in Iowa is superior to the U.S. average or that care in Manitoba suffers in comparison with care in the rest of Canada. The reversal in ratios therefore suggests that these differences in gross measures of health are determined largely by nonmedical factors, such as personal behavior, the environment, and genetic endowment.

The data on per capita health expenditures (Table 2) show that the ratios between the United States and Canada and between Iowa and Manitoba are much greater for physicians' services than for hospital services or other expenditures. They also show that within the category of physicians' services, procedures account for nearly all the higher spending in the United States. To understand the difference between the ratios for procedures and for evaluation and management, it is necessary to examine the ratios for fees and for the quantity of services separately.

Table 2

Health expenditures per capita, according to type of expenditure, 1985[a]

Expenditure	United States	Canada	Ratio of United States to Canada	Iowa	Manitoba	Ratio of Iowa to Manitoba
Total	$1,780	$1,286	1.38	$1,432	$1,326	1.08
Physicians	347	202	1.72	240	159	1.51
Procedures	193	69	2.78	130	51	2.54
Evaluation and management	154	133	1.16	110	107	1.02
Hospitals	698	520	1.34	541	519	1.04
All other[b]	735	564	1.30	651	648	1.01

[a]Sources: Data were collected from references 20 and 30 through 34. Values are in 1985 U.S. dollars.

[b]Includes expenditures for nursing homes and other institutions, drugs, dentists' services, other professional services, public health, appliances, prepayment administration, construction, research, home care, ambulance services, other personal health care, and miscellaneous expenses.

Fees

Physicians' fees for procedures are approximately 234 percent higher in the United States than in Canada (Table 3); the difference between Iowa and Manitoba is about 199 percent. By U.S. standards, fees for procedures are exceedingly low in Canada. For example, in Manitoba in 1985 total obstetrical care was reimbursed at $245; the fee for a hernia repair was $186 and for a cholecystectomy $311. Canadian surgical fees are much lower across the board than U.S. fees: for the United States and Canada, 27 of the 33 ratios for surgical procedures are between 2.0 and 4.5; and for Iowa and Manitoba, 29 of the 33 ratios are between 1.75 and 4.25.

Fees for evaluation and management are also higher in the United States than in Canada, but the ratios are much smaller: 1.82 for the United States and Canada, and 1.72 for Iowa and Manitoba. Canadian fees for hospital visits are particularly low; in Manitoba physicians received only $7.20 for a "moderate" hospital visit in 1985 (a visit limited in scope and duration).

The overall fee ratio was moderately sensitive to our allocation of expenditures between procedures and evaluation and management. For instance, if the true share of procedures were five percentage points larger than our estimate, the overall fee ratio between the United States and Canada would increase from 2.39 to 2.47. If the share were five percentage points smaller, the ratio would be 2.32. The exchange rate also affected the fee ratio. If we had used the market rate

Table 3

Physicians' fees, 1985[a]

Service[b]	Ratio of United States to Canada	Ratio of Iowa to Manitoba
Surgery	3.21	2.76
Anesthesiology	3.73	2.86
Radiology	3.59	4.19
Procedures (weighted average)	3.34	2.99
Moderate office visit	1.56	1.44
Extensive office visit	1.55	1.50
Moderate hospital visit	4.77	3.56
Extensive hospital visit	2.57	2.70
Consultation	1.60	1.64
Evaluation and management (weighted average)	1.82	1.72
All services[c]	2.39	2.18

[a]Values are in 1985 U.S. dollars.
[b]"Moderate" visits were limited in scope and duration. "Extensive" visits were longer and broader in scope.
[c]Values are weighted averages of the procedures and evaluation-and-management ratios.

($1.00 U.S. equals $1.36 Canadian), which reflects capital movements and speculation as well as the relative purchasing power of the two currencies, the overall fee ratio would be 2.68. Finally, the relation between the fee ratio and our assumption of a 20 percent discount from billed charges for U.S. fees should be noted. If we had assumed a 25 percent discount, the overall ratio would be 2.24; a 15 percent discount would yield a ratio of 2.54.

Quantity of Services per Capita

Table 4 provides striking refutation of the hypothesis that lower spending in Canada is achieved by providing fewer services. On the contrary, the ratio between the United States and Canada for all services is 0.72, and between Iowa and Manitoba the ratio is 0.69. The disparity in use is much greater for evaluation and management than for procedures. These results are sensitive to possible biases in the fee ratios, but the conclusion that the rate of use is greater in Canada than in the United States appears robust. For instance, if the overall fee ratio between the United States and Canada were 2.0 instead of 2.39, the ratio of the quantity of services per capita would be 0.86, still well under 1.0. These results are not sensitive to assumptions about the exchange rate because using a different rate would change the expenditures and fee ratios in equal proportion; the ratio of the quantity of services per capita would not be affected.

Table 4

Estimation of the ratios of quantity of physicians' services per capita, 1985

Service	Ratio of United States to Canada	Ratio of Iowa to Manitoba
Procedures		
Expenditures per capita (Table 2)	2.78	2.54
Fees (Table 3)	3.34	2.99
Quantity of services per capita[a]	0.83	0.85
Evaluation and management		
Expenditures per capita (Table 2)	1.16	1.02
Fees (Table 3)	1.82	1.72
Quantity of services per capita[a]	0.64	0.60
All services		
Expenditures per capita (Table 2)	1.72	1.51
Fees (Table 3)	2.39	2.18
Quantity of services per capita[a]	0.72	0.69

[a]Values are expenditures per capita divided by fees.

Prices of Resources

As a share of total expenditures, the most important resource in both countries is the physician; the physician's net income is 52 percent of gross income in the United States and 66 percent in Canada. In 1985 net income per office-based physician was $112,199 in the United States and $73,607 in Canada (37, 38). After adjustment for differences in the mix of specialties, U.S. incomes were 35 percent higher than those in Canada, and 61 percent higher in Iowa than in Manitoba (Table 5). The price ratio for other personnel was based on the full-time compensation of a registered nurse (16, 39–41). The price of occupying and maintaining an office varies greatly depending on geographic location, and direct estimates were unobtainable. We assumed that the price increases as the relative wealth of an area increases; our calculations were therefore based on regional and state per capita income weighted according to the number of physicians in the area. We assumed that the real prices of equipment and supplies used by physicians are roughly the same in both countries; the ratio was therefore assumed to be 1.0.

We calculated the price ratio for all resources as an expenditure-weighted average of the ratios for the four categories, using the average of U.S. and Canadian weights. Liability insurance is an important item of expenditure for U.S. physicians, but their Canadian counterparts do not incur a similar expense; estimates of liability expenses for Canadian physicians are less than 1 percent of gross receipts. We did not consider expenditures on liability insurance to reflect any real resource used in the practice of medicine; thus, liability insurance was

Table 5

Estimation of the prices of resources, 1985

Resource	Ratio of United States to Canada	Ratio of Iowa to Manitoba
Net income per physician[a]	1.35	1.61
Other resources		
Compensation rate of other personnel	1.09	0.98
Office	1.15	1.05
Medical supplies, equipment, and other	1.00	1.00
All resources[b]	1.24	1.37
All resources, as adjusted for liability insurance	1.30	1.43

[a]Adjusted for mix of specialties.
[b]Weighted average of all ratios.

treated as a tax on the prices of all resources. The ratios of resource prices were therefore increased by the share of all expenditures attributable to liability-insurance premiums. We concluded that the prices of resources are moderately higher in the United States than in Canada (Table 5), but the ratio is small as compared with the fee ratio of 2.39. Most of the excess of U.S. over Canadian fees must be attributable to the fact that Americans use more resources to produce a given quantity of services.

Ratio of Quantity of Resources to Quantity of Services

The results of our estimation of the ratios of resources to services (Table 6) were extraordinary. It appears that the United States uses 84 percent more real resources than does Canada to produce a given quantity of physicians' services. The difference between Iowa and Manitoba is somewhat smaller, with a ratio of 1.53.

Summary and Update

The study's most important results are summarized in Table 7. First, higher expenditures on physicians' services per capita in the United States were entirely explained by higher fees; in fact, the quantity of services per capita is actually lower in the United States than in Canada. Second, the higher fees were attributable primarily to the fact that Americans use more resources to produce a given quantity of services. Third, a small portion of the higher U.S. fees was reflected in higher prices of resources, especially physicians' net incomes. Fourth, the results of the comparison between Iowa and Manitoba were similar to those of the comparison between the United States and Canada, except that a larger proportion of the higher fees in Iowa reflected higher physicians' net incomes. Finally, updating the analysis to 1987 with data on changes in each

Table 6

Estimation of the quantity of resources relative to the quantity of services, 1985

Variable	Ratio of United States to Canada	Ratio of Iowa to Manitoba
Expenditures per capita (Table 2)	1.72	1.51
Prices of resources (Table 5)	1.30	1.43
Quantity of resources per capita[a]	1.32	1.06
Quantity of services per capita (Table 4)	0.72	0.69
Ratio of quantity of resources to quantity of services	1.84	1.53

[a]Values are expenditures per capita divided by the prices of resources.

Table 7

Summary and update of estimates

Variable	1985 Ratio of United States to Canada	1985 Ratio of Iowa to Manitoba	1987 Ratio of United States to Canada
Expenditures per capita	1.72	1.51	1.75
Fees	2.39	2.18	2.61
Quantity of services per capita	0.72	0.69	0.67
Prices of resources	1.30	1.43	1.32
Ratio of quantity of resources to quantity of services	1.84	1.53	1.98

country from 1985 to 1987 yielded results similar to those obtained for the 1985 comparisons between countries.

DISCUSSION

Two striking conclusions emerged from our statistical analysis of the difference between the United States and Canada in spending for physicians' services. First, the data firmly reject the view that Canadians save money by delivering fewer services. On the contrary, the quantity of services per capita is much higher in Canada than in the United States. Second, as compared with Canada, the United States uses appreciably more real resources to produce a given quantity of services. We will discuss eight possible explanations for these findings: the effects of insurance on demand, the effects of physicians on demand, billing costs, amenities, other administrative costs, overhead accounting, the workloads of procedure-oriented physicians, and the quality or intensity of care.

Effects of Insurance on Demand

Canadians have universal coverage and face no out-of-pocket expenses, whereas U.S. patients pay coinsurance rates ranging from 0 (full insurance) to 100 percent (for the uninsured). Thus, lower rates of use in the United States must reflect in part the price sensitivity of the demand for physicians' services. If, on average, Americans face the equivalent of 25 percent coinsurance, the results of the Rand Health Insurance Experiment predict that there will be 27 percent fewer visits and 33 percent less outpatient expenditure per capita than if they had full coverage (42). We found that the use of evaluation and management services in the United States was 36 percent less than in Canada, and the difference between

Iowa and Manitoba was 40 percent. Another source has estimated per capita contacts with a physician at 7.1 in Canada in 1985 and at 5.4 in the United States in 1986 (43).

Effects of Physicians on Demand

To the extent that higher rates of use in Canada are not fully explained by more complete insurance coverage, they may be explained by demand induced by Canadian physicians (44). The number of general practitioners and family physicians is very high in Canada, and their fee per visit is low. They may thus be more inclined to recommend additional evaluation and management services.

Billing Costs

In each Canadian province there is only one source of payment for physicians' services. Physicians typically submit one bill, and payment is usually punctual and complete. In contrast, American physicians must bill a myriad of private and public third-party payers, and often must also bill patients directly. Numerous complex forms must be filled out, there are frequently delays in payment as well as disagreements concerning the amount to be paid, and collection efforts impose additional costs. The differences in billing undoubtedly account for some of the additional resources reflected in the U.S. data, but we do not know exactly how much. The order of magnitude can be inferred from the fact that approximately 16 percent of the gross receipts of physicians are devoted to personnel who are not medical doctors. If one-fourth of those personnel are needed for billing tasks that are not required in the Canadian system, then 4 percent of U.S. expenditures can be explained by this factor. There are also additional billing costs for physicians' time, computers, stationery, and postage.

Amenities

Fragmentary data from one Canadian province and the American Medical Association suggest that U.S. physicians spend considerably more than their Canadian counterparts for rent and related office expenses, possibly twice as much. It is unlikely that this large difference is primarily the result of higher prices for identical offices. Some portion, probably a considerable portion, reflects a higher level of amenities in the average U.S. office. This may take the form of a more desirable location, more space per patient, newer furnishings, or more elaborate decor. Why would this occur? One reason is that real per capita income in the United States is 10 to 15 percent higher than in Canada; Americans are therefore accustomed to a somewhat higher level of amenities in most aspects of life. But the income difference would probably explain only about a 10 to 15 percent difference in amenities. More important may be the fact that competition for well-insured patients is more intense in the United States, especially among procedure-oriented physicians, many of whom have lower workloads than they desire. Physicians usually do not compete for insured patients by lowering fees, but they can try to attract such patients by offering a higher level of amenities.

Other Administrative Costs

There are numerous other costs incurred by many U.S. physicians that are lower or nonexistent for their Canadian counterparts. For instance, concern over possible malpractice suits (much rarer in Canada) may cause U.S. physicians to keep additional notes and records, or to undertake other activities that require their time and other resources but that are not reflected in the measures of quantity of services. (If concern over possible malpractice suits leads U.S. physicians to order additional visits and tests, the ratio between resources and services is not affected, because both the additional services and resources required to produce them are accounted for.) Other administrative costs that are more likely to be incurred by American than Canadian physicians involve maintaining contractual relations with preferred-provider organizations, dealing with third-party use reviews, and marketing.

Overhead Accounting

Overhead makes up 48 percent of expenditures in the United States, but only 34 percent in Canada (37, 38). Some of this difference undoubtedly reflects the greater use of resources in the United States, as discussed above. Some, however, may reflect more stringent scrutiny of overhead accounting by the Canadian government, because the overhead percentage is part of the background for negotiations between the provincial governments and physicians' organizations over fees. This constraint is not present in the United States. If identical accounting practices were applied in both countries, the overhead percentages might be slightly closer to each other and the difference in net income might be slightly larger. Such an adjustment would increase the ratio of the price of resources in the two countries by a few percentage points and decrease the ratio of resources to services by an equivalent amount.

Workloads of Procedure-Oriented Physicians

There can be little doubt that the average Canadian physician who specializes in procedures does more of them during a year than his or her counterpart in the United States. We estimated that there are about 40 percent more procedure-oriented physicians in the United States than in Canada (relative to the population), but the number of procedures performed appears to be about 20 percent higher in Canada. For some specialties the difference in workloads may be of the order of magnitude of two to one. This explanation is not as relevant for the comparison between Iowa and Manitoba, because the per capita supply of procedure-oriented physicians is about the same in both places. The difference in the supply of physicians may help explain why the ratio of resources to services is much higher between the United States and Canada than between Iowa and Manitoba.

Quality or Intensity of Care

The most uncertain and potentially controversial explanation concerns possible differences in quality or intensity of care. This question required that evaluation and management and procedures be considered separately. We estimated that approximately two-thirds of the evaluation and management services in Canada are delivered by general practitioners and family physicians, and one-third is delivered by internists, pediatricians, psychiatrists, and other specialists. In the United States the proportions are reversed. Should this be interpreted as a difference in quality of care? Some would argue that care provided by physicians with specialty training should be considered as "more" care. But there are others who believe that in most cases the quality of care provided by general practitioners or family physicians is as high, and may even be superior because of their greater familiarity with the patient and his or her circumstances. The question of intensity of care arises because of the possibility that some of the additional evaluation and management services provided in Canada are for patients with minor problems such as colds or upset stomachs. Some visits of this type may be deterred in the United States because insurance coverage is not as complete and because patients have been urged by employers and insurance companies not to visit physicians for minor problems. If the category of moderate office visits included fewer patients with minor problems in the United States, an adjustment for intensity would result in a slight increase in the ratio of the quantity of services per capita and a slight decrease in the ratio of resources to services.

With respect to procedures, the question of possible differences in the quality of care arises for other reasons. The technical competence of the specialists performing the procedures in the two countries is probably not an issue. A comparison of surgical mortality in Manitoba and New England concluded that the differences were small (45) (see Chapter 12). Timeliness and convenience, however, may differ. Because on a per capita basis there are so many more procedure-oriented specialists in the United States than in Canada, it is likely that Americans with insurance find it easier to have procedures performed when and where they want. From the patient's perspective, this may offer an additional source of satisfaction with the service provided. Whether such differences exist, how large they are, and how they are valued by patients are subjects for further research. These issues are much more muted in the comparison between Iowa and Manitoba than in that between the United States and Canada, because there are so few physicians per capita in Iowa as compared with Manitoba.

This discussion points up the need for additional studies to determine the magnitude of the many factors affecting fees, use of services, and use of resources to produce those services. Further refinements in the ratios of physicians' fees and the prices of resources would be particularly valuable, given the central role of these ratios in the statistical analysis. Such studies and refinements, however, are not likely to alter the principal lesson of this study: U.S. fees are more than double those of Canada, but physicians' net incomes are only about a third higher. The disparity is explained in part by much greater overhead expenses in the United States and in part by the lower workloads of American procedure-oriented physicians as compared with their Canadian counterparts.

REFERENCES

1. Iglehart, J. K. Canada's health care system faces its problems. *N. Engl. J. Med.* 322: 562–568, 1990.
2. Doherty, K. Is the Canadian system as good as it looks for employers? *Bus. Health* 7(7): 31–34, 1989.
3. Moloney, T. W., and Paul B. A new financial framework: Lessons from Canada. *Health Aff. (Millwood)* 8(2): 148–159, 1989.
4. Andreopoulos, S. (ed.). *National Health Insurance: Can We Learn from Canada?* Wiley, New York, 1975.
5. Evans, R. G., and Stoddart, G. L. (eds.). *Medicare at Maturity: Achievements, Lessons, and Challenges.* Proceedings of the Health Policy Conference on Canada's National Health Care System. Calgary, Alb.: University of Calgary Press, 1986.
6. Iglehart, J. K. Canada's health care system. *N. Engl. J. Med.* 315: 202–208, 778–784, 1623–1628, 1986.
7. Barer, M. L., and Evans, R. G. Riding north on a south-bound horse? Expenditures, prices, utilization and incomes in the Canadian Health Care System. In *Medicare at Maturity: Achievements, Lessons, and Challenges.* Proceedings of the Health Policy Conference on Canada's National Health Care System, edited by M. L. Barer and R. G. Evans, pp. 53–163. University of Calgary Press, Calgary, Alb., 1986.
8. Detsky, A. S., Stacey, S. R., and Bombardier, C. The effectiveness of a regulatory strategy in containing hospital costs: The Ontario experience, 1967–1981. *N. Engl. J. Med.* 309: 151–159, 1983.
9. Detsky, A. S., et al. Global budgeting and the teaching hospital in Ontario. *Med. Care* 24: 89–94, 1986.
10. Fulda, T. K., and Dickens, P. F. Controlling the cost of drugs: The Canadian experience. *Health Care Financ. Rev.* 1(2): 55–64, 1979.
11. McRae, J. J., and Tapon, F. Some empirical evidence on post-patent barriers to entry in the Canadian pharmaceutical industry. *J. Health Econ.* 4: 43–61, 1985.

12. Scherer, F. M. Post-patent barriers to entry in the pharmaceutical industry. *J. Health Econ.* 4: 83–87, 1985.
13. McPherson, K., et al. Regional variations in the use of common surgical procedures: Within and between England and Wales, Canada and the United States of America. *Soc. Sci Med. [A]* 15: 273–288, 1981.
14. Vayda, E., Mindell, W. R., and Rutkow, I. M. A decade of surgery in Canada, England and Wales, and the United States. *Arch. Surg.* 117: 846–853, 1982.
15. Himmelstein, D. U., and Woolhandler, S. Cost without benefit: Administrative waste in U.S. health care. *N. Engl. J. Med.* 314: 441–445, 1986.
16. American Hospital Association. *Hospital Statistics.* Chicago, 1986.
17. American Medical Association. *Physician Characteristics and Distribution in the U.S.* Chicago, 1986.
18. Health and Welfare Canada. *Active Civilian Physicians by Type of Physician, Canada, by Province, December 31, 1987.* Ottawa, Ont., 1988.
19. Iowa Development Commission. *Statistical Profile of Iowa.* Des Moines, 1987.
20. Statistics Canada. *Canadian Economic Observer, Historical Statistical Supplement, 1988/89.* Catalog 11-210. Ottawa, Ont., 1989.
21. Statistics Canada. *Canada Year Book 1985.* Ottawa, Ont., 1985.
22. Statistics Canada. *Canada Year Book 1988.* Ottawa, Ont., 1988.
23. Statistics Canada. *Hospital Annual Statistics, 1984–85.* Catalogue 83-232 annual. Ottawa, Ont., 1987.
24. Statistics Canada. *Life Tables, Canada and Provinces, 1985–1987.* Catalogue S41-044. Ottawa, Ont., 1988.
25. Statistics Canada. *Postcensal Annual Estimates of Population by Marital Status, Age, Sex, and Components of Growth for Canada, Provinces, and Territories, June 1, 1985,* Vol. 3, 3rd issue. Catalogue 91-210 annual. Ottawa, Ont., 1988.
26. Bureau of the Census. *Statistical Abstract of the United States: 1987,* 107th ed. Government Printing Office, Washington, D.C., 1987.
27. Bureau of the Census. *Statistical Abstract of the United States: 1988,* 108th ed. Government Printing Office, Washington, D.C., 1988.
28. Bureau of the Census. *Statistical Abstract of the United States: 1989,* 109th ed. Government Printing Office, Washington, D.C., 1989.
29. Bureau of the Census. *City and County Data Book.* Government Printing Office, Washington, D.C., 1986.
30. Health and Welfare Canada. *National Health Expenditures in Canada, 1975–85.* Ottawa, Ont., 1987.
31. Levit, K. Personal health expenditures by state, 1976–82. *Health Care Financ. Rev.* 6(4): 1–49, 1985.
32. Organisation for Economic Co-operation and Development. *National Accounts. Vol. 1. Main Aggregates, 1960–1985.* Organisation for Economic Co-operation and Development, Paris, 1987.
33. Department of Commerce, Bureau of Economic Analysis. *Survey of Current Business, May 1988.* (No. 337-790.) Government Printing Office, Washington, D.C., 1988.
34. Waldo, D., Levit, K. R., and Lazenby, H. National health expenditures, 1985. *Health Care Financ. Rev.* 8(1): 1–21, 1986.

35. Medical Group Management Association. *The Cost and Production Survey Report: 1986 Report.* Denver, 1986.
36. Health Care Financing Administration. *Average Allowed Charges for Selected Procedure Codes by Type of Service, 1985: Part B Medicare Annual Data Procedure File.* Baltimore, 1985.
37. Health and Welfare Canada. *Physicians' Income by Specialty Study 1985.* Ottawa, Ont., 1988.
38. American Medical Association. *SMS Detailed Tables.* AMA Center for Health Policy Research, Chicago, October 1987.
39. Department of Commerce, Bureau of the Census. *Current Population Survey, March 1985,* Public Use Tape.
40. Health and Welfare Canada. *Salaries and Wages in Canadian Hospitals, 1962 to 1985.* Ottawa, Ont., 1988.
41. Statistics Canada. *Annual Return of Hospitals—Hospital Indicators, 1984–85,* Catalogue 83-233. Ottawa, Ont., 1987.
42. Manning, W. G., et al. Health insurance and the demand for medical care: Evidence from a randomized experiment. *Am. Econ. Rev.* 77: 251–277, 1987.
43. Sandier, S. Health services utilization and physician income trends. *Health Care Financ. Rev.* 11(1): 33–48, 1989.
44. Ginzberg, E. *Men, Money, and Medicine.* Columbia University Press, New York, 1969.
45. Roos, L. L., et al. Postsurgical mortality in Manitoba and New England. *JAMA* 263: 2453–2458, 1990.

Hospital Spending
in the United States
and Canada: A Comparison

Joseph P. Newhouse, Geoffrey Anderson,
and Leslie L. Roos

Numerous health policy analysts on both sides of the border have discussed the Canadian method of financing medical care as a possible model for the United States (1–3). Canada not only has achieved universal coverage but spends substantially less per capita on health than the United States. Those favoring the Canadian model have tended to assume that the savings in cost come with minimal or no effect on the quality of care or health outcomes. On the contrary, because of universal coverage, health outcomes averaged over the Canadian population as a whole may even exceed those in the United States. However, the U.S. debate over whether the Canadian system is superior has paid less attention to health outcomes than to differences in cost and coverage levels. In Canada, by contrast, there is no serious advocate of the U.S. system.

In this chapter, we do not examine differences between the two countries in health outcomes, but we do examine the differences in the use of acute care hospitals—the largest single component of health care expenditures in both countries. We compare the countries in terms of three measures of hospital utilization: (*a*) admissions, (*b*) length-of-stay, and (*c*) case-mix, measured using the weights attached to the diagnosis-related groups (DRGs) of the U.S. Medicare program. We limit the analysis to the care provided to individuals age 65 and

Published by *Health Affairs,* Winter 1988, pp. 6–16. Copyright 1988, The People-to-People Health Foundation, Inc., Project HOPE.

older because they receive universal public insurance in both countries.[1] Thus we can attribute differences in use to factors other than differences in insurance coverage and can compute rates of use for defined populations. While our analysis does not compare the ultimate effects of differences in health care expenditures between the two countries, it does provide a first step toward a better understanding of the factors that drive those differences.

HOSPITAL USE IN THE UNITED STATES AND CANADA

We compare utilization in two Canadian provinces with both the United States as a whole and selected states geographically close to the two provinces. We chose the two provinces because of data availability. However, they contain 40 percent of the Canadian population; also, results for the two provinces are similar, suggesting that our conclusions may hold for a comparison of all of Canada with the United States.

Data Sources and Numbers

For the United States, our data come from a 20 percent sample of all Medicare hospital claims in calendar year 1981 and fiscal years 1984 and 1985. From this file we deleted claims from the four states that at that time had waivers from the prospective payment system (PPS)—Maryland, Massachusetts, New Jersey, and New York. Thus, references to the entire United States mean only 46 states. We also deleted claims from Puerto Rico and the Virgin Islands, although including them would have negligible effects because they are so small. We also deleted claims for those under age 65.

For Canada, the data come from a 100 percent sample of claims from Ontario and Manitoba. Although we compare both provinces with the entire United States, we also compare Ontario with Michigan and Ohio, and Manitoba with North Dakota and Montana. The samples from each of the two-state areas are about half as large as the comparable provinces.

Type of Provider and Case-Mix

The goal of our analysis was to compare the use of acute care hospital services in the two countries. However, differences in the definitions of institutions and units exist. To make our comparisons as similar as possible, we excluded cases in

---

[1] In the United States, the widespread nature of so-called Medigap policies makes cost sharing for hospital services among those over 65 unimportant. Approximately 75 percent of people over 65 were covered by Medigap policies, and another 8 percent were covered by Medicaid, although not all Medigap policies cover all cost sharing. The remaining sixth face a deductible equal to the average cost of one day in the hospital (4).

rehabilitation and long-term care hospitals and units. We used the following methods to define use of acute care beds.

In Ontario, each discharge abstract contains a variable that identifies the institution from which the individual was discharged. Each institution is assigned a unique identifier. Long-term care and rehabilitation units within acute care hospitals are assigned identifiers that are distinct from the number assigned to the acute care section of the hospital. A transfer from an acute care section to a rehabilitation or long-term care section of the same institution produces a discharge abstract. A discharge was included in the analysis only if it was from an identical acute care institution. Discharges from acute care psychiatric units were included.

In Manitoba, each discharge abstract contains a service code indicating the type of care received by the patient during the admission. Patients receiving personal care, physical medicine and rehabilitation, geriatrics, and extended treatment were excluded from the analysis. Patients receiving psychiatric or psychogeriatric care were included.

In the United States, certain hospitals—rehabilitation, chronic or long-term, psychiatric, and children's—were exempt from PPS, which began in October 1983. Unfortunately, we cannot identify these exempt hospitals in 1981. We have therefore estimated 1981 admission and case-mix figures using the relationship between acute care hospitals (and psychiatric hospitals) and all hospitals in 1984 and 1985. Specifically, to estimate a figure for admissions and the case-mix index for 1981, we used the admission (case-mix) figure for all hospitals for 1981 and multiplied it by the ratio of admissions (case-mix) in all hospitals other than long-term and rehabilitative to admissions (case-mix) in all hospitals. This ratio was available for both 1984 and 1985; we averaged the two values.

Only around 5 percent of all admissions occurred in rehabilitative and long-term care hospitals and units in both 1984 and 1985, and, if anything, the value was probably lower in 1981 because of fewer such units. Our method for estimating a 1981 rate therefore effectively decreased the admission rate to all hospitals (including rehabilitative and long-term) in 1981 by about 5 percent. The resulting 1981 admission rate for the United States may be slightly too low, but any error is almost certainly not serious enough to affect the comparisons with Canada.

The value for the case-mix index is about 1 percent higher in both 1984 and 1985 if cases in rehabilitation and long-term hospitals and units are excluded. Hence, our methods led us to increase the case-mix index for all hospitals in 1981 by about 1 percent. That adjustment also does not affect any of our comparisons.

Length-of-Stay

Unlike admissions and the case-mix index, the 1981 length-of-stay values are sensitive to the adjustment process, because of the long lengths-of-stay in rehabilitation and long-term care hospitals and units (mean values in the United

States of 50 days in 1984 and 35 days in 1985). To reduce the sensitivity of our length-of-stay comparisons to errors in classification of cases, we began by computing not only the usual mean but also a trimmed mean by setting all stays of over 60 days equal to 60 days. This reduced the influence of very long-stay cases. However, when we then adjusted the 1981 U.S. values in the same way that we adjusted admissions and case-mix, we obtained the anomalous result that the adjusted trimmed length-of-stay exceeded the adjusted untrimmed length-of-stay. Hence, we have followed the simple step of reporting the length-of-stay values for all U.S. hospitals for 1981 (both untrimmed and trimmed). Although this will overestimate length-of-stay in hospitals other than rehabilitation and long-term, the values are still well below the Canadian values, so that our qualitative conclusions are unaffected. In the U.S. data, we have excluded discharges from skilled nursing facilities.

Population Data

U.S. enrollee data come from the Health Care Financing Administration (HCFA). These data are for 1984 and come from aggregating enrollees by zip code. To project the number of enrollees for 1981 and 1985, the total number of Part A enrollees over age 65 in 1981, 1984, and 1985 in the entire country was used (5). The number of enrollees in each of the two subregions analyzed in 1981 and 1985 was assumed to change proportionally the same as the national number (0.9439 for 1981 and 1.0211 for 1985, both relative to 1984). In Canada, federal support for the provincially administered health care systems is contingent upon universal coverage of the population. Therefore, census data were used to identify the eligible populations in Ontario and Manitoba.

We have not age- and sex-adjusted our figures because the age-sex distributions are virtually identical. Using five-year age groups for each sex (through age 85), the percentage of the population in each group in North Dakota and Montana is always within one percentage point of the group in Manitoba; similarly, the percentage for Michigan and Ohio is almost always within one percentage point of the group in Ontario (one case differed by 1.3 points). We cannot compare costs or charges at the case level directly because Canada does not associate costs or charges with a particular case in its global budgeting method.

RESULTS OF THE COMPARISON

As is commonly known, real personal health expenditure per person is substantially higher in the United States than in Canada; we estimate that the United States spent about 50 percent more per person throughout the first part of the 1980s (Table 1). Similar percentage differentials also applied to hospital services. Hospital expenditure per capita in Manitoba is identical to that in all of Canada.

Table 1

Health expenditure per capita in the United States and Canada,
1981–1985, 1985 U.S. dollars[a,b]

| | United States | | Canada | | Manitoba |
Year	Personal health expenditure per capita	Hospital expenditure per capita	Personal health expenditure per capita	Hospital expenditure per capita	Hospital expenditure per capita
1981	$1,260	$590	$ 800	$380	$380
1984	1,440	670	1,010	470	470
1985	1,500	680	1,010	460	460

[a]Sources: Data for United States 1981, 1984: K. R Levit et al., National Health Expenditures, 1984, *Health Care Financing Review,* Fall 1985; for 1985: D. Waldo et al., National Health Expenditures, 1985, *Health Care Financing Review,* Fall 1986. Data for Canada: *National Health Expenditures in Canada, 1975–1985; National Health and Welfare, 1987; Quarterly Economic Review,* Annual Reference Tables, Department of Finance, Canada, June 1987; Manitoba Health Services Commission, Annual Reports. Converted to U.S. dollars at exchange rates of 1.199 for 1981, 1,295 for 1984, and 1,366 for 1985.

[b]Uses United States gross national product (GNP) consumption deflator.

To examine in more detail what might account for these differences in the level of hospital expenditure, we examined admission rates and lengths-of-stay between 1981 and 1985 (Tables 2 and 3). Admission rates were comparable between Michigan/Ohio and Ontario in 1981 and 1984, and were lower in Michigan in 1985. Although admission rates in Montana/North Dakota fell 15 percent from 1984 to 1985, they remained about 10 percent above those in Manitoba and well above those for the United States. On the whole, by 1985, admission rates in the two countries seem approximately the same. In contrast, length-of-stay differs markedly between the two countries. Length-of-stay in Manitoba was approximately double the length-of-stay in Montana/North Dakota, while length-of-stay in Ontario was notably longer than in Michigan/ Ohio, especially by 1985. North Dakota/Montana had somewhat shorter stays than the U.S. average, and Michigan/Ohio had somewhat longer stays.

To determine how length-of-stay might be affected by very long-stay patients, we recomputed the mean length-of-stay by trimming stays at 60 days (that is, patients with stays longer than 60 days were set equal to 60 days). The results are shown in Table 4. Stays in Manitoba are particularly affected, falling by three to four days. Values for the United States are not much changed. Nonetheless, even after reducing the effect on the mean of these very long-stay patients, there remain substantial differences between the countries in mean length-of-stay.

Results for the case-mix index are somewhat difficult to interpret because of the rapid increase in the U.S. index, much of which has been attributed to better coding procedures (Table 5) (6). By contrast, the values for Canada have

Table 2

Hospital admission rates for people over age 65, selected states and provinces

Year	Ontario	Michigan/ Ohio	Manitoba	North Dakota/ Montana	All United States[a]
1981	.33	.33[b]	.32	.41[b]	.34[b]
1984	.35	.36	.32	.44	.37
1985	.35	.32	.34	.38	.33

[a]Excludes waiver states of Maryland, Massachusetts, New Jersey, and New York.
[b]Estimated; see text.

Table 3

Length-of-stay for people over age 65, selected states and provinces, in days

Year	Ontario	Michigan/ Ohio	Manitoba	North Dakota/ Montana	All United States[a]
1981	14.43	11.11[b]	15.88	8.35[b]	9.90[b]
1984	14.48	9.40	15.38	7.64	8.66
1985	14.25	8.60	15.77	7.16	8.07

[a]Excludes waiver states of Maryland, Massachusetts, New Jersey, and New York.
[b]Value is overestimated because it includes stays at rehabilitation and long-term care hospitals and units; see text.

Table 4

Length-of-stay for people over age 65, selected states and provinces, stays trimmed at 60 days

Year	Ontario	Michigan/ Ohio	Manitoba	North Dakota/ Montana	All United States[a]
1981	13.27	10.98[b]	11.07	8.23[b]	9.75[b]
1984	13.43	9.25	12.29	7.41	8.48
1985	13.32	8.48	12.16	6.77	7.96

[a]Excludes waiver states of Maryland, Massachusetts, New Jersey, and New York.
[b]Value for all hospitals; see text.

Table 5

Case-mix index for people over age 65, selected states and provinces

Year	Ontario	Michigan/ Ohio	Manitoba	North Dakota/ Montana	All United States[a]
1981	1.10	1.08[b]	1.07	0.96[b]	1.01[b]
1984	1.11	1.13	1.08	1.10	1.12
1985	1.12	1.19	1.09	1.20	1.19

[a]Excludes waiver states of Maryland, Massachusetts, New Jersey, and New York.
[b]Estimated; see text.

increased at a rate of half a percent to a percent a year, which is similar to the pre-PPS trend of a half percent a year that Grace Carter and Paul Ginsburg estimated for the United States (6).

WHAT ACCOUNTS FOR THE DIFFERENCE?

In the early 1980s, the United States spent nearly 50 percent more per person on hospital services than Canada; the important question is what, if anything, the United States bought for that additional expenditure. To shed light on that question, we have decomposed hospital spending in two provinces and compared the anatomy of that spending with two comparable areas in the United States and the United States as a whole.

Overall, our findings, which apply only to the elderly, somewhat deepen the puzzle of what the United States might be buying. By 1985, admission rates were roughly comparable in the two countries, being somewhat higher in North Dakota and Montana than in Manitoba, but somewhat lower in Michigan and Ohio than in Ontario. The U.S. admission rate was marginally below that of the two provinces. Hence, the differences in spending between the two countries cannot be attributed to a higher rate of hospital admissions in the United States.

In each of the three years we examined, lengths-of-stay were markedly longer in Canada. The considerable fall in length-of-stay in the United States was not matched in Canada. By 1985, lengths-of-stay in Ontario were more than two-thirds again as long as in Michigan and Ohio, and in Manitoba were more than double the lengths-of-stay in North Dakota and Montana. Because admission rates were roughly similar (in 1985), the number of patient days per person over age 65 in the United States are only 50 to 60 percent of the corresponding number in Canada. It follows from the values in Table 1 that spending per patient day is perhaps three times as great in the United States as in Canada.

Case-Mix

To understand why the United States might be spending half again as much per case and three times as much per day, we examined the case-mix index for the two countries. Comparison between the two countries is complicated by the rapid rate of increase in the U.S. index that can be attributed to PPS. Coding now affects the hospital's reimbursement; this has resulted in both a substantial increase in the accuracy of the coding and an incentive to code cases in higher-weighted DRGs. Neither of these effects was present in Canada.

If we judge the comparability of case-mix using data from 1981, a time when coding incentives in the two countries were more nearly similar, the case-mix index is higher in Canada; this is especially true of the comparison between Manitoba and North Dakota/Montana. In 1984 the two countries were roughly comparable, although by 1985 the United States had a somewhat higher case-mix index. If one could adjust for upcoding, however, it is likely that the 1985 U.S. value would be equal to or below the Canadian (6). The similarity of the annual change in case-mix in Canada with the annual U.S. change prior to PPS strongly suggests that most of the change in the United States was not true change. Even if the 1985 difference between the United States and Canada is true (which we think is unlikely), case-mix, as measured by DRGs, can at best account for only a small portion of spending differences.

Thus, the difference in hospital spending between the two countries, which may account for around 40 percent of the difference in total expenditure between the two countries, must be accounted for primarily by differences in the cost of a "case-mix index unit" per beneficiary. With admissions and the case-mix index in the two countries at approximately the same level, the cost of a case-mix unit in the United States was approximately 50 percent higher than in Canada. What might account for such a difference? The Canadian method of global budgeting of course, makes it easier to control costs, and some discussions appear to assume that the additional American costs are pure inefficiency. However, other factors ought to be considered.

Severity of Illness

Differences in severity or complexity within DRGs could be such that American patients are sicker. There is no reason, however, to think that this is the case; indeed, the similar admission rates and longer lengths-of-stay in Canada, if anything, point in the other direction. Lack of insurance coverage, which could lead to increased severity of illness in some under age 65 admitted to a U.S. hospital, should not play an important role in the Medicare population.

Volume of Services

American patients could have more done to or for them when in the hospital. Not only could there be more tests and other ancillary procedures, but staffing ratios could be higher. Indeed, staffing ratios per patient day in the United States appear to be almost double those in Ontario. There were 3.47 employees per adjusted census in nonfederal short-term general and other special hospitals in the United States in 1981, and 1.87 per inpatient day in 1980–1981 in Ontario (7, 8). However, staffing ratios per stay or per person in the population are not very discrepant between the two countries.

Higher-Paid Staff

Employees of American hospitals could be paid more than similar employees at Canadian hospitals. We do not have data on wages. Hospital inputs other than personnel (for example, beds) tend to be traded in international markets, so their costs should not much differ between the two countries.

Administrative Costs

Certain overhead or administrative costs may differ. For example, malpractice premiums no doubt are higher in the United States than in Canada. (Note, however, that one justification of the malpractice system is deterrence of negligent actions, which, if it were effective, ought to lower U.S. hospital costs relative to Canadian.) Administrative costs to cope with multiple sources of financing and various utilization review mechanisms also may be higher in the United States. However, it is unlikely that such differences could begin to account for the magnitude of the overall difference in spending, because total administrative and accounting costs are estimated to account for only 18 percent of U.S. expenditure on personal health care versus 8 percent in Canada.[2]

A CLOSER LOOK AT LENGTH-OF-STAY DIFFERENCES

Our work points up the methodological difficulties of making comparisons across countries. Although our major conclusions do not appear sensitive to definitional differences, the difficulties in developing comparable definitions of hospitals may be a problem for more detailed analysis of the two countries. Indeed, even within each country there are difficulties with hospital definition.

---

[2] These numbers are suspect because definitions may not be comparable; even so, they demonstrate that it is unlikely that differences in administrative costs could account for a majority of the difference (9).

Table 6

Percentage of patients over age 65 staying over 60 days

	1981	1984	1985
United States			
All hospitals	0.5	1.4	1.0
All excluding rehabilitation and long-term	—	0.4	0.2
Ontario[a]	2.7	3.0	2.9
Manitoba[b]	5.0	5.0	5.0

[a]All patients excluding rehabilitation and long-term.
[b]Excludes stays in personal care units, geriatrics, and extended treatment hospitals.

For example, the figures often cited to show the decline in length-of-stay caused by PPS do not compare patients in the same hospitals over time (10). As a result, the well-known fall in length-of-stay resulting from PPS is overstated. If one includes patients in exempt hospitals in 1981 and 1984, average length-of-stay actually rose among those age 65 and over, from 9.9 days to 10.7 days in 1984; in 1985, however, length-of-stay fell to 9.5 days.[3]

Because of the importance of hospital definition in the number of long-stay patients and the importance of such patients in the overall length-of-stay figures, we compared the percentage of patients in the two countries with stays of over 60 days. Two conclusions emerged (Table 6). First, U.S. data for all hospitals show a substantial increase in long-stay patients between 1981 and 1985. At the same time, long-stay patients in PPS-covered hospitals have decreased. (Of course, PPS gives a considerable reward for caring for long-stay patients in exempt hospitals or units.) Hence, average length-of-stay figures will be sensitive to the definition of hospital used and to the nature of patients in those hospitals.

Second, comparing the United States with Ontario and Manitoba shows that the proportion of patients with very long stays is considerably greater in Canada, especially in Manitoba; this proportion has been increasing in Ontario as well as in the United States (though not in Manitoba). The proportion of elderly with very long stays also has been increasing in British Columbia (11). The reasons for this increase remain to be explored, but a small increase can cause a dramatic change in the average length-of-stay. For example, the average U.S. length-of-stay for patients staying over 60 days in 1985 was 130 days. Hence, a one percentage point increase in such patients will raise average length-of-stay 1.3 days. Given

---

[3] The trimmed mean (trimmed at 60 days) fell from 9.7 days in 1981 to 9.5 days in 1984 to 8.9 days in 1985. Standard errors on the untrimmed means are around 0.01 to 0.02.

the increases in long-stay patients, government insurers might well want to investigate ways to reduce length-of-stay.

Although this is only a first look at comparing Canada and the United States, patients at U.S. hospitals appear to use either more inputs or more highly paid inputs (or both) than do patients at Canadian hospitals. This difference in intensity appears to account for the bulk of the difference in hospital spending between the two countries. If so, the ultimate question is what the United States buys with the additional intensity, if anything. That question can best be addressed with data that pertain to outcomes. The most readily available outcome data are mortality data, but they are too crude to answer the question. Readmissions data for complications and other poor outcomes following surgery are another available indicator of outcome. Lacking comprehensive measures of outcome, one reasonable next step is to pursue the type of analysis used here at the level of specific diseases and treatments.

REFERENCES

1. Andreopoulos, S. (ed.). *National Health Insurance: Can We Learn from Canada?* Wiley, New York, 1975.
2. Iglehart, J. K. Canada's health care system. *N. Engl. J. Med.* 315: 202–208, 1986.
3. Iglehart, J. K. Canada's health care system. *N. Engl. J. Med.* 315: 778–784, 1986.
4. U.S. Department of Commerce. *Statistical Abstract, 1988.* U.S. Government Printing Office, Washington, D.C., 1987.
5. U.S. Department of Commerce. *Statistical Abstract, 1987.* U.S. Government Printing Office, Washington, D.C., 1986.
6. Carter, G., and Ginsburg, P. B. *The Medicare Case-Mix Index Increase: Medical Practice Changes, Aging, and DRG Creep.* Pub. No. R-3292-HCFA. RAND Corporation, Santa Monica, Calif., 1985.
7. American Hospital Association. *Hospital Statistics, 1986.* Chicago, 1986.
8. Detsky, A., Stacey, S. R., and Bombardier, C. The effectiveness of a regulatory strategy in containing hospital costs—The Ontario experience, 1967–1981. *N. Engl. J. Med.,* July 21, 1988, pp. 151–158.
9. Himmelstein, D. U., and Woolhandler, S. Cost without benefit. *N. Engl. J. Med.,* February 13, 1986, pp. 441–445.
10. Newhouse, J. P., and Byrne, D. J. Did Medicare's prospective payment system cause length-of-stay to fall? *J. Health Econ.,* December 1988.
11. Evans, R. G., et al. The Long Good-Bye: The Great Transformation of the British Columbia Hospital System. Discussion Paper HPRU 88: 2. University of British Columbia, March 1988.

CHAPTER 4

Debate on
U.S./Canadian Health Expenditures—I

A
How Well is Canada Doing?

Edward Neuschler

References to the success of the Canadian health care system have become increasingly frequent in the American press. If one measures access by health insurance coverage and health care cost by percentage of gross national product, Canada is doing well. All Canadians have health insurance coverage and Canada spends a smaller percentage of its total economic output on health care than does the United States. But if cost containment is measured by rates of increase in health care spending, and access by prompt availability of needed services, the picture is less clear. An analysis of trends suggests that: (*a*) Canada has done no better than the United States in taming health care cost escalation; and (*b*) Canada may be starting to have problems with access to needed services, particularly when expensive, high-technology care is required.

This chapter examines the evidence on cost containment and reviews the ongoing debate in Canada over access to care.[1]*

Part A reprinted from *Canadian Health Care: The Implications of Public Health Insurance,* Health Insurance Association of America, Washington, D.C., 1990, with permission of the Health Insurance Association of America.

*Editors' note:** In Part A, the notes are listed as endnotes preceding the Reference list (p. 64). The Appendix (pp. 62–63) lists the data used in much of this article, and their sources.

HEALTH CARE COST CONTAINMENT

International comparisons of health care expenditures must be adjusted in some way to account for differences in size among national economies. There are two ways to do this. One is to express health care expenditure as a percent of total economic output—gross national product (GNP) or gross domestic product (GDP).[2] The other is to express expenditure in per capita terms.

Comparisons between Canadian and U.S. health care expenditures often use the former method. On this measure Canada has been more successful than the United States in containing costs: health care expenditures as a proportion of GNP have not grown as fast in Canada as they have in the United States. Canada spent a slightly higher percentage of GNP on health than the United States in the 1960s, but fell below the U.S. level in 1969 and has stayed there. The most recent available figures show Canada spending 8.98 percent of GNP on health care (1987), and the United States spending 11.06 percent (1988).[3] (See the Appendix.) As this chapter demonstrates, however, when health care costs per capita are compared, the two countries have very similar growth patterns. Thus, this chapter argues, the difference in the proportion of GNP going to health care is due not to differences in how the two countries finance and deliver health care but to differences in overall economic growth rates—the Canadian economy grew significantly faster than the U.S. economy over the past two decades.

For this study, we examined the growth rate of per capita health spending[4] in Canada and the United States from 1967 through 1987 (the most recent 20-year period for which health spending totals are available for both countries). Figure 1 plots per capita health care spending in the United States and in Canada during that period, in the currency of each country and in the nominal dollars of each year (i.e., not adjusted for inflation). Canadian spending (CAN $1,869 per capita in 1987—$1,520 after conversion to U.S. dollars[5]) is lower than U.S. spending ($2,004 per capita in 1987) in absolute terms, but the similarity of the growth trend is striking. During the 20-year period, Canada's health care spending per capita grew at an average annual rate[6] of 11.50 percent, compared to a U.S. rate of 10.75 percent.

Because general inflation was greater in Canada than in the United States during this period, however, comparing growth in nominal dollars does not accurately measure the increase in real economic resources devoted to health care. To gain a more accurate picture of differences in the resources going to health care in the two countries, Figure 2 displays health spending per capita in constant 1981 dollars.[7] To remove any distortion in the comparison due to the varying relative value of the two currencies, Canadian expenditures are shown in both 1981 Canadian dollars and 1981 U.S. dollars.[8] The similarity in growth patterns remains striking, whichever measure is used. In fact, on an inflation-adjusted basis, the average growth rate over the 20-year period is slightly lower in the United States: 4.38 percent per year compared to 4.58 percent per year in

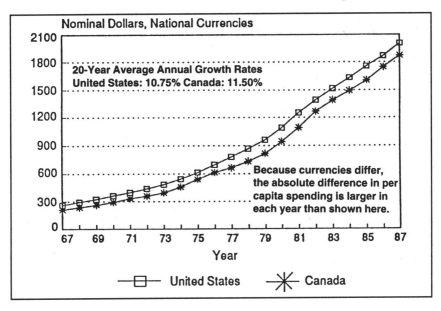

Figure 1. Total per capita health care spending in the United States and Canada, 1967–1987.

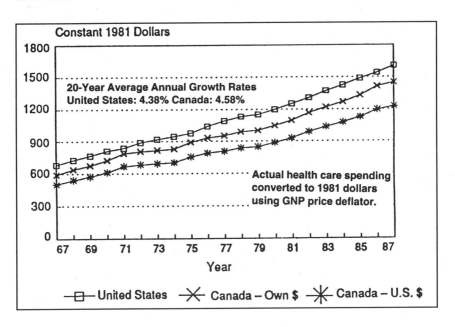

Figure 2. Total per capita health care spending in the United States and Canada, 1967–1987.

Canada. In Figure 3, each country's real health spending per capita is displayed as the ratio of spending in that year to spending in 1967, such that the graph represents the cumulative growth of real per capita spending over the 20-year period. With the visual distortion caused by the difference in base-year spending thus removed, the almost precise coincidence of the trend lines is absolutely clear.

But does the similarity of long-term trends mask some significant change during the 1967 to 1987 period? In particular, did Canada's growth rate slow after universal public health insurance was implemented fully, as some analysts have argued (4)? To examine this question, Figure 4 presents average annual growth rates in U.S. and Canadian health care spending per capita over successive 5-year periods, beginning in 1967. As shown, health care costs grew more rapidly in Canada than in the United States between 1967 and 1972. Canada's provinces implemented universal public medical insurance between 1968 and 1971,[9] so its somewhat more rapid escalation of costs in this period may be due to increased demand for services from newly insured individuals. After full implementation of public insurance, the rate of increase slowed significantly in Canada. But, despite the 1972 expansion of U.S. Medicare to include disabled persons under age 65, the U.S. growth rate fell as well, suggesting that the advent of the public insurance system in Canada was not the only factor affecting health care costs at that time. Since 1977, real health spending per capita has grown a bit more slowly

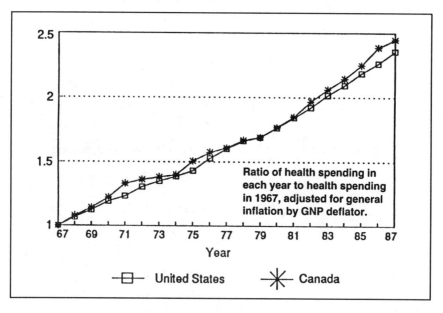

Figure 3.   Ratio of real per capita health care spending, 1967–1987, with 1967 = 1.0.

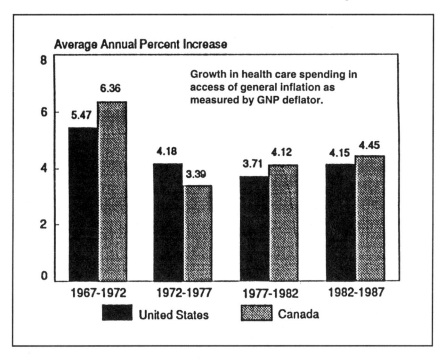

Figure 4. Average annual growth rates in per capita health care spending in 5-year periods, 1967–1987.

in the United States than in Canada. The average growth rate during 1977 to 1987 was 4.28 percent per year in Canada and 3.93 percent in the United States.[10]

It may be argued that health spending would have grown somewhat faster in the United States if the number of uninsured Americans had not increased between 1977 and 1987. One way to adjust for this factor is to re-estimate U.S. health spending in 1977 and 1987, under the assumption that all U.S. residents had health coverage in each year, and then recompute the growth rate from the new spending totals. Carrying out these calculations raises the estimated real U.S. growth rate per capita to about 4.4 percent per year, only slightly higher than the Canadian rate.[11]

Growth rates, of course, fluctuate from year to year. Figure 5 plots the yearly growth rates in real health care spending per capita over the entire 20-year period, yielding similar year-to-year patterns.

A final way of looking at the growth rate issue is displayed in Figure 6, which plots per capita healths pending in Canada as a percentage of per capita U.S. spending (in constant 1981 U.S. dollars) from 1967 through 1987. As can be seen, the percentage fluctuated in a very narrow range over the period. Canada

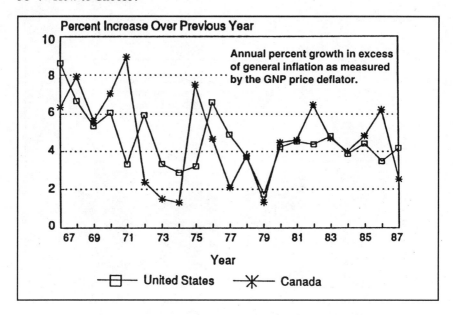

Figure 5. Yearly growth rates in per capita health care spending, 1967–1987.

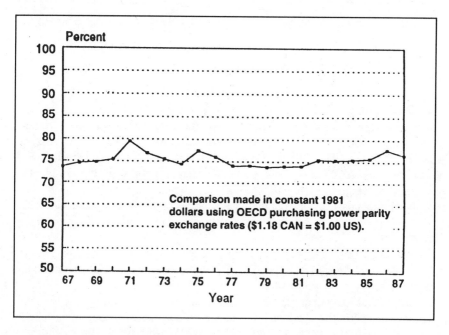

Figure 6. Per capita health spending in Canada as percent of U.S. spending, 1967–1987.

was spending about 75 percent of what the United States spends per capita on health care before implementation of universal public health insurance and has continued to do so since. The factors leading to different levels of health care spending in the two countries, therefore, must be more basic than the difference in health care financing arrangements.

The analysis presented here is consistent with work published by a pair of international experts. Writing in the Fall 1989 *Health Affairs,* Schieber and Poullier (5) compared growth rates of health care spending per capita between the United States and Canada (along with five other large democracies), using price indices specific to medical care.[12] In this way, they were able to divide overall growth in health care spending for 1960 to 1970, 1970 to 1980, and 1980 to 1987 into real growth in consumption of health care resources and medical price inflation in excess of general price inflation. In each period, excess medical price inflation and growth in real consumption of health care resources per capita were very similar in the two countries (Table 1).

If per capita health spending is growing as fast in Canada as in the United States, why does health spending continue to consume a smaller proportion of total Canadian economic output than of U.S. output? A major reason appears to be that Canada's economic output per capita has grown faster than ours,

Table 1

Annual growth rates of health care spending, 1960–1987[a,b]

	1960-70	1970-80	1980-87	1960-87
	Nominal health spending per capita			
United States	8.1%	11.5%	9.4%	10.2%
Canada	9.3%	12.5%	9.9%	10.7%
	Real[c]-expenditures per capita			
United States	4.6%	3.9%	1.7%	3.9%
Canada	7.0%	3.8%	1.5%	3.5%
	Excess medical-specific inflation			
United States	−0.9%	0.0%	3.0%	1.1%
Canada	−1.0%	0.0%	2.9%	1.2%

[a]Source: reference 5, Exhibit 5, p. 174.

[b]All entries are annual compound growth rates.

[c]In this chapter, we have used the term "real" health spending to denote comparisons made in constant (i.e., GNP-deflated) dollars. Schieber and Poullier had available to them price indices specific to the heatlh care sector in each country. They were therefore able to separate increases in health spending into three components: general inflation (not shown), medical (price) inflation in excess of general inflation, and real growth in the consumption of health care resources. The entry "real expenditures per capita" in this table reflects the last of the three components.

particularly from 1967 through 1976. In 1967, Canada and the United States spent virtually identical proportions of GNP on health care (6.33 percent in the United States, 6.38 percent in Canada). Two years later, the Canadian figure had fallen slightly below the U.S. figure; the gap widened noticeably after 1971 (Figure 7).

Because universal insurance was implemented in Canada between 1968 and 1971, some analysts have attributed Canada's slower increase in health spending as a percent of total economic output after 1971 to improved cost controls made possible by a universal government-financed system (4). But an alternative explanation is possible, one more consistent with our observation that Canada's provincial health plans have not been more effective than the pluralistic U.S. health system in controlling per capita health spending. As Figure 8 shows, beginning in 1968 Canada's economy grew faster than the U.S. economy (on a per capita basis) for a sustained period of 9 years. In 6 of those years, the difference in growth rates was more than 2 percentage points per year. Over the entire 20-year period (1967 to 1987), Canada's real GNP per capita grew 74 percent; U.S. real GNP per capita grew only 38 percent.[13] Given very similar growth rates of per capita health spending, the country that expands economic output more rapidly will spend a smaller proportion of that output on health care.

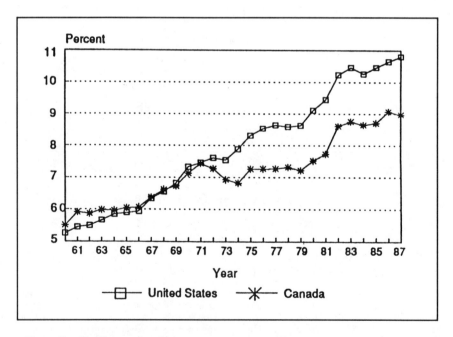

Figure 7.   Health care spending as percent of GNP, 1960–1987.

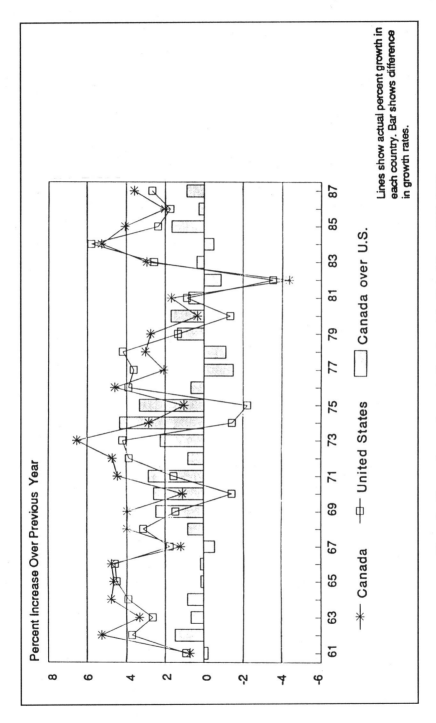

Figure 8. Economic growth rates in Canada and the United States, 1960–1987.

61

APPENDIX
Data and Sources

United States[a]

Year	Gross national product, current U.S.$ in billions	Total population, thousands	Total national health expenditures, current U.S.$ in billions	Implicit price deflator for GNP, 1982 = 100.0	Implicit price deflator for GNP, 1981 = 100.0 (calculated from 1982)
1960	515.3	180,671	27.1	30.9	32.9
1961	533.8	183,691	29.1	31.2	33.2
1962	574.6	186,538	31.6	31.9	34.0
1963	606.9	189,242	34.4	32.4	34.5
1964	649.8	191,889	38.0	32.9	35.0
1965	705.1	194,303	41.6	33.8	35.9
1966	772.0	196,560	45.9	35.0	37.2
1967	816.4	198,712	51.7	35.9	38.3
1968	892.7	200,706	58.5	37.7	40.2
1969	963.9	202,677	65.7	39.8	42.3
1970	1015.5	205,052	74.4	42.0	44.7
1971	1102.7	207,661	82.3	44.4	47.2
1972	1212.8	209,896	92.3	46.5	49.5
1973	1359.3	211,909	102.5	49.5	52.7
1974	1472.8	213,854	116.1	54.0	57.4
1975	1598.4	215,973	132.9	59.3	63.1
1976	1782.8	218,035	152.2	63.1	67.1
1977	1990.5	220,239	172.0	67.3	71.6
1978	2249.7	222,585	193.4	72.2	76.9
1979	2508.2	225,055	216.6	78.6	83.6
1980	2732.0	227,757	249.1	85.7	91.2
1981	3052.6	230,138	288.6	94.0	100.0
1982	3166.0	232,520	323.8	100.0	106.4
1983	3405.7	234,799	356.1	103.9	110.5
1984	3772.2	237,001	387.0	107.7	114.7
1985	4014.9	239,279	402.1	110.9	118.1
1986	4231.6	241,625	450.5	113.8	121.1
1987	4524.3	243,934	488.8	117.4	124.9
1988	4880.6	246,329	539.9	121.3	129.1

[a]Sources: U.S. Dept. of Commerce, Bureau of Economic Analysis, *Survey of Current Business* 69: 9, Tables 1 and 3, pp. 53 and 57, September 1989. U.S. Dept. of Commerce, Bureau of the Census, *Statistical Abstract of the United States: 1989,* 109th ed., (Table) No. 2. Population: 1900 to 1988, 1989. U.S. Dept. of Commerce, Bureau of the Census, *Current Population Rep.,* Series P-25, No. 1045, Table D, January 1990. Office of National Cost Estimates, U.S. Health Care Financing Administration, revised national health expenditure series through 1988, DHHS Press Release May 3, 1990; and personal communication.

			Canada[a]		
Year	Gross national product, current CAN $ in millions	Total population, thousands	Total national health expenditures, current CAN $ in millions	Implicit price deflator for GDP, 1981 = 100.0	OECD purchasing power parity currency conversion factor
1960	38,832	17,909.0	2,141.7	29.7	1.02
1961	40,164	18,271.0	2,375.5	29.9	1.03
1962	43,637	18,614.0	2,561.4	30.3	1.02
1963	46,830	18,964.0	2,801.5	30.9	1.03
1964	51,283	19,325.0	3,059.9	31.7	1.04
1965	56,531	19,678.0	3,415.5	32.8	1.05
1966	63,268	20,048.0	3,837.5	34.4	1.06
1967	67,824	20,412.0	4,324.4	35.8	1.07
1968	74,197	20,729.0	4,911.9	37.1	1.06
1969	81,819	21,028.0	5,505.3	38.8	1.05
1970	87,765	21,324.0	6,253.8	40.6	1.04
1971	95,784	21,591.7	7,118.7	41.9	1.02
1972	107,168	21,821.7	7,787.7	44.3	1.04
1973	125,642	22,072.3	8,699.4	48.2	1.06
1974	149,873	22,395.4	10,223.9	55.1	1.11
1975	169,002	22,726.9	12,267.8	60.6	1.11
1976	194,388	23,017.9	14,119.9	65.8	1.13
1977	213,308	23,295.0	15,500.0	69.9	1.13
1978	235,654	23,534.6	17,248.0	74.2	1.12
1979	268,941	23,768.3	19,412.1	81.6	1.13
1980	302,064	24,070.1	22,703.9	90.2	1.15
1981	344,657	24,362.1	26,650.0	100.0	1.18
1982	361,772	24,603.5	31,150.2	108.7	1.20
1983	394,114	24,803.3	34,511.5	114.1	1.22
1984	431,249	24,995.1	37,310.3	117.7	1.22
1985	463,656	25,181.3	40,407.9	120.7	1.22
1986	488,083	25,372.9	44,285.7	123.6	1.22
1987	533,812	25,643.9	47,934.8	129.1	1.23

[a]Sources: Statistics Canada, *National Income and Expenditure Accounts: Annual estimates 1926–1986,* Tables 4 and 7, Minister of Supply and Services Canada. Statistics Canada, *National Income and Expenditure Accounts: Annual estimates 1977–1988,* Tables 4 and 7, Minister of Supply and Services Canada, Ottawa, 1989. Health and Welfare Canada, *National Health Expenditures in Canada 1975–87,* Table 1, Minister of Supply and Services Canada, Ottawa, 1988. Final tables prepared for inclusion in this publication were supplied by the Health Information Division, Health and Welfare Canada. The 1987 figure is provisional. J.-P. Poullier, Health care expenditure and other data: An international compendium from the Organization for Economic Cooperation and Development, *Health Care Financ. Rev.,* 1989 Annual Supplement, Table 67, p. 194.

NOTES

1. Quality of care is obviously the other major consideration, but the science of measuring quality is in its infancy. We are just beginning to learn how we might compare outcomes of care across hospitals. Collecting the volumes of data that would be necessary for a reasonably valid cross-national comparison of medical outcomes is a task that no one yet has attempted. Even if data were available, it would be difficult to prove that any observed differences in outcomes were due to differences in financing mechanisms. The gross health status measures that are available—primarily infant mortality and life expectancy at birth—favor Canada. (For a comparison of the United States with Canada and several European countries, see reference 1.) These measures are so influenced by factors other than the quality of medical care, however, that they can shed little light on that issue.

2. Gross domestic product (GDP) measures the total value of production originating within the geographic boundaries of the country, regardless of whether the factors of production are owned by residents or nonresidents. Gross national product (GNP) measures income received by resident factors of production, regardless of where the production takes place. GNP is used here to measure total economic output because the United States traditionally has kept its national accounts in this form and it is therefore familiar to American readers. Using GDP as the basis, as is usually done for international comparisons, would change the apparent differences between the United States and Canada only slightly. In Canada, GDP exceeds GNP by about 3 percentage points. In the United States the reverse is true: GNP exceeds GDP by about 1 percentage point.

3. The U.S. figure for 1987, recently revised downward, is 10.80 percent of GNP. If GDP is used to measure total economic output instead of GNP, the figures are 8.71 percent for Canada (1987) versus 10.88 percent (1987) and 11.14 percent (1988) for the United States. The basic data used in this section and the sources thereof are documented in the Appendix.

4. Per capita health spending is defined as total national health expenditures divided by total population (including armed forces).

5. The conversion to U.S. dollars was made using the OECD's purchasing power parity currency conversion factor for 1987: $1.23 CAN = $1.00 U.S. The OECD defines purchasing power parity (PPP) as "Rates of currency conversion that equalize the purchasing power of different currencies. This means that a given sum of money, when converted into different currencies at the PPP rates, will buy the same basket of goods and services in all countries. Thus, PPPs are the rates of currency conversion which eliminate differences in price levels between countries" (2). The Canadian per capita health spending figure given here is slightly higher than the figure ($1,483) reported in other recently published work (see note 12, below) because more recent revised estimates of total Canadian health spending and population were obtained from Health and Welfare Canada. The U.S. per capita health spending figure given here is higher than the figure ($1,941 in 1987) published by the Office of National Cost Estimates, U.S. Health Care Financing Administration (3), because population figures from the U.S. Census Bureau were used rather than the higher Social Security Administration population estimates used by HCFA. The U.S. per capita figure is lower than the one shown by Schieber and Poullier (note 12, below) because a new

revision of the U.S. national health expenditures totals was used, as shown in the Appendix.

6. "Average annual rates" are calculated as annual compound growth rates (ACGR), rather than as the average of the observed yearly growth rates. The ACGR is the single annual growth rate which, if it had been the actual rate for each year during the period in question, would have produced the same total growth over the entire period.

7. The conversion to constant 1981 dollars was made by dividing health care spending by the GNP implicit price deflator for the United States and by the GDP implicit price deflator for Canada, both indexed such that 1981 = 1.0. See the Appendix for data used and sources.

8. The conversion to U.S. dollars was made using the OECD's purchasing power parity for 1981: $1.18 CAN = $1.00 U.S. Robert Evans (4) suggested this two-step approach to comparing growth rates between countries (first convert to constant dollars within each country, then convert currencies using the PPP for the "constant dollar" year).

9. Saskatchewan pioneered in 1962, but no other province adopted a universal public program until 1968.

10. The Office of National Cost Estimates, U.S. Health Care Financing Administration, recently completed a thorough revision of the U.S. national health expenditure series from 1960 through 1987. (The Appendix has the revised figures, and the analysis here is based on them.) The revision lowered the 1987 U.S. health spending total significantly—to about $11.5 billion below the previously published figure. If the previously published figures for 1977 and 1987 are used, the U.S. average annual growth rate for the 10-year period becomes 4.31 percent, almost indistinguishable from the Canadian figure. For the 1978 to 1988 period, the U.S. average annual growth rate is 4.15 percent. Canadian figures for 1988 are not yet available [1990].

11. The number of U.S. residents without health care coverage increased from about 26 million in 1977 to over 31 million in 1987. (Estimates range from 31 million to 37 million, depending on which data source is being used.) Essentially all residents of Canada were covered under the provincial health insurance plans in both years. People who lack health care coverage use fewer services than people who have coverage. Therefore, it could be argued that the rate of increase in U.S. health care costs over the 1977 to 1987 period would have been higher if the number of uncovered people had remained the same.

    To remove the effects of changes in the number of uninsured U.S. residents from the calculation of the growth rate of health care costs, we reestimated U.S. health care spending in both 1977 and 1987 under the assumption that all Americans had health care coverage, and then recalculated the annual compound growth rate over the 1977 to 1987 period. These calculations produced a revised U.S. average growth rate of 4.42 percent per year—about one-half of one percent higher than actually observed and still very close to the Canadian growth rate. Thus, the 1977 to 1987 increase in the number of Americans without health care coverage slowed the growth of health care costs only slightly. Details of this calculation are available upon request.

12. This article by Schieber and Poullier (5) was published before the latest U.S. and Canadian national health expenditure data became available. Therefore, the article underestimates Canadian spending and overestimates U.S. spending.

13. Calculations are based on figures given in the Appendix.

REFERENCES

1. American Medical Association, Center for Health Policy Research. *Chartbook of Cross-National Health Care Comparisons: Demographics, Expenditures, Utilization and Resources.* December 1989.
2. Organization for Economic Cooperation and Development. *National Income and Expenditure Accounts,* Volume 1. Paris, 1988.
3. U.S. Department of Health and Human Services. Press release, May 3, 1990.
4. Evans, R. G. Perspectives: Canada—Split vision: Interpreting cross-border differences in health spending. *Health Aff.* 7(5): 17–24, Winter 1988.
5. Schieber, G. J., and Poullier, J.-P. [Data Watch] International health care expenditure trends: 1987. *Health Aff.* 8(3): 169–181, Fall 1989.

B

Canadian/U.S. Health Care: Reflections on the HIAA's Analysis

Morris L. Barer, W. Pete Welch, and Laurie Antioch

The monograph entitled *Canadian Health Care: The Implications of Public Health Insurance,* by Edward Neuschler of the Health Insurance Association of America (HIAA), is really three different pieces of work living together uneasily between common covers. Taken together, the pieces describe the Canadian system and suggest that (*a*) Canadian and American health care cost control experiences have been much less different than is suggested by comparing their relative percentages of gross national product (GNP); (*b*) Canada's cost control has come at the expense of a variety of access problems, most notably unreasonably long waiting lists for necessary (mostly surgical) interventions; and (*c*) the dramatic increase in public funding and the increased government role implicit in a wholesale U.S. adoption of a Canadian-style system would be unacceptable to Americans.

The three pieces differ in content, rigor, and tone. The first is a superb and objective description of the Canadian health care system. It deserves to be used

Parts B and C were published by *Health Affairs,* Fall 1991, pp. 229–239. Copyright 1991, The People-to-People Health Foundation, Inc., Project HOPE.

widely as a convenient summary description of Canadian health care financing, physician and hospital reimbursement, and recent health policy.

In the second, analytic piece, Neuschler compares Canadian and American real health care costs per capita during 1967–1987. He concludes that the perception of relative cost control success in Canada arises from an inappropriate base of comparison (percentage of GNP or gross domestic product (GDP) rather than real costs per capita) and the fact that real GNP rose more rapidly in Canada. The claim is that health care's share of GNP rose less rapidly in Canada not because of any cost control advantage in the numerator but because of more rapid growth in the denominator. In the second part of this analytic section, Neuschler considers fiscal impact in the United States of a Canadian-style funding system.

The third piece deals with access to health care issues, including a broad-ranging (largely rhetorical) discussion of the social and political impediments to Canadian-style health care financing in the United States. We limit our critique to Neuschler's comparisons of health care costs and discussion of access to health care.

ASSESSING COST CONTAINMENT

Neuschler argues that relative success with cost control should be measured not relative to growth in GNP, but in terms of real per capita health care costs. He finds Canada's experience with the latter very similar to that in the United States. Canada's percentage of GNP going to health care has grown far less rapidly than that in the United States, while the two countries' real per capita costs have moved in parallel. Thus, Neuschler attributes the former difference "not to differences in how the two countries finance and deliver health care but to differences in overall economic growth rates—the Canadian economy grew significantly faster than the U.S. economy" (1).

We suggest that there are three types of problems with Neuschler's analyses and conclusions. First, in making international comparisons of cost control, there are compelling theoretical reasons to use percentage of GNP going to health care rather than real per capita health care costs. Second, the suggestion that Canada's cost control has been an illusion created by its relatively rapid real growth in GNP is inconsistent with the body of empirical research that has examined the income elasticity of health care costs. Third, we show that Neuschler's real per capita cost results are products of two strategic analytic choices—the time period of analysis and the lack of selectivity in sectors chosen for comparison—both of which ignore fundamental institutional facts about Canadian health care.

Share of GNP or Real Per Capita Costs

The choice between these two measures has a major impact on one's assessment of the relative health care cost control success of Canada and the United

States. As the monograph notes, if one measures "health care cost by percentage of [GNP], Canada is doing well. . . . But if cost containment is measured by rates of increase in health care spending . . . the picture is less clear."

Neuschler is not alone in using real health care costs per capita to assess relative success in health care cost containment. George J. Schieber noted recently that although (among the industrialized nations) the United States had the largest increase in health care costs as a percentage of GDP since 1960, "much of this phenomenon can be explained by the slower growth of U.S. GDP relative to U.S. health spending" (2). Similarly, in the context of the debate over Canada's cost-control experience, Judith Feder, William Scanlon, and John Clark concluded that "[f]aster GNP growth, then—not slower health spending—explains why health's share of the GNP has stayed lower in Canada" (3).

In fact, a nation's relative success in containing health care costs can only reasonably be measured in terms of health care costs as a percentage of GNP; rather, it cannot be measured by comparing trends in real costs per capita. In the long run, rising real GNP per capita increases real wages in the health care sector, *causing* health care costs per capita to rise. In judging the comparative international performance of one sector of the economy, such as health care, it is inappropriate to use a measure that is heavily influenced by the comparative performances of entire economies.[1]

Theory

Consider this simple example. Suppose that the real wages of all workers in the economy increase by 10 percent; that labor is the only factor of production; and that wages are the only source of income.[2] Even if health care use is unchanged, real health care costs per capita will still increase by 10 percent. Yet only an unusual definition of health care cost containment could lead one to conclude that this increase in real expenditure was evidence of a country's failure to contain its health care costs.

In this example, real GNP per capita would increase by 10 percent, as would real health care costs per capita. Health care costs as a percentage of GNP would

---

[1] Analogously, one should not use unadjusted expenditures to evaluate the efficiency of hospitals, some of which are in high-wage areas and some in low-wage areas. Just as each hospital must take the areawide wage levels as given, each sector of the economy must, to a larger extent, take economywide wage levels as given. Recognizing this, the U.S. Medicare system varies its payment to hospitals according to area wages.

[2] In the United States, three-quarters of income is received as wages, a ratio that has remained constant since 1970. A minor assumption here is that the number of wage earners per capita remains constant or at least is the same in the two countries. In 1971, civilian employment as a percentage of the population was 38.2 in the United States and 37.6 in Canada. In 1987 (the latest year for which data are available [as of 1991]), this percentage was 46.1 in the United States and 46.7 in Canada (4).

not change, because increases in its denominator (GNP per capita) would cancel out those in its numerator (health care costs per capita). Given that nothing has occurred in the health care sector per se, an appropriate measure of cost containment would not be expected to change in this situation. Hence, health care costs as a percentage of GNP is conceptually a more appropriate measure for comparison.

While GNP can be thought of as the value of all final goods and services, it can also be thought of as the sum of the incomes of all factors of production, including labor. In the long run, increases in real output per capita will raise wages in all sectors of the economy. The mechanism by which this occurs can be described most simply by supposing otherwise: that wages increase in some sectors of the economy but not in the health care sector.

In the short run, workers in the health care sector—physicians, nurses, administrators, and so forth—would find that their wages, relative to those in other employment opportunities, had fallen. This would cause some of these personnel to switch sectors, forcing the health care sector to raise the wages it pays. This "employment adjustment" would not occur at the same rate for all occupational groups. In the long run, however, the wages of all occupational groups in the health care sector would be expected to rise at the same rate as those in the rest of the economy. Note that in real terms, nothing has changed in the health care sector. There are no new labor or capital inputs in the sector, no new technology has been introduced, and there have been no improvements in health outcomes. The only change is that the opportunity costs of the sector's inputs have increased.

In sum, Neuschler's contention that relatively rapid economic growth is likely to be associated with relatively less rapid growth in health care expenditures has no obvious theoretical basis. In the extreme, his explanation implies that no matter how much faster Canadian real per capita GNP growth had been over the 20-year period, U.S. health care cost control would have been at least as "successful" as in Canada unless Canada's real growth in per capita health care costs had been less rapid than that in the United States.

Empirical Evidence

Several analysts have investigated the relationship between health care costs and GNP (5–9). In principle, such investigations capture both input price effects and changes in health care use as a function of changes in national income. Relying primarily on a macroeconomic framework and downplaying the input price effects, analysts have labeled this relationship the "income elasticity" of health care expenditure. Empirical analyses incorporate the impact of returns to nonlabor inputs as well as labor income. Hence, they relax the assumptions of the theoretical analyses above.

An income elasticity of, say, 0.5 would indicate that an increase of 10 percent in GNP per capita would be associated with (result in) an increase of 5 percent in health costs per capita. An elasticity of one would imply equal percentage increases in GNP and health costs per capita and would be associated with an unchanged ratio of health costs to GNP. An elasticity of zero would indicate that a 10 percent increase (or decrease) in GNP per capita would typically have no effect on health costs.

An income elasticity near zero would suggest that general macroeconomic activity has no systematic impact on health care, in which case one could reasonably use trends in real per capita costs to compare cost containment. On the other hand, an elasticity closer to one would lend support to use of the health care share of GNP to compare relative cost containment experiences.

Most of these analyses have involved simple, cross-sectional regressions, involving as many as 20 developed nations. To our knowledge, no one has seriously suggested that income elasticity is close to zero. Rather, the issue is whether health care has an income elasticity a little less than one or a little greater than one. This body of research supports our argument that real health care cost per capita is a poor measure of relative cost containment performance.

Short Run Versus Long Run

Even if long-run elasticity is in the neighborhood of one, in the short run, the share of GNP devoted to health care might rise or fall as a result of sharp turns in general economic fortunes. If, for example, health care prices, wages, and use are relatively insulated from the early effects of broader business cycles, then the share might increase at points of economic downturn and decrease in the early growth phases of the cycles. For example, in the early 1980s, the share jumped sharply in both Canada and the United States as a result of the onset of the common recession.

But these are short-run phenomena. Neuschler and others have argued implicitly that the numerator is not a function of the denominator, that factor prices in health care (for example) are not a function of real GNP per capita. Such an argument inappropriately uses a short-run model to explain a long-run phenomenon.[3]

---

[3] It is understandable that analysts focus on health care costs, whether or not adjusted for population and price level. In the short term, the public policy problem is how to control those expenditures. Expenditures appear in public budgets and must be compared to available revenues, whereas health care expenditures as a percentage of GNP do not appear in those budgets. Whether in a provincial parliament or the U.S. Congress, the immediate focus is necessarily on expenditures (costs). The same holds for an American firm that offers health insurance to its employees. As often is the case in macroeconomics, the perspective of one component of the economy is different from the perspective of the economy as a whole.

Measurement Problems

Of less importance in this particular context is the fact that international comparisons of real per capita costs require an explicit analytic effort to make the figures in each country comparable. Costs in each country must first be converted to "constant (base) year" values through the use of general expenditure (for example, GNP) deflators, comparably constructed for international comparisons. Furthermore, to compare absolute levels of cost per capita at particular points in time, figures from each country must be made commensurable through the use of a purchasing power parity (PPP) conversion for the base year. The accuracy of such statistical adjustments is a consideration not encountered with the use of the ratio of health care costs to GNP in each country.[4]

REVISITING THE HIAA ANALYSIS

Choice of Period

Neuschler chose the period 1967–1987 because it was "the most recent 20-year period for which health spending totals are available for both countries." The "magic" of using 20 years would seem to be outweighed by the pragmatic fact that Canadian Medicare was not fully in place until early 1971. Worse yet, during 1967–1971, the Canadian provinces were in the process of developing and implementing their universal medical care insurance programs.

Whereas Neuschler found expenditures to have risen slightly faster in Canada over the 1967–1987 period (Canada, 4.58 percent; United States, 4.38 percent), Table 1 illustrates clearly that this results from Neuschler's inclusion of the four years during which the Canadian system was still evolving. During 1971–1987, U.S. real per capita costs rose 0.3 percent a year faster than those in Canada. Extending the period to take advantage of more recent data indicates that Canadian real cost growth has declined since 1987, while that in the United States has increased. Over the longer 18-year period, the gap in rates of real per capita growth is a more substantial 0.7 percent annually (about 14 percent cumulative).

This suggests a quite different conclusion than Neuschler's: namely, that despite the fact that one might have anticipated more rapid growth of real per capita expenditures in Canada because of its more rapid real economic growth, one finds quite the opposite. U.S. real per capita health care costs have grown more rapidly than those in Canada since the inception of Canadian universal

---

[4] On the problems with attempting such comparisons using exchange rates in each year, see reference 10. The appropriate procedures do appear to have been adopted in Neuschler's analysis.

Table 1

Real health care costs per capita, Canada and United States, 1971, 1987, and 1989[a]

	1971	1987	1989	Average annual percent change	
				1971–1987	1971–1989
Canada	$786.3	$1,442.1	$1,499.1	3.86%	3.65%
United States	839.7	1,616.5	1,819.0	4.18	4.39

[a]Sources: Real expenditures are reported in the currency of each country and were computed using the GNP deflator for each country and 1981 as the base year. For Canada, the GNP deflator was derived from series published in the *Bank of Canada Review,* Bank of Canada, Ottawa, November 1990, and health care expenditure and population data for 1987 are taken from *National Health Expenditures in Canada, 1975–1987,* Health and Welfare Canada, Ottawa, 1990. The preliminary (unpublished) estimate of health care expenditures for 1989, and revised data for 1971, were kindly provided by the Health Information Division, Health and Welfare Canada. For the United States, the GNP deflator and the population were taken from the 1990 *Statistical Abstract of the United States,* 110th ed., U.S. Department of Commerce, Bureau of the Census, 1990, and the health care expenditure data were provided by the Office of National Health Statistics, Health Care Financing Administration (but can also be found in various issues of the *Health Care Financing Review*).

hospital and medical insurance, and recent data suggest that the gap in rates of growth is widening.[5]

Choice of Expenditure Categories

But even this revised picture is misleading. An examination of the relative cost control record of the Canadian national health insurance program should exclude health care subsectors for which it was not designed (such as dental care, pharmaceuticals, long-term care, and medical devices). Again, failure to take note of the institutional details creates quite misleading results.

In Figure 1 we plot the share of total health care expenditures represented by hospital services, physician services, and administration in each country during 1971–1987. This figure illustrates the dramatic effect of the Canadian system. The share of total Canadian health care costs represented by hospital, medical, and administrative expenditure fell from about 64 percent at the beginning of the period to under 57 percent in 1987. Cost control in these three sectors has been

[5] Of course, one could play endless games with shorter periods. For example, in his executive summary, Neuschler points out that real per capita costs rose faster in Canada than in the United States over the period 1977–1987. But the reverse is true for the period 1979–1989 (Canadian annual costs rose an average 4.12 percent, while those in the United States increased 4.68 percent annually) and for 1975–1985 (Canada, 4.08 percent; United States, 4.3 percent). This instability in results from shorter periods points to the need to view comparative cost experiences over the long run. When overall experiences have been relatively similar, it will always be possible for those with a particular agenda to pick beginning and end points to meet specific purposes.

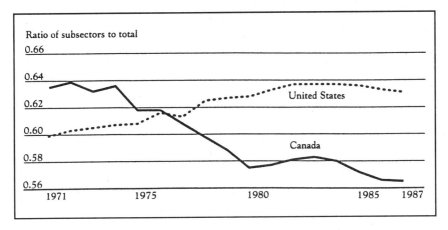

Figure 1. Ratio of hospital, physician, and administrative costs to total health care costs, 1971–1987. Sources: Health care expenditure subsector data for Canada are taken from *National Health Expenditures in Canada, 1975–1987*, Health and Welfare Canada, Ottawa, 1990, and from unpublished revised data for 1971 from Health Information Division, Health and Welfare Canada. U.S. data are from Office of National Health Statistics, Health Care Financing Administration.

relatively more successful than the absence or patchwork of control mechanisms in the rest of the sector. At the same time, the comparable U.S. share rose, from about 60 percent to about 63 percent.

The trends in per capita cost data underlying these dramatically different internal health care sector reallocations in the two countries suggest no basis for doubt about relative cost control success, even using real per capita health care costs as the basis of comparison (Table 2). Average real U.S. increases in these three subsectors outran those in Canada by 1.4 percent annually, or by over 20 percent cumulatively over the 16 years. In particular, average annual growth in real per capita costs for administering the U.S. system was over 5 percent; in Canada, this figure was about 1.6 percent.

In principle, services not covered by the single-payer Canadian system could have been increasingly substituted for the included services over this period. However, comparisons of medical and hospital services use suggest that Canada has contained physician costs by controlling fees, not use (11) (see Chapter 2).

Similarly, Canada has controlled hospital costs not because of lower rates of hospital utilization but through less intensive servicing associated with each day of hospital care (12, 13) (see Chapter 3). While there has been considerable growth in the relative share of total costs going to "other institutions" in Canada, the nursing home sector in the United States also grew over this period, and a large share of the "other institutions" sector in Canada is funded from the same public budgets. Thus, it seems unlikely that the single-payer funding of hospital

Table 2

Average annual rates of growth in real health care costs per capita,
Canada and United States, selected subsectors, 1971–1987[a]

	Canada	United States	Difference
Hospitals	3.09%	4.48%	1.35%
Physician services	3.27	4.41	1.10
Administration	1.58	5.23	3.59
Subsectors total	3.10	4.52	1.38
Total health care	3.86	4.18	0.30

[a]Sources: *National Health Expenditures in Canada, 1975–1987*, Health and Welfare Canada, Ottawa, 1990; Health Information Division, Health and Welfare Canada; and Office of National Health Statistics, (U.S.) Health Care Financing Administration. Population data are from the sources noted in Table 1.

and medical care in Canada has shifted costs from the relatively more to the relatively less controlled subsectors.

Updating the Share of GNP Comparison

In Figure 2 we compare the share of GNP going to total health care and to the three subsectors (hospital, physician, and administration) in the two countries during 1971–1989. This illustrates two important trends. First, even viewed in terms of overall health care costs, the gap has widened dramatically over the most recent two years for which data have become available since Neuschler's analysis. The Canadian share appears to have stabilized at just under 9 percent, while the U.S. share was 11.6 percent in 1989. Second, the gap for the three subsectors affected by Canadian national health insurance is both wider (in proportionate terms) and growing faster.

THE ACCESS DEBATE

Neuschler's contribution to the debate over access to health care is, in our view, the weakest section of his monograph. It suffers from two major methodological problems. First, unlike the cost analysis, the treatment of access to necessary health care drops the comparative approach and focuses only on Canada. If, as Neuschler suggests, the motivation for his study was to contribute to informed policy discussion about whether "public insurance fashioned on the Canadian model . . . [might be] an approach that would work well [in the United States]," then surely an analysis of access ought to be undertaken in a similar comparative context. The relevant question is, of course, whether a Canadian-style system would represent an improvement in, or an erosion of, the access situation in the

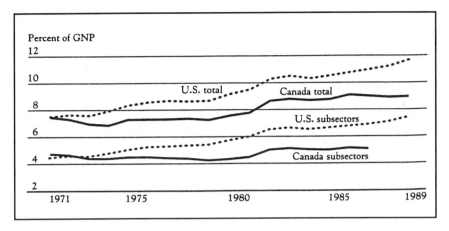

Figure 2. Health care costs as a percentage of GNP, total and subsectors, Canada and United States, 1971–1989. Sources: *National Health Expenditures in Canada, 1975–1987,* Health and Welfare Canada, Ottawa, 1990; Health Information Division, Health and Welfare Canada; and Office of National Health Statistics, (U.S.) Health Care Financing Administration. Preliminary data for Canada for 1988–1989 were provided by Health Information Division, Health and Welfare Canada. Data on Canadian subsectors were not yet available for 1988 and 1989. Note: The subsectors represented are hospitals, physicians, and administration, shown here in combined form.

United States, and for whom. Neuschler's approach precludes addressing that question.[6]

Second, Neuschler's analysis of access to health care in Canada is based almost entirely on anecdotal reports from the Canadian popular press. While this may have been about all there was in the public record at the time, it does not sit well in a monograph described in its preface (by HIAA President Carl Schramm) as based on "thorough research and objective presentation." Newspapers and weekly newsmagazines are a particularly suspect source of information in Canada because, as Neuschler notes, "creating a sense of imminent crisis helps the health care industry argue for additional resources or fend off deeper cuts. . . . Media reports become part of the political infighting and are, therefore, all the more difficult to evaluate." We agree.

Some serious analyses, at least of queues in Canada, are now beginning to engage researchers on both sides of the border (15, 16). Of course, queues for

---

[6] Neuschler's claim (1, p. 53) that "it is impossible to quantify the extent of [access] problems or to compare them in any meaningful sense with the problems in other health care systems" seems an unconvincing justification for not having at least considered "evidence," of equivalent "quality," on access problems in the United States. Some of this even appears in the Canadian press (see, for example, 4).

particular high-profile procedures (such as cardiac surgery) are only one small part of access to effective health care, and we do not wish to imply that there are no access problems in Canada. But Neuschler's treatment of the issue does not represent a contribution to any reasoned debate about relative problems of access to appropriate health care interventions in the two systems.

SOME FINAL THOUGHTS

For two decades, a major "natural" experiment on health care financing has been conducted in North America. Canada has had a single-payer system for the major components of health care, while the United States has employed a multi-payer system. The results on cost containment are available, although the results on access to and quality of care are not (17).

In analyzing relative international cost containment records, the appropriate measure is the proportion of GNP devoted to health care, not real costs per capita. Furthermore, when Neuschler's cost analysis is refocused only on the sectors commonly understood to be governed by Canadian national health insurance, even real health care costs per capita—biased against the Canadian experience by the more rapid real economic growth—are found to have grown much less rapidly in Canada than in the United States. The North American experiment demonstrates conclusively that the Canadian single-payer system has contained costs more effectively than has the U.S. multipayer system.

It seems time for the American debate to move beyond attempts to cast the U.S. health cost control record in a favorable international light. Many comparative questions are of interest both to Canadians and Americans, but they have nothing to do with whether American health care costs are really as high in relative terms as everyone knows they are, or whether the latest cardiac waiting list death in Canada might have been averted in the United States.

REFERENCES

1. Neuschler, E. *Canadian Health Care: The Implications of Public Health Insurance.* Health Insurance Association of America, Washington, D.C., 1990.
2. Schieber, G. J. Health expenditures in major industrialized countries, 1960–87. *Health Care Financ. Rev.,* Summer 1990, pp. 159–167.
3. Feder, J., Scanlon, W., and Clark, J. Canada's health care system (letter to the editor). *N. Engl. J. Med.* 317: 320, 1987.
4. Organization for Economic Cooperation and Development. *Labour Force Statistics, 1967–1987. Paris,* 1989.
5. Parkin, D., McGuire, A., and Yule, B. Aggregate health care expenditures and national income: Is health care a luxury good? *J. Health Econ.* 6: 109–127, 1987.
6. Newhouse, J. P. Cross national differences in health spending: What do they mean? *J. Health Econ.* 6: 159–162, 1987.

7. Parkin, D., McGuire, A., and Yule, B. What do international comparisons of health expenditures really show? *Community Med.* 11: 116–123, 1989.
8. Schieber, G. J., and Poullier, J. P. International health care expenditure trends: 1987. *Health Aff.,* Fall 1989, pp. 169–177.
9. Gerdtham, U. *Essays on International Comparisons of Health Care Expenditure.* Linkoping Studies in Arts and Science 66. Department of Health and Society, Linkoping University, Linkoping, Sweden, 1991.
10. Evans, R. G. Split vision: Interpreting cross-border differences in health spending. *Health Aff.,* Winter 1988, pp. 17–24.
11. Fuchs, V. R., and Hahn, J. S. How does Canada do it? A comparison of expenditures for physicians' services in the United States and Canada. *N. Engl. J. Med.* 323: 884–890, 1990.
12. Newhouse, J. P., Anderson, G., and Roos, L. L. Hospital spending in the United States and Canada: A comparison. *Health Aff.,* Winter 1988, pp. 6–16.
13. Barer, M. L., and Evans, R. G. Riding north on a south-bound horse? Expenditures, prices, utilization, and incomes in the Canadian health care system. In *Medicare at Maturity: Achievements, Lessons, and Challenges,* edited by R. G. Evans and G. L. Stoddart, pp. 53–163. University of Calgary Press, Calgary, 1986.
14. Silversides, A. Technology serves the rich while the poor wait for care. *Toronto Globe and Mail,* September 16, 1986, pp. A1, A10.
15. Naylor, D. *Health Aff.,* Fall 1991.
16. Katz, S. J., Mizgala, H. F., and Welch, H. G. Bypassing the queue in Canada? British Columbia sends patients to Seattle for coronary artery surgery. *JAMA,* 1991.
17. Evans, R. G., Barer, M. L., and Hertzman, C. The twenty year experiment: Accounting for, explaining, and evaluating health care cost containment in Canada and the United States. *Annu. Rev. Public Health* 12: 481–518, 1991.

C

Debating the Canadian System:
A Response from the Author

Edward Neuschler

Morris Barer, Pete Welch, and Laurie Antioch have two main complaints about my monograph on the Canadian health care system. First, they question the methods I used to compare health spending trends of the United States and Canada. Second, they complain that my discussion of access problems in Canada was one-sided and not objective because it omitted discussion of similar problems in the United States and relied primarily on press reports.

In the context of an ongoing policy debate, which is certainly what we are engaged in here, all potential ramifications of a proposed policy change must be explored. At the time I began my research on this topic (in 1989), the Canadian health care system was being actively promoted in both the academic literature and the popular press (1, 2). Canada was praised for its universal access to care and its apparent success in controlling costs. One would have thought, from reading many of these articles, that there were no drawbacks whatsoever to Canadian-style public health insurance and that the United States ought to adopt such an approach forthwith. In this context, it seemed to me perfectly appropriate and, in fact, a necessary contribution to the debate to look for flaws in the prior published analyses and to examine the potential drawbacks of the Canadian approach. Simply put, no one else was doing so at the time.

As for relying on press reports about access problems, the commentators acknowledge that at that time, reports in the popular press were, indeed, "about all there was in the public record." But the sheer volume of these reports was sufficient to establish that, while Canada may have universal coverage, prompt access is by no means guaranteed for all services. I agree that more primary research on the nature, extent, and consequences of access problems, in both the United States and Canada (and in various other countries), would be a useful contribution to the U.S. debate about health care reform.

EFFECTIVENESS
OF COST CONTAINMENT

Regarding my analysis of the relative effectiveness of health care cost containment in Canada and the United States, the commentators have two main criticisms. First, they argue that per capita spending is an inappropriate base for international comparisons. Second, they complain that my results are skewed by the choice of time period for the analysis and by the use of total national health expenditures as the basis of comparison.

Methods of Comparison

Comparing health care costs between countries is a difficult business (3, 4) (see Chapter 5). Accounting systems differ between countries. Different ways of financing hospitals' capital requirements mean that the extent to which the cost of capital is measured and recorded varies across countries. Different demographic, sociological, and disease profiles place varying demands on the health care systems in different nations. (The last area, in particular, deserves further investigation, in my view.)

Against this background, it seems obvious that no single approach will yield a full understanding of how the factors driving health care costs differ across nations. In my analysis, I chose to focus on a comparison of the rate of growth of per capita health care expenditures in the two countries, because the percent-of-GNP (gross national product) argument had already been thoroughly presented. Moreover, the approach of comparing per capita growth rates is well established in the literature, as Barer and colleagues note. (In fact, it is used by one of them in a comparison of U.S. and Canadian health spending (1).)

The latest comparative figures (for the period 1970–1989) on the percentage of gross domestic product (GDP) devoted to health care and on the income elasticity of health care costs suggest that Canada is doing better than the United States but not as well as Germany, Japan, the United Kingdom, and many other members of the Organization for Economic Cooperation and Development (OECD) (5). Some advocates (not necessarily Barer and colleagues) tend to look at this kind of analysis and proclaim a Canadian-style approach the "silver bullet" that will magically solve all of America's health care woes. In this context, comparing per capita growth rates sounds a cautionary note for policymakers. We do not understand as well as we would like all of the structural factors that drive health care costs. If Canada's per capita growth rate is essentially the same as ours (and, in particular, remains the same as ours well after the introduction of government-run health insurance), prudence suggests that we evaluate advocates' claims of a massive fiscal dividend with a large dose of skepticism.

Choice of Time Periods

As to the second set of issues, choice of time period does indeed affect the results of a per capita growth rate comparison. If 1967 is used as the base year, the increased utilization associated with Canada's move to universal coverage (during, roughly, 1968–1971) raises the apparent growth rate of Canadian health care costs per capita.[1] If 1971 is used as the base year, that large utilization increase is in the past, and the growth rate for subsequent years is lower. But the United States enacted Medicare coverage for the disabled in 1972, which presumably increased health care use for this very expensive population. So it is not entirely clear that using 1971 as the base year is "fair" to the United States. Moreover, the fact that Canada experienced higher annual rates of increase (relative to U.S. experience at the time) while implementing universal coverage is by no means irrelevant to the policy debate here. Analyses that start with 1971 (as does every "pro-Canada" analysis I have seen) completely ignore this aspect of the issue.

The charts and tables in my monograph cover the 20-year period from 1967 to 1987, but my analysis specifically considered and compared average growth rates

[1]Between 1967 and 1971, health care costs per capita grew noticeably faster in Canada than in the United States. Presumably, this faster growth reflects increased use of services by the previously uninsured and the switch to billing for services that physicians previously provided free to uninsured indigents.

for each of four five-year subperiods. Growth of per capita costs was higher in Canada than in the United States between 1967 and 1972, as could be expected. The reverse was true between 1972 and 1977. From 1977 to 1982 and from 1982 to 1987, the per capita growth rate was slightly higher in Canada. Although final figures for the United States are now available through 1989, Canadian figures for 1988 and 1989 are still preliminary estimates [as of fall 1991], subject to change.

Categories of Expenses

As to the selection of categories of expenses to be compared, the use of total national health expenditures is commonplace for international comparisons. Canada's cost containment record does appear stronger if hospital and physician expenditures only are considered, as one would expect from the virtually complete government control over hospital budgets and physician fees. What is surprising to me is that Canada's overall cost containment record is not better, given the degree of control the provinces have over these two major components of health spending.

THE AUTHOR'S REJOINDER

In their comment, the authors give little attention to the rest of my monograph, which estimated the tax cost of implementing a Canadian-style system in the United States. They dismiss it as a "broad-ranging (largely rhetorical) discussion of social and political impediments to the emergence of a Canadian-style system" in the United States. They chose to focus their comment as they did, I suspect, because they have already decided that the United States is unlikely to adopt a pure Canadian system. They are therefore free to focus on narrower "what can we learn" questions. I remain more concerned with the larger issue.

However unlikely U.S. adoption of a "pure" Canadian-style public health insurance system may be, there is no doubt that several advocacy groups are strongly urging adoption of a government-run, single-payer system in the United States. These advocates focus on the apparent positives of a government-run system—universal coverage, allegedly lower costs. They give little attention to the potential long-run consequences of complete government control over the financing of medical care or to the realities of how the sociopolitical environment and institutions differ between the United States and Canada. In the context of the broader debate, those consequences and realities deserve to be raised and considered.

REFERENCES

1. Evans, R. G., et al. Controlling health expenditures: The Canadian reality. *N. Engl. J. Med.* 320(9): 571–577, 1989.
2. Himmelstein, D. U., and Woolhandler, S., and the Writing Committee of the Working Group on Program Design. A National Health Program for the United States. *N. Engl. J. Med.* 320(2): 102–108, 1989.
3. Krasny, J., and Ferrier, I. R. A closer look at health care in Canada. *Health Aff.,* Summer 1991, pp. 152–158.
4. Waldo, D. R., and Sonnefeld, S. T. U.S./Canadian health spending: Methods and assumptions. *Health Aff.,* Summer 1991, pp. 159–164.
5. Schieber, G. J., and Poullier, J. P. International health spending: Issues and trends. *Health Aff.,* Spring 1991, pp. 106–116.

CHAPTER 5

Debate on U.S./Canadian Health Expenditures—II

A

A Closer Look at Health Care in Canada

Jacques Krasny and Ian R. Ferrier

A simple comparison of U.S. and Canadian health care spending suggests that the Canadian system provides universally available health care at a lower cost than the U.S. system. Thus, it is not surprising that a number of observers have called for the United States to consider adopting Canadian-style national health insurance. However, a fair comparison of the two systems suggests that wholesale adoption of the Canadian system will not result in a satisfactory decline in U.S. health care costs.

First, a number of significant differences between the United States and Canada make it difficult to compare the percentage of gross national product (GNP) spent on health care in the two countries. Second, while Canada has achieved a slower rate of growth of health care costs, this has come with a profound limitation in access to institutional services and new health care technologies. Third, the Canadian system is made workable by a culture that accepts greater government intervention and constraint of individual rights. These cultural aspects would be generally unacceptable to U.S. citizens.

Parts A, B, and C published by *Health Affairs,* Summer 1991, pp. 152–165. Copyright 1991, The People-to-People Health Foundation, Inc., Project HOPE.

COMPARISONS

We make the following adjustments to avoid comparing "apples and oranges." The analyses are intended to indicate the nature and proportion of adjustment necessary for fair comparison, not definitive numbers. Calculations throughout represent conservative, middle-ground estimates.

Capital Costs

U.S. business is accustomed to perceiving health care as a system in which, as in any other business, the cost of working capital represents an expense. Hospitals, provider networks, rehabilitation facilities, insurance plans, and others must raise money either through equity markets or by raising debt in the form of bonds or other debt-financing instruments. Whether through equity or debt, individual or institutional investors expect returns when they advance these funds. By contrast, the capital structure of the Canadian health care system is largely invisible. Thus, the country's 1,400 hospitals were created, for the most part, through a combination of one-third community (local government) contributions matched by a two-thirds federal contribution. Also, there are no real working capital needs in the Canadian system, since global budgets are advanced in a way that precludes the requirement for net cash outflows for such items as payroll and medical supplies.

However, capital does not come free in Canada. The capital cost of the health care system is largely buried in the total "financing" cost of the Canadian government. Undoubtedly, this cost contributes significantly to Canada's substantial national debt (roughly 50 percent higher per capita than in the United States).

To determine the level and amount of capital employed by the Canadian system, we extrapolated from U.S. experience the ratio of capital employed to annual operating costs for health care institutions (67 percent). We then multiplied this by the percentage of total health care expenditures attributable to institutions (47 percent) and, using a conservative 10 percent cost of money (this is substantially below current Canadian costs), determined the net annual cost.[1] This calculation suggests that total Canadian health care expenditures must be increased by 3.15 percent to allow for the cost of capital. Applying this increase to the 9 percent of GNP that was determined as the level of health spending in Canada in 1987 increases the Canadian percentage of GNP figure by 0.3 percentage points.

---

[1] Ratio of Canadian government cost components used to determine total health care costs.

Health Benefits

The U.S. health care system is a major employer, with labor costs constituting approximately 75 percent of all health spending. The costs of U.S. health care employers that are associated with "health benefits" are included in the operational costs of the health facilities. These costs in turn are included in the total operating costs of the U.S. health care system. In the United States, these expenses constitute a measured component of the cost of operating the health care system and are included when it is measured as a percentage of GNP. In Canada, where health costs are overwhelmingly absorbed by and paid for out of general taxation, these costs are not included in health care operating costs and thus are excluded from calculations of health spending as a percentage of GNP.

We developed an adjustment to account for differences in labor costs of health benefits. First, we analyzed federal statistics to determine the percentage of overall health spending that is made up of labor costs. We then multiplied this by 10 percent to approximate conservatively what health insurance benefits would be as a percentage of payroll. A small proportion of health benefits are absorbed in government-levied health insurance premiums in Canada (Ontario Health Insurance Program premiums account for 17 percent of total health spending). Consequently, determining the portion that is not directly charged requires multiplying the projected total health benefit by 0.83 percent (the ratio of costs not directly charged to employers and employees). The product of these numbers determines the amount by which Canadian health expenditure totals must be increased to make them comparable to U.S. costs. This figure is 6.3 percent and, when applied to the stated cost of Canadian health care as a percentage of GNP, increases this number by 0.6 percentage points.

Population Mix

In comparing Canada and the United States, it is important to account for the disproportionate share of health care consumption by the elderly in the two nations. This adjustment is difficult to do, and precise data are lacking. While estimates vary, it is generally accepted that while the elderly make up just over 12 percent of the U.S. population, they account for well over 50 percent of health care consumption. In the United States, the cohort age 65 and over is 1.2 percent larger than in Canada (as a percentage of the population), with a resulting net impact on U.S. health care costs of 5.3 percent. That is, if the Canadian system were required to look after a population with the same demographic profile as in the United States, it would face a 5.3 percent increase in its health care costs.

When this is applied to the reported 9 percent of GNP that is the cost of the Canadian health care system, it results in an increase of 0.5 percentage points.[2]

Other demographic considerations also make the United States a more demanding population to serve. For example, the impact of past military actions—particularly the Vietnam and Korea experiences—greatly increase demand for medical care.[3] No equivalent experience exists in Canada since World War II. Inner-city phenomena such as crimes of violence, substance abuse, sexually transmitted disease, and teen pregnancy also have greater impact on health costs in the United States than in Canada.

Research and Development

Whether research and development (R&D) expenditures should constitute any part of the calculation of current health spending is arguable. One perspective is to consider R&D expenditures as investments since these expenditures have nothing to do with satisfying current health care demands. If all of the differences in health spending as a percentage of GNP between the United States and Canada were accounted for by expenditures on R&D, it is unlikely that many voices in the United States would argue for "closing the gap" by eliminating U.S. health care research. However, both countries elect to include R&D expenditures in health care GNP calculations.

We examined the absolute dollar expenditures for R&D in the United States and Canada as a ratio of respective health spending. This analysis indicates that, if Canada were to spend proportionally as much on health R&D as the United States spends, it would face a 2.4 percent increase in health expenditures. When this is applied to the reported 9 percent of GNP that is the cost of the Canadian health care system, it results in an increase of 0.2 percentage points.

---

[2] The population base of the "old-old" (those age 65 and older) further highlights this disparity in populations. While the ratio of those age 65 and over for Canada is 12.2 percent versus 11 percent (or a 10 percent difference in ratios), the ratios of those age 85 and over is 1.18 percent versus 0.89 percent (a ratio difference of 33 percent). While the comparative size of this "old-old" group is small, the proportionate demand and impact on the health care system is exceptionally large. Since the universally accepted definition of *elderly* is over age 65, there are very few data to determine the net impact of the difference of the ratio of those age 85 and over. However, since in both cases Canada has a relatively younger population, the two cohort comparisons can be considered as indicating the same basic reality.

[3] This amount is as important as it is difficult to determine. For example, the Department of Veterans Affairs (VA) designates approximately 20 percent of its patients as "Vietnam-era veterans" (those who served between 1964 and 1975, but not necessarily in Vietnam). While the 1990 VA budget is $12.3 billion, it is unlikely that a straight prorating of 20 percent of this cost would be attached to Vietnam veterans. As in the population at large, health care costs are disproportionately skewed to the elderly, and the Vietnam veterans have not yet entered the "senior" category. A recent study by the Centers for Disease Control that examined 15,000 veterans concluded that Vietnam veterans were substantially more prone to problems of alcohol abuse or dependence, clinical depression, and general anxiety. To quote William Eaton, a psychiatric epidemiologist at The Johns Hopkins University, "Vietnam raises the risk of enduring psychological problems by a factor of 2.5."

Adjusted Comparison

The combined net impact of these adjustments is significant. They increase the Canadian amount from 9 percent of GNP to 10.6 percent, converting an apparent advantage of 2.1 percent of GNP reported by the Canadian health care system to a difference of 0.5 percent. They do not, however, take into account additional factors that increase the costs of the U.S. health care system. For instance, we did not adjust for (*a*) the large number of U.S. Vietnam veterans; (*b*) the inner-city phenomena of more intense urbanization in the United States; (*c*) the substantially greater cost of malpractice liability and insurance in the United States than in Canada; (*d*) substantial hidden administrative costs of the Canadian health care system that are absorbed into general, federal, and provincial government expenditures (the government system collects the revenue, through both general taxation and direct health premiums, and administers the programs but does not allocate the costs associated with these administrative functions back to health care revision); and (*e*) the significant but currently unmeasured use of the U.S. health care system by Canadian citizens. Each dollar spent by a Canadian in the United States has the numerical impact of appearing to increase the cost of the U.S. health system (since total expenditure is measured) and to decrease the apparent cost of the Canadian health system (by reducing expenditure in the system).[4] Given the intensely conservative nature of our adjustment components, more sophisticated numerical analysis would likely yield the result that the Canadian system costs as much as, or slightly more than, the U.S. system.

---

[4] An examination of the methods used by the Canadian federal government in calculating health expenditure to determine the percentage of GNP indicates no allowance for the expenditures of Canadians for health care outside of the country. Rather, expenditures are segmented into categories, then each category's cost is determined by combining payment to it from the various levels of government. Provision is made for private-sector (insurance companies and individuals) participation in the system by balancing the difference between total revenues of each component and the funding made available through documented public sources. That is, the private-sector expenditure is the "plug figure" used to balance the equation. The very few totally private situations in Canada that would attract international clientele (such as the Shouldice Clinic in Toronto) are not measurable by these methods, since private concerns are not required to disclose revenue figures. Moreover, since no public funding whatsoever is provided, there is no reason for measuring these mathematically small phenomena. While Americans do undoubtedly end up using the Canadian health system (because of illness or accident while visiting Canada), there is little reason to believe there is any usage other than that caused by these unforeseen events. There are neither insurance, access, nor technological incentives to persuade any American to ever use Canadian facilities. By contrast, availability of high technology, rapid access, and world-renowned physicians establish both a clear motivation and a regular trail of Canadians to the American health system. Since expenditures by Canadians on health care in the United States are not (in the overwhelming majority of cases) reimbursed by Canadian provincial health care plans, they go largely unmeasured.

Access and Insurance

A dimension of the Canadian health care system that is generally described as superior to the U.S. system is its universal coverage of the population. It is important to distinguish between health *care* and health *insurance*. Universal access to health care is the ability of all the population to obtain stated levels of medical intervention. Universal access to health insurance (health care benefits) deals with paying for these services.

While approximately 31 million U.S. citizens are without health insurance (health care benefits) at any given time, this does not mean that this entire group is denied access to health care. Many in the United States receive needed care, whether or not they have insurance coverage (although needed care may be less than they want). Hospitals, municipal and state governments, charities, and other agencies absorb the costs of these unreimbursed services. Charges are shifted to those patients with insurance, or, in the case of publicly funded facilities, financial deficits are made up through general tax funds. The absence of health insurance for this numerically significant cohort, while not resulting in the denial of required medical services, comes at a profound price. The uninsured recipient of health care is required to spend personal funds, becoming indigent before these services are provided free through one of the agencies or mechanisms described above. In Canada, it is a fundamental tenet of the Canada Health Act that all residents are covered by the various provincial health plans. While health insurance is universally provided, access to care itself is limited.

SHORTCOMINGS OF THE CANADIAN SYSTEM

One demonstrable benefit of the Canadian health care system has been its ability to control the rate of growth of health costs, particularly when compared to recent experience in the United States. However, this benefit has come at the substantial price of limited access to resources, services, and new treatment regimens and technologies.

Cost Containment

While Canadian health care costs have been rising as a percentage of GNP, this rate of growth has been slower than that in the United States. However, adjusting for cost of capital, health labor, health insurance benefits, R&D, and demographics shows a different picture of cost containment "success" in Canada.

Canadian health spending in the 1960s was characterized by a period of relatively free spending (Figure 1). At that time, the legislation surrounding the Canada Health Act granted provincial governments 50 cents on the dollar for all health expenditures. This enabled the provincial health ministries to spend relatively cheap dollars on health care with the political benefit of providing highly

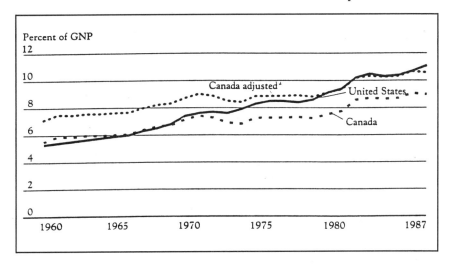

Figure 1. Health care costs as percentage of gross national product, United States, Canada, and Canada adjusted, 1960–1987. Sources: *Health, United States, 1989,* Table 100; *National Health Expenditures in Canada, 1975–1987.* Health and Welfare Canada, unpublished report, Table 6; and adjustments by the authors.
[a]Adjustment of Canadian GNP figures adds 1.6 percentage points to reflect a fair comparison between Canada and the United States in the areas of (1) cost of capital; (2) health benefits and health care-related costs of labor; (3) different emphases on research and development; and (4) population mix, especially regarding number of elderly citizens.

visible community activity and selectively creating jobs in jurisdictions where social or political considerations indicated the need. Recognizing the fiscal consequences of this legislation, the federal government in Ottawa instituted cost containment procedures in the 1970s. No longer were 50-cent dollars available to the provincial governments of Canada. Instead, the funding provided to provincial governments now became pegged to growth of the Canadian economy.

As a consequence, the provincial health ministries faced a significantly reduced formula for securing matching health funding from the federal government while having to deal with provincial health care providers that had grown accustomed to relatively easy funding. The 1970s represented a period of rigorous management control in Canadian health care that resulted in removal of fiscal softness and lax management in the Canadian system. For example, early versions of global hospital funding had the perverse incentive of rewarding hospitals that provided minimal acute medical care but allocated a high proportion of their activities to "hotel days" (simply looking after the basic human needs of patients without providing any substantial medical intervention). Provincial health management could legitimately argue that costs were being contained without fundamentally impairing quality of care as these reverse anomalies were corrected and the system was made more efficient.

By contrast, the 1980s represented a troublesome era for health care in Canada. The bulk of cost constraint now accomplished in Canada comes at the direct expense of accessibility of health care resources and new medical procedures and technologies.

Resource Constraint

Perhaps nothing illustrates the problem of resource constraint in Canada so dramatically as the comparison of access to higher technologies between the United States and Canada. The per capita ratio of accessible higher (or newer) technology resources between the United States and Canada ranges from 200 to 800 percent. The comparison of the availability of these resources is not a commentary on what the absolute level of resources should be for a population, given a specific medical need or indication. Rather, it highlights the important principle that people clearly have greater ease of access, a larger range of choices, and more timely access in the United States than in Canada.

Management Skill

While there are pockets of management genius in the Canadian health care system, the system is not managed in an effective manner, particularly when compared to U.S. models. Ironically, while examination of the Canadian system has recently become topical in the United States, Canadians are studying U.S. models, particularly health maintenance organizations (HMOs).

While the fundamental economic support and character of the Canadian health care system derives from the federal government, the Canadian system is, in fact, a collection of ten distinct provincial plans. Ten Canadian provinces have a population base of one million or less. By comparison, seven HMOs in the United States each provide health care services to an enrollment of over one million subscribers. With the exception of the Ontario and Quebec programs, the Canadian system has no programs or insights on economies of scale to offer U.S. providers that can serve as templates for amortizing costs of care across large population groups. Moreover, examination of discrete, large-volume health care systems (considering the entire Canadian experience as one) demonstrates that U.S. managed systems designed to control costs in fact do so far better than the Canadian system. In 1987, three of the larger U.S. HMOs provided a full range of health care services with per capita cost on the order of $900 to $1,000. By contrast, the provision of the same services in Canada involved per capita cost of approximately $1,400 (U.S.).

CULTURAL ISSUES

Meaningful comparisons of the cost of different health care systems must correct for a variety of differing social factors. Canada and the United States appear to be culturally similar. However, social attitudes toward the direct authority of government in everyday life and individual rights are substantially different. Canada has never experienced a revolution, evolving gradually from a colonial into a democratic society. Canada has kept many of the centralized characteristics of the colonial administration from which it grew. It uses a parliamentary form of government exported from Great Britain and continues to have a nominal monarch as its head of state—although it now elects Her Majesty's government.

These cultural differences affect the consumption of health care by creating limitations on individual rights, which would be generally unacceptable or even culturally repugnant to most U.S. citizens. For example, Canadians wronged by a medical practitioner do not have access to punitive damages since, for all intents, none are awarded by Canadian courts. There are no contingent legal fees in Canada; consequently, those wishing to pursue legal remedy must have the necessary financial resources at hand. With minor exceptions, there are no class-action suits. Consequently, there is no mechanism for pursuing legal remedy in situations in which large numbers of people have been wronged. There is no right to sue government officials, or ministries of health, for medical negligence. Indeed, there is no right to sue the Canadian government without first obtaining permission from the government to do so.

Also, there is portability of the health care system within Canada, but the provincial systems are variations of the same basic health care delivery system available throughout the country. There is no effective choice of which system to use. Finally, there is no real ability to opt out of the public system and find alternative avenues for care.

In some respects, the accessibility to U.S. health care enables the Canadian system to cope with demand. The United States is the principal source of new medical technologies for Canada. It is, for an increasing number of Canadians, the only available source of prompt access to advanced medical technologies and procedures. If the United States were to adopt the Canadian health care system with its limitation of resources, it would not only affect the availability of resources to U.S. consumers but would also remove the "safety valve" for Canadians.

SATISFACTION OF CITIZENS

A recent Harris poll showed that the overwhelming majority of Canadians prefer their system to the U.S. or the British systems (by 95 percent and 91 percent) (1). By contrast, more than 60 percent of U.S. citizens indicate that they would prefer the Canadian system to their own. Clearly, some attributes of the Canadian system make it popular with Canadians and appealing to Americans and Britons.

Undoubtedly, the first and most significant characteristic is that Canadians live secure in the belief that a catastrophic medical event will not be compounded by a financial catastrophe. Canadians routinely read about U.S. citizens left destitute by major health calamities. Another important element that has contributed to the perceived success of the Canadian health care system has been its ability to recruit popular support by coopting community opinion leaders.

While the Canadian health care system is showing signs of strain, the continued overall satisfaction of Canadians with their system reflects their perception that scarce resources have been allocated in a manner sensitive to community needs and that they are financially risk free. In marked contrast to the situation in the United Kingdom (where formalized community involvement ultimately proved to be a procedural impediment), Canada seems to have succeeded in involving the community. Each province has determined its own way to decentralize the decision-making process. Smaller provinces have adopted planning methods that are compatible with their methods of provincial decision-making and that reflect the diversity of their population base and scarcity of communities.

Of perhaps more importance is the fact that these various bodies deal with the issue of finite resources, and the competing demands for them, at the beginning phase of a budgeting and planning process, when the decisions are still in their hands. Consequently, when crises do emerge, negative public opinion can be legitimately countered by the understanding that resource priorities were established by public decision rather than through a central bureaucracy or through heartless and invisible market forces. For example, lack of acute care beds is made more acceptable when elected leaders and the citizens they serve recall the choice that was made to make additional funds available to long-term care and home care programs rather than acute care beds.

The Canadian health care system does not operate less expensively or more effectively than the U.S. system. The Canadian mechanism for funding health care does constrain expenditure effectively. However, it comes at the price of limiting access to resources and technologies. This results in decreased accessibility to medical procedures and the use of procedures that are substantially inferior. The domestic and international popularity of the Canadian system stems largely from the perception that there is a safety net against the financial consequences of medical catastrophe. It is also a measurement of the effectiveness of a politicized system that enjoys sensitive community-based involvement in making difficult health resource trade-offs.

Moreover, this system can be executed only in an environment that would be legally and culturally unacceptable to U.S. citizens. What Canada offers U.S. health planners are important insights into the efficient proactive involvement of stakeholders in its resource rationing decisions and the tremendous popular value of a safety net against the financial consequences of medical catastrophe.

REFERENCE

1. Blendon, R. J., and Taylor, H. Views on health care: Public opinion in three nations. *Health Aff.*, Spring 1989, pp. 149–157.

B

U.S./Canadian Health Spending: Methods and Assumptions

Daniel R. Waldo and Sally T. Sonnefeld

In their comparison of Canadian and U.S. health spending statistics, Jacques Krasny and Ian Ferrier draw three conclusions. First, accounting and other differences exaggerate the spread between the two countries' spending as a share of gross national product (GNP). Second, slower growth in Canadian expenditures as a percentage of GNP is attributable to restricted access to care. Third, cultural differences preclude the wholesale adoption of a Canadian-type system in the United States.

We have reservations about the first two of these conclusions. Specifically, the adjustments Krasny and Ferrier make to the two countries' accounts are too large, and Canadian expenditures as a percentage of GNP remain significantly lower than in the United States even after adjustment. Further, the authors have not adequately made the case that limited access has negative implications for health.

DIFFERENCES IN HEALTH SPENDING

Krasny and Ferrier adjust the Canadian figures to allow for institutional differences in the two health care systems and conclude that the adjusted proportion of GNP accounted for by health is virtually the same in the two countries. We believe that only three of the adjustments they make are warranted, and the adjustments themselves should be much lower.

Fringe Benefits

Unlike their Canadian counterparts, U.S. health care providers must pay a fringe benefit to workers in the form of private health insurance premiums; recent U.S. figures peg that fringe benefit at about 7.5 percent of total payroll (1). Krasny and Ferrier argue that this raises the unit labor cost of U.S. health services relative to that in Canada, warranting an adjustment equal to 10 percent of payroll or 6.3 percent of total Canadian health expenditures.

We feel that this adjustment is invalid. In economic theory, labor receives a total compensation package, part of which comes in the form of wages and part in the form of fringes. All other things being equal, the lower the fringe benefit, the higher the wage. Failing evidence to the contrary, the assumption must be that Canadian workers receive higher money wages (again, all other things equal) than their colleagues in the United States, and that they then pay taxes to receive the health benefits that U.S. workers receive through fringe benefits. In that case, the market has adjusted for this difference, and any further adjustment would involve double counting.

In a September 1990 *Issue Brief,* the Employee Benefit Research Institute (EBRI) used U.S. Labor Department data to show that fringe benefits (including private health insurance contributions) in the United States averaged 27 percent of average hourly compensation in 1989, compared to 22 percent in Canada (2).[1] However, average hourly pay in Canada was greater than in the United States, making total average hourly compensation in the two countries almost identical. The study did not adjust for industrial composition of the work forces, but it does provide plausible empirical support for the theory embedded in labor economics.[2]

Levels of Research

Krasny and Ferrier observe that the United States spends a far greater proportion of its health dollar on research than does Canada. They increase Canadian health expenditures a total of 2.4 percent to show what Canadian experience would be were Canada to spend the same proportion of its health dollar on research as does the United States.

Rather than adjusting for research, it is appropriate to exclude it, and construction as well. Both types of expenditure are directed at the development of the health sector's infrastructure. Although directly related to the future ability of the

[1] The abstract cites the U.S. Labor Department's *International Comparisons of Hourly Costs for Production Workers in Manufacturing, 1975, 1980, and 1982–89.*

[2] The adjustment made by Krasny and Ferrier must be held to be too high in any case. The Canadian tax expenditure program covers only hospital and physician services; private insurance covers other types of spending. Thus, the 10 percent adjustment made to Canadian payroll is far greater than U.S. data suggest.

system to provide care, they do not affect current levels of care. We recognize that there are counterarguments to this position. For example, colleagues have argued that higher construction costs in the United States are part and parcel of the problems caused by the U.S. system. However, for the sake of comparing delivery systems alone, we feel comfortable eliminating from consideration both research and construction.[3]

In the U.S. national health accounts, this reduced scope of expenditure, called "health services and supplies," is published annually, along with the more comprehensive national health expenditures. In 1987, U.S. spending for health services and supplies was $475.2 billion, an amount equal to 10.6 percent of gross domestic product (GDP) (3, 4). The comparable figure for Canada was $45.4 billion, or 8.2 percent of GDP (5).[4]

Capital-Related Expenses

Krasny and Ferrier assert that because working capital in Canada is advanced by provincial governments out of general funds, interest on that capital is not allocated to health care costs. By contrast, private U.S. providers must find their own working capital, interest on which is booked as part of the cost of the health care system. Further, the authors claim, hospital construction in Canada is financed mainly through public funds, so that—again in contrast to the U.S. system—amortization costs are not considered. To compensate for these differences, they impute a cost of capital (interest and depreciation) to the Canadian accounts that raises total Canadian health expenditures by 3 percent.

We agree that there is a difference in treatment of capital costs in the two countries, but only a partial difference. First, depreciation is, in fact, booked by Canadian hospitals except in Quebec (and possibly additional provinces in the future). Second, Quebec hospitals (which account for about a quarter of all Canadian hospital spending) borrow funds and, as a result, report interest payments. Consequently, one needs to make only a partial adjustment of published expenditures to fully allocate capital-related expenses to Canadian institutions.

However, a similar adjustment must be made to U.S. hospital spending. Federal hospitals in the United States book neither interest nor depreciation expenses. Further, state government operation of hospitals frequently is subsidized by general revenue, and interest is not allocated back to the various end users of that revenue.

---

[3] The research excluded is only noncommercial research. U.S. drug manufacturers tend to recoup R&D costs through U.S. sales rather than sales in Canada, but we have made no adjustment for that.

[4] GDP is used in making these comparisons, rather than the more familiar GNP. Unlike GNP, GDP includes production by foreigners in the host country and excludes production by citizens outside their home country. GDP provides a more comparable base in comparing health expenditures across countries. In Canada, GDP exceeds GNP, while the opposite is true in the United States.

Demographics

We feel that the correction Krasny and Ferrier made to account for the difference in the demographic composition of the two populations is mathematically incorrect and incomplete.[5] To capture the effect of the demographic distribution, we applied an age/sex cost matrix to the two countries' populations. The matrix was derived from the National Medical Care Expenditure Survey (NMCES) conducted in the United States in 1977, augmented by other survey data.[6] Expenditures per capita were tallied for five-year age cohorts by sex, and the resulting distribution was smoothed using actuarial tools of analysis. These expenditure factors were applied to the U.S. and Canadian populations as of 1986. The difference in per capita expenditure, which is due solely to the difference in the age/sex profiles of the two populations, was 3.3 percent. That is, had the U.S. population of 1986 exhibited the same age/sex profile as did the Canadian population, U.S. expenditures would have been 3.3 percent lower than was actually the case.

A startling result of extending this analysis to other years is that the demographic effect on differences in health spending between Canada and the United States is in the process of reversing sign. The adjustment was as high as 6.9 percent as recently as 1966 but will drop to –8.4 percent in 2031. That is, 40 years from now [1991] we can expect U.S. spending per capita to be 8.4 percent lower than in Canada on the basis of age and sex alone. This phenomenon is due to the different shape of the two countries' population distributions. Currently, Canada is characterized by a larger middle-aged group, while the United States has more young and aged people. This difference, especially the presence of a larger U.S. aged population, accounts for the relatively higher U.S. expenses at this point in time (6). However, as the Canadian middle-aged group ages, the relative positions of the two countries will be reversed. In 1961, people age 65 and older accounted for 9.2 percent of the U.S. population and for 6.6 percent of the Canadian population. In 1986, the respective proportions were 11.9 and 10.7 percent; in 2031, they are projected to be 21.0 and 23.8 percent.

Net Effect of Adjustments

The data in Table 1 summarize our adjustment of the difference between U.S. and Canadian health expenditures as a percentage of their respective countries'

---

[5] For complete methodology, contact the authors at Office of the Actuary, Health Care Financing Administration, Room L1-EQ05, 6325 Security Boulevard, Baltimore, Maryland 21207.

[6] Although the NMCES data are over ten years old, they serve as an excellent tool for making the kind of analysis described here. When data become available from the 1987 National Medical Expenditure Survey (NMES), the age/sex matrix will be updated.

GDP. Where Krasny and Ferrier find only half a percentage point difference in 1987 after adjustment, we find a difference of 1.9 percentage points. Further, we find that the gap between the U.S. and Canadian shares of GDP has been widening over time, suggesting that Canada has successfully restricted growth of health expenditures relative to GDP. In fact, prior to the full implementation of universal insurance in 1972, Canada's adjusted share of GDP for health was higher than the U.S. share; since 1972, its health-to-GDP ratio has been lower than in the United States.

Growth Rates

Canadian health expenditures per capita have grown more rapidly than have U.S. expenditures (Figure 1). This is true in both nominal terms and opportunity cost. Yet Canadian GDP has grown much more rapidly than has U.S. GDP, which accounts for the finding that the share of GDP consumed by health has risen more slowly in Canada than in the United States.

Unquantified Adjustments

Krasny and Ferrier cite additional national differences that could contribute to a distorted comparison of U.S. and Canadian health spending.

1. The United States has more military veterans, who incur higher costs than nonveterans. This may be a factor, yet we were unable to estimate the effect of the difference with data at hand.

2. The United States has more inner-city crime, substance abuse, sexually transmitted disease, and teenage pregnancy than Canada has, all of which raise spending. Again, we were unable to quantify the effect with available data. Krasny and Ferrier neglect to mention the effect of population density itself upon access to and use of care, but it undoubtedly contributes to cross-national differences in spending as well.

3. The U.S. professional liability climate leads to higher consumption of services than in Canada. This is almost certainly true, but once again we were unable to quantify the effect. The evidence that exists tends to be anecdotal.

4. Administrative costs of the Canadian system are hidden in general government figures and do not appear in health expenditures. This may be true, but the effect probably is not significant. The U.S. system generates "hidden" administrative costs as well, since large employers incur directly much of the administrative expense of their group policies.

5. Canada "imports" health services from the United States. Given the way in which national health expenditures are measured, services provided by the U.S. providers to foreigners are reflected in U.S. expenditure data. Overall, this overstatement is probably small, although individual providers may find otherwise.

Table 1

Comparison of U.S. and Canadian health expenditures as percentage of gross domestic product, before and after adjustment for national differences, selected years, 1960–1987 (amounts in millions of national currency)[a]

	1960	1965	1970	1975	1980	1985	1987
Published national health expenditures							
Canada							
National health expenditures	$ 2,142	$ 3,416	$ 6,254	$ 12,268	$ 22,704	$ 40,408	$ 47,935
Health-to-GDP ratio	5.4%	5.9%	7.0%	7.2%	7.3%	8.5%	8.7%
United States							
National health expenditures	$27,135	$41,615	$74,377	$132,944	$249,054	$420,058	$492,498
Health-to-GDP ratio	5.3%	6.0%	7.4%	8.4%	9.3%	10.6%	11.0%
Exclusion of research and construction							
Canada							
Research	$ 12	$ 31	$ 70	$ 101	$ 215	$ 391	$ 411
Construction	197	256	365	612	1,234	1,863	2,133
Health services and supplies	1,933	3,128	5,819	11,555	21,255	38,154	45,391
United States							
Research	$ 692	$ 1,523	$ 1,956	$ 3,326	$ 5,444	$ 7,795	$ 9,029
Construction	1,006	1,928	3,366	4,954	5,831	7,600	8,244
Health services and supplies	25,437	38,164	69,055	124,664	237,779	404,663	475,225

Imputation of capital expenses[b]	1.0%	1.0%	1.0%	1.0%	1.0%	1.3%	1.3%
Canada	0.4%	0.4%	0.4%	0.5%	0.4%	0.4%	0.5%
United States							
Imputation of demographic effects[b]							
Canada	—	—	—	—	—	—	—
United States	–6.6%	–6.9%	–6.4%	–6.1%	–5.1%	–3.3%	–3.3%
Adjusted health services and supplies (HSS)							
Canada							
HSS adjustment factor	1.0%	1.0%	1.0%	1.0%	1.0%	1.3%	1.3%
Adjusted HSS	$ 1,952	$ 3,160	$ 5,877	$ 11,670	$ 21,468	$ 38,650	$ 45,981
Adjusted share of GDP	4.9%	5.5%	6.6%	6.8%	6.9%	8.1%	8.4%
United States							
HSS adjustment factor	–6.2%	–6.5%	–6.0%	–5.6%	–4.7%	–2.9%	–2.8%
Adjusted HSS	$23,860	$35,683	$64,912	$117,683	$226,603	$392,928	$461,919
Adjusted share of GDP	4.7%	5.1%	6.4%	7.4%	8.4%	9.9%	10.3%
Difference between U.S. and Canadian health-to-GDP ratios							
Unadjusted	–0.1%	0.0%	0.4%	1.3%	2.0%	2.1%	2.3%
Adjusted	–0.3%	–0.4%	–0.2%	0.6%	1.5%	1.8%	1.9%

[a]Sources: Data from Canadian Department of National Health and Welfare and U.S. Health Care Financing Administration, developed by the authors.
[b]Percent of health services and supplies.

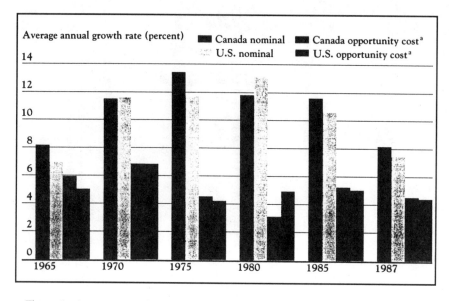

Figure 1. Average annual growth in adjusted health expenditures per capita, United States and Canada, 1965–1987. Source: U.S. and Canadian governments; data developed by the authors.
[a]Opportunity cost is the value of other goods and services that could have been bought with dollars spent for health.

6. In the United States, some 33 million people do not have health insurance, and almost nobody has true catastrophic coverage; Canada's universal insurance includes coverage of catastrophic expenses. Although not mentioned by the authors, the extent to which universal coverage induces demand in Canada may well narrow artificially the gap between the two countries' spending.

7. In addition to the differences mentioned by Krasny and Ferrier, we feel that GDP per capita plays an important role in creating differences in health expenditures across countries. Data collected by the Organization for Economic Cooperation and Development show a correlation between health expenditures per capita and GDP per capita. Analysis of a simplistic regression suggests that U.S. expenditures should have been 3 percent higher than Canadian expenditures in 1987, based on differences in GDP per capita (7). The actual gap (after the adjustments discussed above) was 29 percent. Figure 2 shows how the narrowing gap in GDP per capita in the two countries should have caused health expenditures per capita to converge, and how in fact the gap in health expenditures per capita has remained nearly unchanged. As noted above, the gap between expected and observed expenditures widened once the Canadian universal insurance program reached full implementation in the early 1970s. Of course, this regression

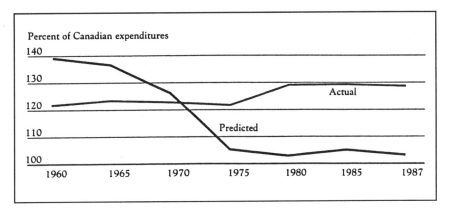

Figure 2. U.S. adjusted health expenditures per capita as percentage of Canadian expenditures, actual and predicted by gross domestic product per capita, 1960–1987. Source: U.S. and Canadian governments; data developed by the authors.

analysis is merely suggestive. The expenditure model makes no provision for income distribution, access to care, or any other determinants of health expenditure, but the results are thought-provoking.[7]

LIMITS ON ACCESS

The second major conclusion of Krasny and Ferrier is that Canada has accomplished slower growth rates by restricting access. They distinguish between the rationing systems of the two countries. Although the uninsured are not locked out of the U.S. delivery system, they probably receive less care than they desire. Further, uninsured Americans are liable for larger expenses out of pocket for health care. This is troublesome to many Canadians. By contrast, all Canadians are covered for basic hospital and physician services. In that system, access is limited for everybody, and queues form for nearly everything. Krasny and Ferrier see the 1980s in Canada as a period characterized by diminishing returns to productivity and efficiency, reductions in access, and retarded adoption of new technology. They state, "People clearly have greater ease of access, a larger range of choices, and more timely access in the U.S. than in Canada."

In response, it is important to clarify the meaning of "slower growth." While Canadian expenditures have grown more rapidly than U.S. expenditures in nominal terms, the Canadian share of GDP has grown more slowly than in the United States. In other words, Canadian income has grown even more rapidly

---

[7] The income distribution in Canada appears to be quite similar to that in the United States, so that factor may not be particularly relevant here.

than has U.S. income. Also, it is not clear that restricted access is inherently bad. Unfettered access has both positive and negative sides. Anecdotal evidence suggests that many medical procedures performed in the United States are of doubtful efficacy. In those cases, increased access has led to increased cost without concomitant increases in health status.

Krasny and Ferrier also believe that the Canadian administrative system may have lessons to learn from the United States. They point out that several large health maintenance organizations (HMOs) in the United States deliver care at a lower cost than the Canadian system. To verify this point, it is important to adjust the HMO experience for demographic mix (and geographic dispersion). Krasny and Ferrier did not do so, and until the adjustment has been made, little can be said about the relative merits of the various systems.

REFERENCES

1. Levit, K. R., and Cowan, C. A. The burden of health care costs: Business, households, and governments. *Health Care Financ. Rev.,* Winter 1990, pp. 127–137.
2. *Medical Benefits,* October 15, 1990.
3. Lazenby, H. C., and Letsch, S. W. National health expenditures, 1989. *Health Care Financ. Rev.,* Winter 1990, pp. 1–26.
4. U.S. Commerce Department, Bureau of Economic Analysis. GDP data for 1987. Washington, D.C.
5. Health and Welfare Canada. *National Health Expenditures in Canada, 1975–1987.* Ottawa, Ont., September 1990.
6. Waldo, D. R., Sonnefeld, S. T., and McKusick, D. R. Health expenditures by age group, 1977 and 1987. *Health Care Financ. Rev.,* Summer 1989, pp. 111–120.
7. Waldo, D. R. Financing health care: Who pays the bill? *Q. Rev. Econ. Business,* Winter 1990, pp. 101–113.

C

U.S./Canadian Comparison: The Authors Respond

Jacques Krasny and Ian R. Ferrier

With the exception of "limited access," which we deal with below, we feel that Dan Waldo and Sally Sonnefeld have been unable to substantiate any material argument to support their contentions. Rather, what they have done is to engage in illusory precision; they have measured that which they found measurable, while unfortunately not addressing that which is in fact germane.

Demographics

A vivid example of this is the recalculation of our analysis of the impact of demographic differences in the two countries. Waldo and Sonnefeld conclude that our calculations were "mathematically incorrect and incomplete." They then recalculate them and come to the conclusion that if one adjusted for the two populations as we did, the U.S. health care burden would have been 3.3 percent lower. We have no point of view on the validity of this number, since we made no reference to it at all. Rather, what we presented was what Canada's increased cost would have been if it had the same demographic population as the United States. If Waldo and Sonnefeld are suggesting that a reduction in U.S. costs based on Canadian demographics should be roughly the same as an increase in Canadian costs if it dealt with U.S. demographics, then inherent in this assumption is the belief that both countries use the same practice patterns for all age groups (particularly the elderly). This assumption would simply be untrue.

Benefit Costs

The authors imply, through a series of cross-border salary references, that even though health care benefits are largely not paid on behalf of health care employees, they are implicitly paid through the salary and taxation system. This supposition might in fact be true if the entire society presented a perfectly balanced, closed economic system. In fact, notwithstanding a gross national product growing at a rate faster than in the United States, Canada has developed a relatively higher per capita gross national debt.

To put this into an American context, it would be as though a large imprudent insurance company elected to provide health insurance for all health care workers and charged them only 17 percent of actual total cost (the percentage that the Ontario Health Insurance Plan actually charges as premiums). The method this insurance company would use to fund its profound losses would be external borrowings. Any calculation as to the health benefit cost of these employees would identify only the 17 percent being paid directly. And, as such, it would have to be adjusted upward exactly as we have done to reflect true cost.

Capital

In looking at the capital expense of the two systems, there is no escaping the fundamental reality that the U.S. system is predominantly private and the Canadian system is predominantly public. In Canada, public facilities do not "change hands," and there is no gross-up of values reflecting inflation and real estate price changes. Since hospitals and most other facilities are tax free, there is no benefit to identify incremental depreciation opportunities. While hospitals do have depreciation accounts, they bear no relationship whatsoever to the full extent of capital involvement in the facility. In the same perspective, while hospitals in Quebec can in fact borrow funds, the amounts again bear no relationship to full capital involvement. Fully aware of these minor anomalies, we deliberately used a conservative interest rate of 10 percent on an equally conservative estimate of the extent of capital involvement in the system. Waldo and Sonnefeld provide no factual basis for concluding that this projection is anything other than valid for its purpose.

Research and Development

In comparing expenditures on research and development, Waldo and Sonnefeld concede that an adjustment (or, in their case, a total removal) of these figures is in order. They then discuss the involvement of "construction" expenses in the various calculations. Since we did not introduce this concept, we see no need to address the incremental accounting confusion it would bring.

In summary, the logical development we provided of making Canada's health care expenditures comparable to U.S. expenditures has not been adequately or materially challenged by Waldo and Sonnefeld. We do concede that we have not proved that limited access has negative implications for health. We have accepted as axiomatic that the pain, fear, and risk endured while waiting for access to facilities are of themselves inherently negative. No doubt, those Canadians who use the American health care system to meet their medical needs would agree. As well, we feel that is unnecessary to prove that a market environment that provides abundant and varied resources—ranging to the best available technology—is inherently better than one that does not.

CHAPTER 6

An Economist's Brief Guide to the Recent Debate on the Canadian Health Care System

Robert Chernomas and Ardeshir Sepehri

As U.S. health care costs continue to grow out of control, the adoption of a Canadian-style universal insurance system has become more attractive to the public, policymakers, and segments of the business community in the United States as a means of containing health care costs and providing universal health insurance coverage. Arguments in favor of the Canadian system usually emphasize its universal coverage coupled with its cost-containment advantages. A comparison of the U.S. and Canadian health care cost trends suggest that the Canadian system has been relatively more successful at cost containment than the U.S. system. Before the full implementation of the Canadian system in 1971, the funding system and the health costs as a share of gross national product (GNP) were virtually identical in both countries at about 7 percent of GNP. After 1971 the health trends of the two countries diverged considerably. Current estimates (for 1992) indicate that the United States spends approximately 13 percent of its GNP on health care, while Canada spends approximately 9.5 percent. Advocates suggest that these cost-containment advantages persist in spite of the fact that the Canadian system provides universal coverage whereas the U.S. system fails to provide full coverage for approximately 35 percent of its population (1) (see Chapter 7).

Recently, economists have aimed a number of criticisms at the purported advantages of the Canadian system. These arguments have been widely disseminated by a broad spectrum of opponents of the Canadian system in the political and business community, and have engendered a reaction by other economists who believe that the evidence still warrants support for the Canadian system's cost and coverage advantages.

Published in *International Journal of Health Services,* 24(2), pp. 189–200, 1994.

It is the cost advantage and the kind of coverage Canadians receive that is being challenged by the critics. The purpose of this chapter is to provide an overview of some aspects of this debate on the Canadian health care system's merits and deficiencies relative to the U.S. health care system. For ease of presentation we have chosen, despite its simplicity and possible overgeneralization, to review this critical literature under two general headings, loosely representing two distinct groups of critics: one raises questions about how to measure inter-country comparisons of health cost trends, and the other asks what is to be included in the measurement.

HOW SHOULD WE MEASURE INTER-COUNTRY HEALTH COST TRENDS?

Real versus Nominal GNP

In a 1987 article in the *New England Journal of Medicine,* Feder, Scanlon, and Clark argued that it was a mistake to suggest that health spending had risen far less rapidly in Canada than in the United States (2). The essence of their argument was that while health care spending from 1970 to 1984 rose faster in Canada than in the United States, GNP in Canada grew even faster. They concluded that it was not that the Canadian health care system was more effective at cost containment, but that because Canadian GNP grew at a more rapid rate, there was the *appearance* of relative health care cost containment. Therefore, while the health care share of GNP in Canada (*H*/GNP) was stable, *H* itself actually grew at a rate more closely resembling the U.S. rate because GNP was growing more rapidly in Canada.

In a 1989 *New England Journal of Medicine* article, Evans and coauthors (3) challenged this conclusion by pointing out that Feder and associates confused nominal with real rates of GNP (see Chapter 1). While Canadian GNP did outgrow the U.S. GNP by 2 percent per year during 1970–1984, the inter-country growth rate of real GNP amounted to only 0.7 percent, not enough to account for the divergence in the share of GNP spent on health.

Health Costs Per Capita versus Health Costs as a Share of GNP

More recently, Neuschler (4), in a monograph published by the Health Insurance Association of America, raised an empirical doubt about the Canadian cost-containment success and its underlying measure of comparison, *H*/GNP. Neuschler argued that it was the relatively more rapid growth in real GNP in Canada during the period 1967–1987 that resulted in a lower health care share in GNP, creating the illusion that the Canadian system was more effective at cost containment. He argued that cost containment can be more accurately measured by real per capita health expenditures and their growth rate. Using real health per capita health expenditures, he concluded that Canada's single-payer system was no more effective at cost containment than the U.S. system over the entire period from 1967 to 1987 because the real health expenditures per capita grew slightly faster in Canada than in the United States. Moreover, he argued that Canada's cost control has come at the expense of a variety of access problems, and the wholesale adoption of the Canadian system would not be acceptable to Americans as it implies, among other things, a dramatic increase in public funding and increased government intervention.

Choice of Time Period, Expenditure Categories,
and the Theoretical Advantage of H/GNP

Barer, Welch, and Antioch (5) have questioned Neuschler's analysis for his (*a*) claim of the superiority of real per capita health expenditures over *H*/GNP as a basis of inter-country comparisons; (*b*) choice of time period of analysis; and (*c*) selectivity of sectors chosen for comparison (see Chapter 4). They argue that real health costs per capita is a poor measure of relative cost-containment performance and Neuschler's conclusions are not sustained once the appropriate expenditure categories and time period are used. Barer and associates argue that a comparison based on the per capita real expenditures has certain intrinsic defects that make it difficult to draw any meaningful conclusion about the trends in resources allocated to the health care sector over time. The theoretical superiority of *H*/GNP over the real health expenditures per capita is skillfully demonstrated through a simple example. If real GNP per capita increased by 10 percent along with health costs per capita, health costs as a percentage of GNP would not change, because increases in the denominator (GNP per capita) would cancel out those in the numerator (health care costs per capita). If in a comparison country there was no change in health care per capita or GNP per capita, this would create the illusion that health cost per capita in the growth country had grown 10 percent faster than in the no-growth country. As Barer and associates note: "Yet, only an unusual definition of health care cost containment could lead one to conclude that this increase in real health expenditure was evidence of a country's failure to contain its health care costs" (5, p. 230). Given that nothing has changed in the health care sector of the growth country per se, Barer and associates argue that health care costs as a percentage of GNP—*H*/GNP—is conceptually a more appropriate measure for comparison.

Moreover, Barer and colleagues question Neuschler's choice of the 20-year period 1967–1987. During the late 1960s Canadian universal health care insurance was still evolving, and only in 1971 was it fully implemented by all provinces. Beginning in 1971 and extending the period until 1989, they find that real health expenditures per capita grew 0.7 percent a year faster in the United States than in Canada. This suggests "a quite different conclusion than

Neuschler's: namely, that despite the fact one might have anticipated more rapid growth of real per capita expenditures in Canada because of its more rapid real economic growth, one finds quite the opposite" (5, pp. 232–233).

This revised picture is still, as argued by Barer and colleagues, misleading unless one takes note of the institutional details, namely, that the Canadian national health system was not designed to control subsectors such as dental care, pharmaceuticals, long-term care, and medical devices. Examination of the relative cost-control effectiveness of the Canadian system should focus exclusively on hospital services, physician services, and administration. Their results suggest a dramatic effect of the Canadian universal health care system on both the internal health care sector reallocations and the growth of resources allocated to health care. The share of total Canadian health care costs represented by the three subsectors (physicians, hospitals, and administration) as a percentage of total health expenditures between 1971 and 1987 fell from about 65 percent at the beginning of the period to below 57 percent in 1987, while the comparable U.S. share rose from about 60 percent to about 63 percent. The inter-country gap between the health care costs trends in the three subsectors is wide and growing faster, even when using the real health expenditures per capita as a basis of comparison. The U.S. real health expenditures per capita for the three subsectors outran those in Canada by 1.4 percent annually, or by over 20 percent cumulatively over the 16 years.

Adjusting for Fluctuations in Real GNP

H/GNP is not, however, a perfect measure of resource utilization. A comparison of relative cost based on H/GNP is sensitive to cyclical fluctuations in real GNP. The sensitivity of the growth rate of H/GNP to economic fluctuations is more severe for the 1970s and 1980s compared with the rapid and stable growth of GNP during the 1960s. However, the inter-country differences in GNP growth rates are not, as we have demonstrated elsewhere (6), sufficient to account for the widening gap between the two countries' health cost trends. Canada's relatively high rate of growth of GNP accounted for only 38 percent of the gap between the two countries' health cost trends during the entire period 1971–1988, and for as little as 11.8 percent of the gap during the period 1982–1988.

A Resource Usage Model

Coyte (7) also raises empirical doubts about the way in which the Canadian system's health expenditures success has been measured, in particular when expenditures are compared with those in the United States. One problem with a simple inter-country comparison of health costs trends based on H/GNP is, as pointed out by Coyte, its sensitivity to cyclical variations in GNP caused by variation in both the unemployment rate and labor force participation rate (defined as the percentage of working age population working or looking for work). An increase in labor force participation that increases GNP and leaves H unchanged would appear to reduce society's resources devoted to the health care industry, while all that has really changed is a reallocation of time from areas of the economy where effort is not captured (e.g., the labor of homemakers) in measures of total income to areas where effort is captured. Coyte proposes an alternative measure of resource usage according to which the conventional measure H/GNP is adjusted for the cyclical variations in both unemployment and labor force participation. Applying this new measure to the Canadian–U.S. data for the period 1960–1988, he concludes that (a) the growth rate of the share of society's resources allocated to health is higher in the United States than in Canada, though the gap between the two countries' cost trends is much smaller than suggested by the unadjusted H/GNP; and (b) the full implementation of universal health care insurance had no discernible effect on the share of resources allocated to the health care industry. Coyte attributes the rising gap between the two countries' adjusted H/GNPs to a more rapid increase in labor force participation rate in Canada than in the United States.

A Critique of the Resource Model

In a 1991 article we cast doubts on Coyte's statistical analysis and conclusions (8). Coyte's main conclusions are reversed once structural changes, especially the full introduction of universal health care insurance in Canada in 1971, are incorporated into the calculation of health care costs trends. Both adjusted and unadjusted H/GNP suggest that the share of resources devoted to health *were affected* dramatically by the introduction of the Canadian insurance system in 1971; that is, the gap in the resources devoted to health care in the United States and Canada grew dramatically after 1971. Moreover, an inter-country comparison of cyclical changes in the labor market (i.e., unemployment and labor force participation) reveals no systematic trend, as asserted by Coyte, suggesting that one has to look for factors other than cyclical changes in the labor market to account for the growing gap in the two countries' health care costs trends.

Another Use for Real Per Capita Health Expenditures
and Its Problems

In a more recent article, Coyte (9) abandons H/GNP, in both its unadjusted and adjusted forms, in favor of real per capita health expenditures as a seemingly more appropriate measure of resource usage. In contrast to his earlier results he concludes (a) that the full implementation of the universal health insurance system did reduce significantly the annual growth rate of per capita real health expenditures and (b) that the U.S. health expenditures experience after 1971 is similar to the Canadian experience as per capita real health expenditures declined significantly from 5.56 percent for the period 1960–1970 to 3.84 percent for the period 1971–1990. The similar decline in the rate of growth of health expenditures in both countries suggests that "the trends in health expenditures transcend international borders" (9, p. 245). Coyte speculates that these slowdowns in the rate of growth are due to an array of cost-containment measures taken in both countries since the early 1970s.

We have critically reevaluated Coyte's analysis and his conclusions (10). Coyte's analysis of structural change is flawed with conceptual and technical problems. The incorporation of institutional and policy changes into his simple statistical analysis requires an a priori identification of institutional/policy changes. While it is possible to view 1971 as a pivotal conjuncture in the history of Canadian health policy when the full introduction of universal medical insurance provided provinces with mechanisms to contain costs, it is not so for the United States. This is not to deny the importance of piecemeal cost-containment policies pursued in the United States in the early 1970s. However, these changes cannot fully capture the influence, if any, of the array of cost-containment measures pursued during that period.

Moreover, Coyte's analysis, like Neuschler's, also fails to take note of the institutional details of the Canadian national health care system. An inter-country comparison of the three subsectors affected by the Canadian universal health care system demonstrates not only a wide and growing gap, as noted above, but also a significant decline in the growth rate of resources allocated to health care after 1971. The relative share of GNP allocated to the three Canadian health subsectors dropped from 3.42 percent a year during the 1960s to 0.47 percent during the period 1971–1988, and to a negative rate of –0.43 percent if the abnormal years of 1980–1982 are excluded. The decline in the U.S. rate was much smaller, from an average rate of 3.78 percent annually to 2.66 percent. These findings demonstrate once again how misleading results are when one fails to take note of the institutional details. Finally, Coyte's assertion that real per capita health expenditure is a more reliable indicator of resource utilization than H/GNP is not, as noted above, supported theoretically or empirically.

WHAT IS TO BE INCLUDED IN THE MEASUREMENT?

Up to this point there is little to support the critics of the Canadian system in their efforts to challenge its relative cost effectiveness. Krasny and Ferrier (11) and Waldo and Sonnefeld (12) extended the scope of the debate by questioning what is to be included in the costs of the two countries' health care systems rather than how the systems relative costs are to be compared on an aggregate basis (see Chapter 5).

Krasny and Ferrier make three arguments with respect to their critique of the Canadian system. Most of their effort is focused on the argument that the percentage of GNP spent on health care in the two countries is much closer than conventional measurements would suggest because of what has and has not been added to the calculations of health care costs in the two countries. Second, insofar as the Canadian system has a slower rate of growth of health costs, it has come with a profound limitation in access to institutional services and new health care technologies. And finally, they argue that the Canadian system's limitations on individual discretion would make it culturally unacceptable in the United States.

Waldo and Sonnefeld contest Krasny and Ferrier's adjustments to the two countries' accounts and suggest that the cost differences between them remain significant. In addition, they challenge the claim that limited access to U.S. levels of technologies has negative implications for health.

The following are the debated adjustments to the health cost data.

Capital Costs

Krasny and Ferrier argue that the public financing of the publicly funded Canadian system is buried in its public debt and therefore is largely invisible and unaccounted for. The U.S. privately funded system must account for financing as an expense. In order to reconcile these differences the Canadian accounts must be adjusted upward. Waldo and Sonnefeld counter this claim by arguing that only a partial adjustment is needed for these hidden interest and depreciation costs because some of the depreciation and interest costs in Canada are reported as costs to the health system.

Health Benefits

Krasny and Ferrier argue that since U.S. health care providers pay a fringe benefit to workers in the form of private health insurance premiums and their Canadian counterparts do not, Canadian health expenditure figures should be raised because these are health costs not accounted for. Waldo and Sonnefeld argue that Canadian workers pay higher taxes out of the higher wages they receive in lieu of fringe benefits. The market has made the necessary adjustments and any further adjustment would be double counting.

Research and Development

Krasny and Ferrier argue that the United States spends more on research and development than Canada and therefore the Canadian health expenditures ought to be raised to match U.S. proportional expenditures on research and development. Waldo and Sonnefeld argue that research and development and construction should be eliminated from the calculation because they are the infrastructure for the health sector and do not affect current levels of care.

Population Mix

Krasny and Ferrier argue that if the Canadian system had the same percentage of elderly as the U.S. system, its health expenditures would be higher. Waldo and Sonnefeld did their own more complex calculation based on an age/sex cost matrix and concluded that if the U.S. population for 1986 had had the same age/sex profile as the Canadian population, U.S. expenditures would have been lower than was actually the case.

Net Effect of Adjustments

According to Krasny and Ferrier the combined net effect of these adjustments increases the Canadian *H*/GNP in 1987 from 9 percent to 10.5 percent, reducing the gap between the two countries from 2.1 to 0.5 percent, indicating that the Canadian cost-containment success is at the very least exaggerated. Waldo and Sonnefeld's adjustments found the U.S. *H*/GNP a full 1.9 percentage points higher, with the gap in the shares of GNP widening over time. The two pairs of authors did not agree on any of the adjustments and often qualified their own calculations. Clearly, more technical work needs to be done on the adjustments already enumerated.

Unmeasured Differences

In addition to the contested numerical adjustments suggested by Krasny and Ferrier is their list of unquantified factors that would suggest that the Canadian system is less effective than the U.S. health care system with respect to cost containment. This list would include: (*a*) the large number of U.S. Vietnam veterans, (*b*) U.S. urbanization, (*c*) malpractice insurance, (*d*) Canadian administrative costs hidden in government bureaucracy, and (*e*) the unmeasured use by Canadians of the U.S. health care system, which raises U.S. health expenditures and lowers Canadian costs. The fact that Krasny and Ferrier cannot quantify these adjustments, and Waldo and Sonnefeld are unable to support or dismiss these additions for similar reasons, begs further research.

Krasny and Ferrier argue that the problem with the U.S. system is not that those who are uninsured are denied required services, but that it creates financial pressure for them. This also helps to explain why Americans and Canadians support a Canadian-style system.

Krasny and Ferrier go on to list the shortcomings of the Canadian system. They suggest that Americans have 200 to 800 percent more access to medical technology, which highlights the important principle that Americans have greater access, a larger range of choices, and more timely access. They argue that U.S. health maintenance organizations (HMOs) provide the same service as the Canadian health care system for considerably less expense. Insofar as the

Canadian system constrains expenditures it does so by decreasing accessibility to medical procedures and by using procedures that are substantially inferior.

Waldo and Sonnefeld criticize Krasny and Ferrier for ignoring the possibility that universal insurance in Canada has had the effect of inducing demand, thereby narrowing the gap in health expenditures between the two countries, and for ignoring the fact that uninsured Americans probably receive less care than they desire, which if adjusted for would presumably further widen the gap in expenditures. In addition, they question the efficacy of much of the technology and medical practice to which some Americans have unfettered access.

And finally, as for the cost advantages of U.S. HMOs, Waldo and Sonnefeld raise doubts about their relative merits until the demographic mixes of the two systems are compared.

DISCUSSION

The problem with this qualitative debate is that it is far more one-sided than the known facts warrant. Krasny and Ferrier are bold and uninhibited in their assertions, whereas Waldo and Sonnefeld are careful and understated in their support for the Canadian system, even where there is evidence that would allow for a more spirited defense.

Subsectors

Whatever the merits of Waldo and Sonnefeld's adjustments, they, like Krasny and Ferrier and other critics, fail to take note of the institutional setting and confine their comparison to the three subsectors directly under the control of the Canadian single-payer system. As suggested above, the effects of incorporating these institutional details into the argument are dramatic with respect to health care expenditure trends.

Health Maintenance Organizations

One obvious example of the rather one-sided debate is Krasny and Ferrier's attempt to equate the Canadian Provincial System with large U.S. HMOs with respect to size and services provided, and then suggest there are cost advantages in the HMO system. One problem with this notion (as suggested by Waldo and Sonnefeld) is that there is evidence that the cost-effective HMOs (like U.S. insurance companies) "skim" for patients that are low risk. Canadian provinces, of course, must take the case mix that exists in their entire populations. A second problem with this notion, and ignored in the debate, is that the evidence does not support the idea that treatment in HMOs is on average less costly than the office costs of ambulatory patients treated in the personal physician system. On the contrary, the savings by HMOs occur by and large because HMOs reduce patient use of Krasny and Ferrier's vaunted American technology. In a word, the key to successful cost control by HMOs is dramatically lower hospital days per patient (13, pp. 221–229). Not only are HMOs less likely to hospitalize their patients, their disproportionate numbers of low-risk patients are less likely to need hospitalization and are likely to have shorter stays. In addition, HMOs with millions of patients are likely to be able to negotiate discounts with hospitals, drug companies, and other suppliers. This, of course, does not guarantee savings in the aggregate as suppliers in the U.S. system attempt to compensate for the income given up to the HMOs with higher prices and more services shifted elsewhere. In many ways the Canadian system is like Krasny and Ferrier's lauded HMO. It is the single-payer system that attempts to control its costs by controlling both quantities and prices. Its cost disadvantages include the fact that it covers heart disease, cancer, and AIDS patients, drug and alcohol abusers, and the chronically ill. Arguably the U.S. system cannot control costs because it does not have any one watching the door, only a few people watching a few of the aisles.

Coverage

Krasny and Ferrier's argument that the uninsured and underinsured in the United States received treatment is a heroic assertion. Whether some of them have no access, little access, or less access than they desire, it would be absurd to believe that they have access to the technology that Krasny and Ferrier suggest Canadians are short of. If adjustments are to be made so that Krasny and Ferrier's cost comparison can be made between the two countries, one question that would have to be addressed is what would be the cost of the U.S. system if the nearly 90 million Americans uninsured and underinsured had equal access to the technology that Canadians are supposed to be lacking?

Technology

As for the lauded technology itself, it is not that the Canadian system lacks CAT scans and MRIs, it just has far fewer than the U.S. system. Neither the Japanese nor the Europeans have chosen to employ medical technology with anything near the intensity used by Americans. Eighty percent of this technology has never been through rigorous scientific investigation (13, pp. 70–90). Some of it is potentially iatrogenic. If there is a need, it is not for a more intense use of technology as much as for a more intense application of technological assessment.

CONCLUSION

The attempt by economists critical of the Canadian health system to dispel the belief in its cost advantages over the U.S. system has up until now been unsuccessful. Their attempts to invent alternative measurements to those that result in identifying the Canadian system as more cost effective have floundered on theoretical and/or empirical grounds. The effect of attempts by critics of the Canadian system to add factors to the accounting is more ambiguous, although it is likely that adding a full range of appropriate factors would work against these critics.

This does not mean that the Canadian system is not in need of reform. Untested technologies and treatments, the supply-induced demand effects of the fee-for-service personal physician system (including extraordinarily high hospital days per capita and the concomitant excess surgery and waiting lists), other health sectors never incorporated into the single-payer system, the minimal commitment to prevention, lack of community control and interdisciplinary practice—all suggest reform is needed. Certain parts of the U.S. system may suggest avenues for reform in Canada (13). The trouble with the U.S. system is that the whole is less than the sum of the parts.

REFERENCES

1. Himmelstein, D., Woolhandler, S., and Wolfe, S. M. The vanishing health care safety net: New data on uninsured Americans. *Int. J. Health Serv.* 22: 381–396, 1992.
2. Feder, J., Scanlon, W., and Clark, J. Canada's health care system. *N. Engl. J. Med.* 317: 317–320, 1987.
3. Evans, R. G., et al. Controlling health expenditures: The Canadian reality. *N. Engl. J. Med.* 320: 571–577, 1989.
4. Neuschler, E. *Canadian Health Care: The Implications of Public Health Insurance.* Health Insurance Association of America, Washington, D.C., 1990.
5. Barer, M. L., Welch, W. P., and Antioch, L. Canadian/U.S. health care: Reflections on the HIAA's analysis. *Health Aff.,* Fall 1991, pp. 229–239.
6. Sepehri, A., and Chernomas, R. Further refinements of Canadian/U.S. health cost containment measures. *Int. J. Health Serv.* 23: 63–67, 1993.
7. Coyte, P. Current trends in Canadian health care: Myths and misconceptions in health economics. *J. Public Health Policy,* Summer 1990, pp. 169–188.
8. Chernomas, R., and Sepehri, A. Is the Canadian system more effective at expenditure control than previously thought? A reply to Peter Coyte. *Int. J. Health Serv.* 21: 793–804, 1991.
9. Coyte, P. C. More myths and misconceptions: A reply to comments on an article. *Int. J. Health Serv.* 23: 239–248, 1993.
10. Sepehri, A., and Chernomas, R. The effects of misconceptions and theoretical beliefs on data and measurement tools: A reply. *Int. J. Health Serv.* 23: 249–255, 1993.
11. Krasny, J., and Ferrier, I. R. A closer look at health care in Canada. *Health Aff.,* Summer 1991, pp. 152–158, 164–165.
12. Waldo, D. R., and Sonnefeld, S. T. U.S./Canadian health spending methods and assumptions. *Health Aff.,* Summer 1991, pp. 159–164.
13. Rachlis, M., and Kushner, C. *Second Opinion.* Harper and Collins, Toronto, 1989.

PART II. COMPARING ACCESS AND QUALITY OF OUTCOMES IN THE CANADIAN AND U.S. HEALTH CARE SYSTEMS

CHAPTER 7

The Vanishing Health Care Safety Net: New Data on Uninsured Americans

David U. Himmelstein, Steffie Woolhandler, and Sidney M. Wolfe

The number of people without health insurance is an important indicator of the adequacy of our health care system. Between the 1930s and the late 1970s the number of uninsured Americans declined steadily. Over the past 15 years the ranks of the uninsured have been increasing. This chapter presents data on health insurance coverage during 1990, obtained from the Census Bureau under the Freedom of Information Act.

METHODS

We analyzed data from the March 1991 Current Population Survey (CPS) and comparable CPS data from the 1990 survey. The CPS is a Census Bureau survey of approximately 60,000 households representative of the noninstitutionalized population. Each year's March survey collects data for the previous calendar year. Thus the 1991 survey provides information about health insurance coverage during 1990 and is the most up-to-date, comprehensive information on insurance coverage. The CPS data on health insurance provide an estimate of the number of people who are uninsured at any one time. That is, if two individuals are each uninsured for six months of the year, this results in a CPS estimate of one uninsured person. Thus, a far higher number of people are uninsured for at least some period during the year than is indicated by the CPS data.

We considered people insured if they reported any health insurance coverage, public or private. Population estimates were derived from the CPS sample using the March CPS Final Weight, a multiplier assigned by the Census Bureau to each

Published in *International Journal of Health Services*, 22(3), pp. 381–396, 1992.

individual in the sample to allow accurate extrapolation of the survey results to the U.S. population as a whole, adjusting for the sample design and the failure to obtain interviews with some households.

We obtain data for other years from publications based on the National Health Interview Surveys (NHIS) carried out by the National Center for Health Statistics in 1976, 1978, 1980, 1982, 1984, 1986, and 1989, as well as CPS data for the years 1980–1988.

Because the CPS methodology for estimating health insurance coverage underwent a major change in 1987 (the March 1988 survey), time series estimates prior to 1987 are problematic. We constructed an approximate time series for the period 1976–1990 in the following manner. For 1987–1990 we used the actual CPS estimate. We adjusted the 1981–1986 CPS estimates downward by multiplying them by a correction factor of 0.8764. This correction factor was derived from the 1987 data, which we analyzed using both the old and the new methodologies. For years prior to 1981, we used data from the NHIS with small corrections in 1978 and 1980 for missing data on uninsured seniors.

RESULTS

The number of Americans without any health insurance rose by 1.3 million between 1989 and 1990. In 1990, 34.7 million were uninsured, more than at any time since the implementation of Medicare and Medicaid in the 1960s. The increase affected all areas of the nation except the West South Central region (Arkansas, Louisiana, Oklahoma, and Texas), though the rate of uninsurance in that region continued to be by far the highest in the nation: 20.9 percent.

In seven states (Pennsylvania, Ohio, Illinois, Maryland, Virginia, Florida, and California) the number of uninsured rose by more than 100,000 people, while the number of uninsured fell by more than 100,000 in only one state, Texas (though Texas still had the second highest rate of uninsurance in the nation). The figures for each region and for individual states (including the District of Columbia) are shown in Table 1, and the rankings for individual states in Table 2. Small differences in state figures should be interpreted cautiously because of the margin of error inherent in the survey design.

The net increase in the number of uninsured was most marked among men, who accounted for 1 million of the 1.3 million additional uninsured. Most of the additional uninsured were white (1.1 million), though the percentage increase was about the same for whites and blacks. The increase affected all income groups, with 26 percent of the additional uninsured from families with annual incomes below $25,000, 42 percent from families with incomes between $25,000 and $50,000, and 32 percent from families with incomes above $50,000. Only 9 percent of the additional uninsured had incomes below the poverty line. The entire increase in the number of uninsured was among working-age adults. Both children and senior citizens showed small (not significant) decreases in the numbers of uninsured, while the number of uninsured working-age adults rose by 1.4 million. Table 3 gives detailed breakdowns by sex, race, income, poverty status, and age.

Although the number of people covered by Medicaid rose by 3.1 million, this increase was more than counterbalanced by a population growth of 3 million and a decrease in the number of people with private insurance. In 1990, 1.3 million fewer people had private coverage than in 1989. This continued a fall that commenced in 1982, when 10 million more Americans had private coverage than in 1990. Figures 1 and 2 show the number of people with private insurance each year since 1960, and the annual change in this number. As illustrated in Figure 3, in 1990 Medicaid enrollment grew more than in any other single year since the program was implemented, reflecting a one-time expansion of eligibility mandated by Congress. In the absence of this Medicaid expansion the number of uninsured would have grown by 4.4 million. Table 4 presents data on insurance coverage by age and source of coverage.

Both employed and unemployed workers suffered increases in the numbers of uninsured. Among the employed, there were 444,000 more uninsured in 1990 than in 1989, while the comparable increase for unemployed and laid-off workers was 649,000. Detailed breakdowns of the number of uninsured workers by labor force participation and work status are given in Table 5.

Analysis focusing on industry of employment revealed striking increases (> 100,000 newly uninsured) among those working in the construction, retail trade, hospital/medical, and business/repair categories. None of the 20 major industry groups showed significant improvements (Table 6). Even many professional workers are uninsured (Table 7). Legislators and judges are virtually the only major categories of workers with universal coverage.

The increase of 1.3 million in the number of uninsured between 1989 and 1990 follows a rise of 700,000 between 1988 and 1989. Overall, about 10 million more people are uninsured today than in 1980. The number of uninsured climbed sharply through the early 1980s, leveled off and then dipped slightly in 1984–1987, and has been climbing for the past three years. Figure 4 shows trends in the number of uninsured since 1976.

DISCUSSION

More Americans are uninsured today than at any time since the passage of Medicare and Medicaid 25 years ago. (The estimate of 37 million uninsured in the mid-1980s was based on the survey methodology used by the Census Bureau prior to 1988. Applying this older methodology would have resulted in an estimate of about 39 million uninsured in 1990. It is unclear which methodology yields a more accurate estimate.) The increase in 1990 is particularly worrisome since it largely predates the current [1992] recession and was cushioned by a massive expansion of Medicaid coverage, which is a one-time phenomenon.

Table 1

Number and percentage of Americans without health insurance,
by region and state, 1989 and 1990

Region/state	No. uninsured, thousands		Percent uninsured		Increase (decrease) in no. uninsured, thousands, 1989–1990
	1990	1989	1990	1989	
U.S. total	34,719	33,385	13.9	13.6	1,355
New England	1,160	1,147	9.0	9.0	13
Maine	139	113	11.2	9.2	26
New Hampshire	107	141	9.9	12.8	(34)
Vermont	54	49	9.5	8.8	5
Massachusetts	530	495	9.1	8.5	34
Rhode Island	105	89	11.1	9.2	16
Connecticut	226	260	6.9	8.3	(34)
Mid-Atlantic	4,166	3,992	11.0	10.6	174
New York	2,176	2,121	12.1	11.8	55
New Jersey	773	782	10.0	10.3	(9)
Pennsylvania	1,218	1,088	10.1	9.0	130
East North Central	4,168	3,932	9.9	9.4	236
Ohio	1,123	912	10.3	8.5	211
Indiana	587	668	10.7	12.3	(81)
Illinois	1,272	1,162	10.9	10.1	110
Michigan	865	776	9.4	8.3	90
Wisconsin	321	414	6.7	8.8	(94)
West North Central	1,810	1,709	10.1	9.7	101
Minnesota	389	366	8.9	8.6	23
Iowa	225	206	8.1	7.3	19
Missouri	665	614	12.7	11.8	51
North Dakota	40	56	6.3	8.7	(15)
South Dakota	81	76	11.6	11.0	4
Nebraska	138	162	8.5	10.1	(24)
Kansas	272	229	10.8	9.4	43
South Atlantic	6,831	6,153	15.7	14.5	678
Delaware	96	104	14.0	15.4	(8)
Maryland	601	467	12.7	10.2	134
District of Columbia	109	120	19.2	21.0	(10)
Virginia	996	699	15.7	11.3	297
West Virginia	249	250	13.8	13.9	(1)
North Carolina	883	889	13.8	14.1	(6)
South Carolina	550	491	16.2	14.2	58
Georgia	971	964	15.3	15.6	7
Florida	2,376	2,169	18.0	17.0	207

Table 1

(Cont'd.)

Region/state	No. uninsured, thousands		Percent uninsured		Increase (decrease) in no. uninsured, thousands,
	1990	1989	1990	1989	1989–1990
East South Central	2,395	2,197	15.7	14.6	198
Kentucky	480	476	13.2	13.3	4
Tennessee	673	619	13.7	12.8	54
Alabama	710	665	17.4	16.3	45
Mississippi	531	436	19.9	16.9	94
West South Central	5,362	5,542	20.3	20.9	(180)
Arkansas	421	410	17.4	17.0	11
Louisiana	797	732	19.7	17.9	66
Oklahoma	574	360	18.6	20.1	(55)
Texas	3,569	3,770	21.1	22.3	(201)
Mountain	2,070	2,005	15.1	14.9	65
Montana	115	120	14.1	14.6	(4)
Idaho	159	158	15.2	15.5	2
Wyoming	58	58	12.5	12.5	0
Colorado	495	443	14.7	13.6	52
New Mexico	339	321	22.2	21.1	18
Arizona	547	580	15.5	16.3	(33)
Utah	156	151	9.0	9.0	5
Nevada	201	176	16.5	15.6	24
Pacific	6,758	6,707	17.3	17.4	51
Washington	557	562	11.4	11.8	(5)
Oregon	360	400	12.5	13.7	(40)
California	5,683	5,577	19.1	19.0	106
Alaska	77	89	15.4	18.3	(12)
Hawaii	81	79	7.3	7.3	1

Without this Medicaid expansion the number of uninsured would have increased by 4.4 million, an all-time record.

All of the increase in the uninsured over the past year (1.3 million) and over the past decade (10 million) is due to the erosion of private insurance coverage. The number of people covered by Medicaid remained about constant through the 1980s (despite a growth in poverty), before rising by 3.1 million in 1990. Medicare enrollment grew steadily throughout the period, due to the rise in the number of Americans over the age of 64. In contrast, according to the Health Insurance Association of America (1), 187.4 million people had private coverage

Table 2

States ranked by percentage, uninsured, 1989 and 1990[a]

	1990		1989	
	Rank	Percent uninsured	Rank	Percent uninsured
North Dakota	1	6.3	8	8.7
Wisconsin	2	6.7	9	8.8
Connecticut	3	6.9	3	8.3
Hawaii	4	7.3	1	7.3
Iowa	5	8.1	1	7.3
Nebraska	6	8.5	16	10.1
Minnesota	7	8.9	7	8.6
Utah	8	9.0	11	9.0
Massachusetts	9	9.1	5	8.5
Michigan	10	9.4	3	8.3
Vermont	11	9.5	9	8.8
New Hampshire	12	9.9	27	12.8
New Jersey	13	10.0	17	10.3
Pennsylvania	14	10.1	11	9.0
Ohio	15	10.3	5	8.5
Indiana	16	10.7	25	12.3
Kansas	17	10.8	15	9.4
Illinois	18	10.9	16	10.1
Rhode Island	19	11.1	13	9.2
Maine	20	11.2	13	9.2
Washington	21	11.4	22	11.8
South Dakota	22	11.6	20	11.0
New York	23	12.1	22	11.8
Wyoming	24	12.5	26	12.5
Oregon	25	12.5	31	13.7
Missouri	26	12.7	22	11.8
Maryland	27	12.7	18	10.2
Kentucky	28	13.2	29	13.3
Tennessee	29	13.7	27	12.8
North Carolina	30	13.8	33	14.1
West Virginia	31	13.8	32	13.9
Delaware	32	14.0	36	15.4
Montana	33	14.1	35	14.6
Colorado	34	14.7	30	13.6
Idaho	35	15.2	37	15.5

Table 2

(Cont'd.)

	1990		1989	
	Rank	Percent uninsured	Rank	Percent uninsured
Georgia	36	15.3	38	15.6
Alaska	37	15.4	46	18.3
Arizona	38	15.5	40	16.3
Virginia	39	15.7	21	11.3
South Carolina	40	16.2	34	14.2
Nevada	41	16.5	38	15.6
Alabama	42	17.4	40	16.3
Arkansas	43	17.4	43	17.0
Florida	44	18.0	43	17.0
Oklahoma	45	18.6	48	20.1
California	46	19.1	47	19.0
District of Columbia	47	19.2	49	21.0
Louisiana	48	19.7	45	17.9
Mississippi	49	19.9	42	16.9
Texas	50	21.1	51	22.3
New Mexico	51	22.2	50	21.1

[a]Includes the District of Columbia. Ranked from 1 to 51 in order of increasing percentages of uninsured.

in 1980. We found that by 1989 this figure had fallen to 178.3 million, and declined to 177.0 million in 1990. The deterioration of private insurance coverage is underlined by the increases in uninsurance among groups that have traditionally been well protected: white, working-age adults, many with middle and even high incomes. Even many professionals are uninsured, with the exception of high government officials.

The primary reason for declining private insurance coverage is the rising cost of insurance. In 1980, business spent 44.4 percent as much for health benefits as they made in profits. By 1989 this figure had risen to 100.5 percent (2), and the employees' share has risen even faster. In Washington, D.C., Blue Cross family coverage through a small business for a 55 year old now costs $12,667.68 annually.

Another important cause of uninsurance is "medical underwriting." According to a Harris Poll, 6 percent of Americans have been denied coverage because they have "preexisting conditions" such as diabetes, high blood pressure, breast

Table 3

Number and percentage of Americans without health insurance,
by sex, race, income, poverty status, and age, 1989 and 1990

	No. uninsured, thousands		Percent uninsured		Increase (decrease) in no. uninsured, thousands,
	1990	1989	1990	1989	1989–1990
Male	18,710	17,680	15.4	14.8	1,030
Female	16,010	15,710	12.5	12.4	300
Whites	26,960	25,860	12.9	12.5	1,100
Blacks	6,093	5,843	19.7	19.2	250
Annual income					
<$25,000	22,190	21,840	22.3	21.6	350
$25,000–$49,999	7,228	6,673	9.0	8.3	555
>$49,999	5,298	4,867	7.7	7.5	431
Poverty status[a]					
<100%	9,696	9,581	28.7	30.2	115
100–124%	3,274	3,238	29.1	29.1	36
125–149%	3,001	2,738	25.9	24.1	263
>149%	18,750	17,830	9.8	9.3	920
Age					
<18 yr	8,504	8,548	13.0	13.3	(44)
18–39 yr	17,640	16,780	20.0	19.0	860
40–64 yr	8,302	7,744	12.7	12.1	558
>64 yr	276	308	1.0	1.0	(32)

[a]These categories refer to incomes as percentages of the poverty line.

cancer, or birth defects and are more likely to need expensive care. Increasingly, insurance companies demand proof that you do not need health care before they will sell you insurance.

The data we analyzed do not include information on the adequacy of coverage for the 214 million people with insurance. Others have estimated that more than a quarter of those with coverage have such inadequate insurance that a major illness would lead to bankruptcy. It is likely that the rate of underinsurance is rising because of increasing copayments and deductibles on many policies.

The futility of patchwork solutions is indicated by the jump in the number of uninsured Americans despite a substantial increase (3.1 million) in the number of people covered by Medicaid. Meanwhile, administrative costs have soared as insurers have augmented their efforts to shift costs to patients and the government, and to regulate the most minute details of clinical care. Bureaucracy now

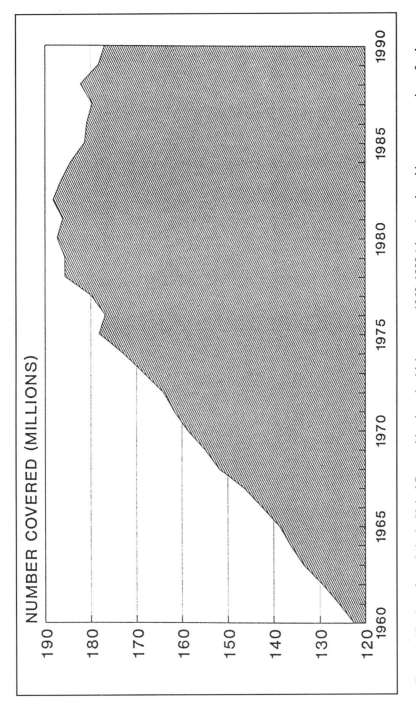

Figure 1. Number of people in the United States with private health insurance, 1960–1990 (above), and total insurance premiums for the same period (below, p. 128). Sources: Health Insurance Association of America, and the National Center for Health Statistics.

NUMBER COVERED (MILLIONS)

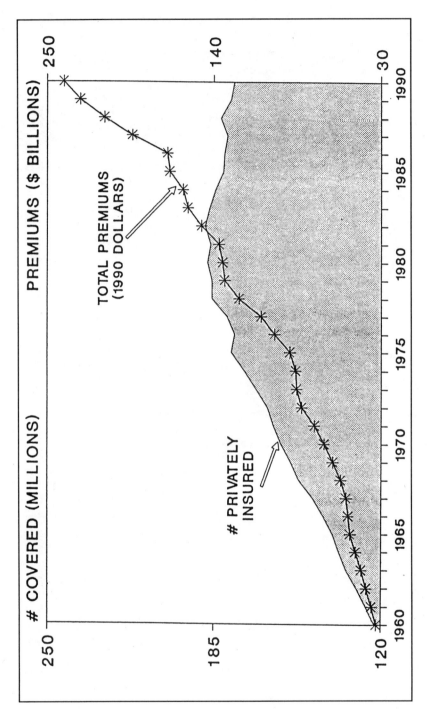

Figure 1. (Cont'd.)

128

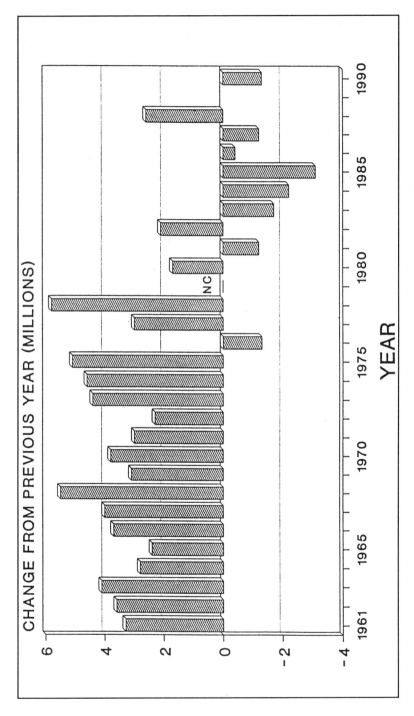

Figure 2. Change in number of people in the United States covered by private health insurance, 1961–1990 (1989 data unavailable). NC, no change. Sources: Current Population Surveys, and Health Insurance Association of America.

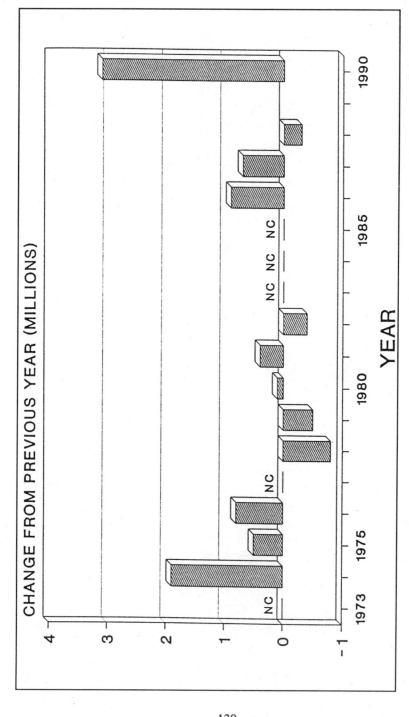

Figure 3. Change in number of people in the United States covered by Medicaid, 1973–1990 (1989 data unavailable). NC, no change. Sources: as in Figure 2.

Table 4

Private insurance and Medicaid coverage, by age group, 1989 and 1990

Type of coverage/ age group	No. (%) covered, millions, 1989	No. (%) covered, millions, 1990	Increase (decrease) in no. covered, millions, 1989–1990
Medicaid			
Total	21.2 (8.6)	24.3 (9.8)	3.1
<18 yr	10.1 (15.7)	12.1 (18.5)	2.0
18–39 yr	5.7 (6.4)	6.5 (7.3)	0.8
40–64 yr	2.8 (4.4)	3.1 (4.8)	0.3
>64 yr	2.6 (8.7)	2.6 (8.6)	0
Private Insurance			
Total	178.3 (72.4)	177.0 (71.1)	(1.3)
<18 yr	42.1 (65.4)	41.3 (63.2)	(0.8)
18–39 yr	64.7 (73.2)	63.0 (71.4)	(1.7)
40–64 yr	51.5 (80.7)	52.1 (79.8)	0.6
>64 yr	20.0 (67.7)	20.6 (68.3)	0.6

Table 5

Number and percentage of workers uninsured,
by labor force participation and work status, 1989 and 1990

	No. uninsured, thousands		Percent uninsured		Increase (decrease) in no. uninsured, thousands,
	1990	1989	1990	1989	1989–1990
Labor force participation					
Working	15,870	15,500	14.3	13.8	370
With job, not at work	703	629	15.8	13.5	74
Unemployed, looking for work	2,556	2,097	35.4	36.1	459
Unemployed, on layoff	493	303	28.1	26.1	190
Work status					
Full time (FT)	11,920	11,820	13.0	12.6	100
Part time (PT) for economic reasons, usually works FT	761	658	32.3	35.3	103
PT for noneconomic reasons, usually works PT	2,446	2,497	13.9	13.7	(51)
PT for economic reasons, usually works PT	1,450	1,155	39.9	38.5	295
Unemployed, usually works FT	2,691	2,120	37.0	38.6	571
Unemployed, usually works PT	359	270	20.9	18.6	89

Table 6

Number and percentage of uninsured, by industry, 1989 and 1990

	No. uninsured, thousands		Percent uninsured		Increase (decrease) in no. uninsured, thousands,
	1990	1989	1990	1989	1989–1990
Agriculture	1,051	999	30.6	29.1	52
Mining	88	94	10.3	11.8	(6)
Construction	2,523	2,351	30.0	27.1	172
Durable goods mfg	1,391	1,303	10.6	9.6	88
Nondurable goods mfg	1,185	1,219	12.6	13.0	(34)
Transportation	815	746	15.2	14.1	69
Communications	105	87	6.4	5.4	20
Utilities/sanitation	90	89	5.3	5.3	1
Wholesale	645	645	12.6	13.4	0
Retail	5,113	4,645	22.8	20.9	468
Finance/insurance/ real estate	740	720	8.9	8.4	21
Household	450	470	38.1	37.5	(20)
Business/repair	1,901	1,765	22.8	21.2	136
Personal services, except household	938	955	22.7	23.3	(17)
Entertainment	356	367	21.7	22.8	(11)
Hospital/medical	1,076	935	10.5	9.5	140
Education	713	644	7.1	6.5	69
Social services	329	368	12.7	15.3	(39)
Other professional	445	431	9.1	8.9	13
Forestry/fishing	63	46	32.5	25.0	17
Public administration	314	309	5.5	5.3	5

consumes almost one-quarter of total health spending, and the number of administrators is rising four times as fast as the number of doctors.

Our figures largely predicate the recession and understate current problems. The 1991 figures are likely to be far worse, close to 40 million uninsured, reflecting the severe economic downturn that has not been cushioned by Medicaid expansion comparable with that implemented in 1990. Moreover, the Census Bureau surveys reflect the number of people who are uninsured at a single moment in time. A far higher number are temporally uninsured at some point during the year.

Fundamental changes in health care financing will be needed to simultaneously contain costs and cover the uninsured. In 1991 we could have saved between

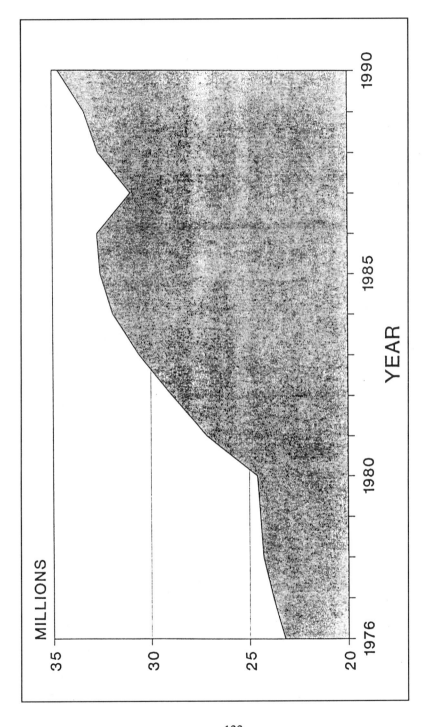

Figure 4. Number of uninsured Americans, 1976–1990. Sources: Current Population Surveys, and National Health Interview Surveys.

133

Table 7

Number and percentage uninsured, under the age of 65,
selected professions, 1989 and 1990

	No. (%) uninsured, 1989	No. (%) uninsured, 1990
Legislators	0	0
Realtors	88,300 (18)	77,300 (20)
Accountants and auditors	75,700 (5)	83,600 (6)
Architects	8,600 (6)	10,300 (8)
Engineers	53,900 (3)	89,900 (5)
Mathematical and computer scientists	32,300 (3)	27,500 (3)
Natural scientists	11,400 (3)	13,100 (3)
College and university professors	49,900 (6)	58,200 (7)
Teachers	276,200 (7)	269,600 (6)
Librarians	13,500 (7)	6,100 (4)
Social scientists	19,200 (5)	42,800 (12)
Clergy	42,000 (14)	52,500 (16)
Lawyers	27,900 (4)	18,600 (3)
Physicians	16,000 (3)	29,000 (6)
Judges	0	0

$115.2 and $135.6 billion on paperwork and bureaucracy by implementing a Canadian-style national health program. These administrative savings are sufficient to cover the uninsured and to improve the coverage of most other Americans by eliminating copayments and deductibles.

REFERENCES

1. Health Insurance Association of America. *Source Book of Health Insurance Data 1990.* Washington, D.C., 1990.
2. *Health Care Financ. Rev.* 12(2): 133, 1990.

CHAPTER 8

Underinsurance in America

Thomas Bodenheimer

On any given day, an estimated 35 million Americans are without health insurance (1). In addition, at least 20 million people have insurance that could prove inadequate in the event of serious illness (2). Coverage by insurance policies that require large out-of-pocket payments has been termed "under-insurance."

Lack of Coverage for Catastrophic Medical Expenses

According to the 1990 report of the Pepper Commission (2),

> a commonly accepted measure of inadequate coverage is health insurance that leaves the person covered at risk of spending more than 10 percent of income on health care in the event of a costly illness. An estimated 13 percent of the under-65 population were underinsured by this definition in 1984—about 20 million people in 1987.

The 13 percent figure, which depends on the definition of underinsurance, could be set far higher (3). According to data from the 1977 National Medical Care Expenditure Survey, projected to 1984, 26 percent of the privately insured population under 65 years of age had no limit on out-of-pocket expenditures for hospital care, leaving this population at risk for a catastrophic level of expenditures (4).

Fourteen percent of insurance plans have a total lifetime benefit of $250,000 or less. A child with congenital heart disease or with anoxic brain damage may exceed this threshold within a few years (2). Two-thirds of insurance plans limit lifetime costs to $1 million or less; thousands of motor-vehicle accidents each

Reprinted by permission of *The New England Journal of Medicine* from 327(4), pp. 274–278, 1992. Copyright 1992, Massachusetts Medical Society.

year cause head injuries for which the cost of medical care exceeds this amount (5). A 1989 survey of 742 working-age people with chronic health problems found that 6.4 percent had exceeded their lifetime benefit caps (5). A ruling by a federal appeals court in 1991 held that employers that insure their workers themselves have the right to reduce total lifetime benefits to as little as $5,000 for employees in whom the acquired immunodeficiency syndrome (AIDS) develops (6); the average lifetime health care costs for a person with AIDS have been estimated at $85,000 (7).

Preexisting-Illness Clauses

In 1990, over 60 percent of group health insurance plans contained exclusions of coverage for preexisting conditions, signifying the denial of benefits for any illness present at the time the insurance is obtained (8). Nine months is the average waiting period before a newly insured person receives coverage for a preexisting condition, but waiting periods can last up to seven years (9). Change of employment often triggers a new restriction on coverage for preexisting illness—a common occurrence, since the average employee remains in a job for only 4.2 years (9). An estimated 81 million Americans under 65 years of age have medical problems (such as hypertension, diabetes, asthma, and chronic back pain) that insurance companies may consider preexisting conditions (5). In 1990, 6 percent of Americans reported that they had been denied all or a part of health insurance coverage because of an existing health problem (10).

Benefits Not Provided

In 1989, 55 percent of employment-based health insurance plans did not provide coverage for basic childhood vaccinations (11), which cost approximately $600 (not including the price of the office visits). In 1986, 17 percent of businesses had health plans that failed to cover visits to physicians' offices (2). In 1989, 58 percent of employer-sponsored health plans did not cover well-baby care, and 56 percent did not cover physical examinations (12). Of women with private insurance, 9 percent are covered by policies that have no maternity benefits (13). According to Dr. Donald Henderson, former dean of the Johns Hopkins School of Hygiene and Public Health, "it has been very difficult to get third-payers to pay for mammograms, Pap smears, or other preventive services" (11).

Deductibles and Coinsurance

In 1987, 75 percent of group health insurance plans featured a deductible and a coinsurance payment of 20 percent or more for physicians' services (14). In 1990, employer-sponsored health insurance plans raised deductibles, copayments, and limits on out-of-pocket payments for their covered workers. For the 62 percent of plans that are not preferred-provider organizations or health maintenance organizations, the mean individual deductible in 1990 was more than $170 (8). The trend toward increased cost sharing will probably continue; the 1990 Foster Higgins survey of employers indicated that 94 percent of employers planned to further increase deductibles and copayments (15).

Medicare

Medicare covers only about 50 percent of the medical expenses of the elderly (16), and 22 percent of Medicare recipients have no supplemental private ("Medigap") or Medicaid coverage (2). Even with Medicare, Medicaid, and Medigap policies, the elderly pay 25 percent of their health care costs out of pocket (16). In 1986, more than one-fifth of the elderly had medical bills exceeding 15 percent of their income (17). Some physicians do not realize that Medicare patients without supplementary insurance face a $628 deductible for hospital care, a daily $78.50 copayment for days 21 through 80 in a skilled nursing facility, and a $100 deductible for physicians' services and have no coverage for most routine screening, immunizations, and care related to eyeglasses and hearing aids (18). Even those with Medigap policies often pay hundreds of dollars each year for prescription drugs (19).

Long-Term Care

Medicare pays less than 2 percent of the nursing home bills of elderly persons, and private insurance policies pick up only an additional 1 percent (16). Many elderly Americans spend their entire life's savings on long-term care, qualifying for Medicaid only after they become impoverished (2). Three-quarters of those 75 years of age or older who live alone would be impoverished in one year if they entered a nursing home (20).

Insecurity about Insurance Coverage

Fear of losing health insurance is a pervasive problem for Americans, although in the strict sense this does not constitute underinsurance (10). Many people see health insurance as a fleeting benefit (21); in the three-year period between the beginning of 1986 and the end of 1988, 63.6 million people lacked health insurance for at least one month—almost twice the number who had no insurance on a given day (1). Thirty percent of Americans surveyed in a 1991 *New York Times*—CBS poll said that someone in their household remained in an unwanted job in order to avoid losing health benefits (22). In the small-group and individual insurance markets, people found to have chronic conditions or who work in occupations considered by insurers to carry high risks face the possibility of denial or cancellation of coverage or large increases in premiums (23). Seven million insured Americans with chronic illnesses would be deemed "medically uninsurable" by insurance companies if they lost their coverage for any reason (24). Growing use of screening tests for chronic illness or risk factors among applicants for jobs and health insurance contributes to the fear of not being able to obtain insurance (25). For many, health insurance is a paradoxical benefit in that "if you use it, you lose it" (9).

A general measure of the lack of insurance and of underinsurance in the United States is the level of out-of-pocket payments. In 1989, 21.4 percent of U.S. health care costs were paid out of pocket. Health care spending by households (which reflects out-of-pocket payments) increased as a percentage of adjusted personal income from 3.9 percent in 1980 to 5.1 percent in 1989 (26).

EFFECTS OF UNDERINSURANCE

Does underinsurance represents a barrier to the receipt of medical care? In answering this question, four factors merit consideration: access to medical care, clinical outcomes, equity, and cost.

Access to Medical Care

From the clinician's perspective, underinsurance makes care more difficult to provide. In my primary care practice, I skimp on ordering needed services for patients who have deductibles of $500 or $1,000. I often prescribe a lower-priced second- or third-choice medication because a Medicare recipient is unable to pay for the drug I would prefer to use. Elderly couples resist long-term care, fearing that they will be forced onto Medicaid as uncovered costs mount into tens of thousands of dollars. Patients sometimes ask me not to specify their true diagnosis on insurance claim forms, because they fear the invocation of preexisting-illness clauses or cancellations of insurance.

Several studies have examined the effect of lack of benefits on access to care. Mammographic screening for breast cancer has the potential to reduce mortality from this disease by as much as 30 percent. Yet in 1990, only 31 percent of women were being screened according to accepted guidelines (27). Studies in Los Angeles and Massachusetts found that cost and lack of insurance coverage were factors preventing women from obtaining mammograms (27, 28).

The proportion of children from one to four years of age who were immunized against measles dropped from 66 percent in 1976 to 61 percent in 1985, and the number of measles cases rose from 2800 in 1985 to 26,500 in 1990 (29, 30). According to the National Vaccine Advisory Committee, one factor contributing to this epidemic is the reluctance of insurers to include childhood immunizations among their health care benefits (11).

In a 1981 survey, Shulman and colleagues found that 36.5 percent of patients with uncontrolled hypertension in Georgia reported difficulty paying for their medications, as compared with 15.5 percent of those whose blood pressure was controlled (31). The authors concluded that the cost of prescriptions contributed to inadequate control of hypertension.

The effects of coinsurance payments and deductibles on access to care were examined in the Rand Health Insurance Experiment, which compared non-elderly persons covered by health insurance plans with no out-of-pocket costs with those covered by plans that required various amounts of cost sharing (32). Overall, the study found that cost sharing reduced the rate of use of ambulatory care, especially among the poor, and that patients in plans that included cost sharing had both fewer appropriate and fewer inappropriate medical visits. Patients with hypertension in the free-care plans were more likely to have their condition diagnosed and more likely to have follow-up visits for blood-pressure control than those who had to pay for part of their health care (33). In a given year, low-income women in the cost-sharing groups had Pap smears 65 percent as often as those in the free-care group (32). Children in the cost-sharing groups had a lower rate of immunization (34).

Using data from the 1986 Robert Wood Johnson Foundation Access to Health Care Survey, Hayward and colleagues studied access to care for the elderly and for insured working-age adults with chronic or serious medical problems. Eight percent of Medicare recipients and 12 percent of insured working-age adults reported that the illness had caused major financial problems. The authors concluded that the elderly face serious problems of access to care because of gaps in Medicare coverage and that "deficiencies in insurance coverage for working-age adults, particularly those with medical problems, constitute an even more serious and as yet unaddressed problem" (35). These conclusions applied both to poor respondents and to those who were not poor.

Clinical Outcomes

Although the Rand Health Insurance Experiment did not uncover widespread differences in health outcomes between the cost-sharing groups and free-care groups, it did identify three specific problems related to outcome in the cost-sharing groups (36). First, for people with hypertension, diastolic blood pressures were significantly higher in the cost-sharing groups, a difference more marked among patients with hypertension whose incomes were lower. This finding is consequential, since the higher blood pressures increased the risk of dying, as calculated by the Rand research group (36). Second, persons who received free care had better visual acuity at the end of the experiment than those who shared costs (36). Third, children in low-income families in the cost-sharing groups had higher rates of anemia (32). The effect of cost sharing on health outcomes in the entire population is probably greater than is evident in the Rand findings because the elderly and chronically disabled persons who use the most medical care were excluded from the Rand study; because the cost-sharing plans, with their income-related cost-sharing caps, were designed to be less onerous for lower-income families than for higher-income families, thereby blunting the extent to which cost sharing affects lower-income people more severely in the real world; and because long-term negative outcomes such as organ damage due to hypertension were not measured in the Rand study (32). Cost-sharing requirements higher than those in the Rand study would be likely to produce worse clinical outcomes for lower-income groups.

Case reports chronicle the fact that underinsurance breeds lack of insurance; people with inadequate health coverage may be forced by the financial consequences of illness and by insurance pricing policies to lose their health insurance coverage altogether (37). The negative clinical outcomes associated with the lack of health insurance have been amply reported in the medical literature (38–40).

Equity

The primary feature of underinsurance is high out-of-pocket expenditures for medical care. Out-of-pocket costs are a regressive method of payment for health services. According to the 1977 National Medical Care Expenditure Survey, the 10 percent of households with the lowest incomes paid 14.0 percent of their income in out-of-pocket expenditures for health care, as compared with 1.9 percent for the wealthiest 10 percent of households (41). The high out-of-pocket costs that characterize underinsurance are a highly inequitable method of financing health care.

Costs

Some analysts contend that underinsurance leads to greater responsibility on the part of patients for medical costs and thereby helps contain health care expenditures. By this line of reasoning, overinsurance is a more serious problem than underinsurance.

This argument flounders on the absence of evidence demonstrating that cost sharing reduces overall health expenditures. Within closed systems, as the Rand study proves, cost sharing cuts the use of health care resources and lowers the costs of care for a relatively healthy population (36). But since 10 percent of the population, with catastrophic acute illness or costly chronic conditions, accounts for 70 percent of health expenditures (42), the reductions produced by cost sharing in the use of health care for less severe illnesses have little effect on overall health care costs. Evans and Barer have pointed out that nations with lower out-of-pocket expenditures devote a smaller percentage of the gross national product to health services than does the United States, with its high level of out-of-pocket payments (43). These findings have been corroborated in the international comparison of health care financing by Glaser, who comments that "American researchers have studied the issue only in controlled and atypical insurance arrangements" (44).

Surveys of households and physicians conducted before and after the introduction of free health care services in Quebec in 1970 demonstrated that the total number of visits to physicians per capita remained constant but that the distribution shifted from higher-income to lower-income patients; the fixed number of physicians was responsible for containing the volume of visits and thereby costs (45). Within the United States, differences in health care use among geographic regions have confirmed that costs are most effectively controlled by limiting the available resources (46).

CONCLUSIONS

Although there are many varieties of underinsurance in America, its essence remains high out-of-pocket expenditures for medical care. Underinsurance is an important problem because it reduces access to health care, especially for lower-income people, it creates an inequitable method of financing care, and when out-of-pocket payments are high, it can contribute to substandard clinical outcomes. Moreover, the out-of-pocket payments inherent in underinsurance cannot be expected to contain costs in the health care system as a whole.

Public attention has focused on the blight of lack of health insurance, with underinsurance receiving far less consideration. Our nation must confront both of these problems in our quest for equitable and affordable medical care.

REFERENCES

1. Friedman, E. The uninsured: From dilemma to crisis. *JAMA* 265: 2491–2495, 1991.
2. Pepper Commission, Bipartisan Commission on Comprehensive Health Care. *A Call for Action.* Government Printing Office, Washington, D.C., 1990.
3. Department of Health and Human Services. *Insuring Catastrophic Illness for the General Population.* Technical report. Washington, D.C., 1987.
4. Farley, P. J. Who are the underinsured? *Milbank Mem. Fund Q. Health Soc.* 63: 476–503, 1985.
5. Citizens Fund. *The Seven Warning Signs: Health Insurance at Risk.* Washington, D.C., 1991.
6. Freudenheim, M. Employers winning right to cut back medical insurance. *New York Times,* March 29, 1992, pp. 1, 14.
7. Hellinger, F. J. Forecasting the medical care costs of the HIV epidemic: 1991–1994. *Inquiry* 28: 213–225, 1991.
8. Sullivan, C. B., and Rice, T. The health insurance picture in 1990. *Health Aff. (Millwood)* 10(2): 104–115, 1991.
9. Cotton, P. Preexisting conditions 'hold Americans hostage' to employers and insurance. *JAMA* 265: 2451–2453, 1991.

10. Blendon, R. J., Edwards, J. N., and Szalay, U. S. The health insurance industry in the year 2001: One scenario. *Health Aff. (Millwood)* 10(4): 170–177, 1991.
11. Skolnick, A. Should insurance cover routine immunizations? *JAMA* 265: 2453–2454, 1991.
12. A. Foster Higgins. *Health Benefits Survey, 1989.* Princeton, N.J., 1989.
13. Braveman, P., et al. Women without health insurance: Links between access, poverty, ethnicity, and health. *West. J. Med.* 149: 708–711, 1988.
14. DiCarlo, S., and Gabel, J. Conventional health insurance: A decade later. *Health Care Financ. Rev.* 10(3): 77–89, 1989.
15. A. Foster Higgins. *Health Benefits Survey, 1990.* Princeton, N.J., 1990.
16. Rice, T., and Gabel, J. Protecting the elderly against high health care costs. *Health Aff. (Millwood)* 5(3): 5–21, 1986.
17. Feder, J., Moon, M., and Scanlon, W. Medicare reform: Nibbling at catastrophic costs. *Health Aff. (Millwood)* 6(4): 5–19, 1987.
18. Social Security Administration. Medicare. SSA publication No. 05-10043. Department of Health and Human Services, Baltimore, 1991.
19. Christensen, S., Long, S. H., and Rodgers, J. Acute health care costs for the aged Medicare population: Overview and policy options. *Milbank Q.* 65: 397–425, 1987.
20. Branch, L. G., et al. Impoverishing the elderly: A case study of the financial risk of spend-down among Massachusetts elderly people. *Gerontologist* 28: 648–652, 1988.
21. Blendon, R. J., et al. Satisfaction with health systems in ten nations. *Health Aff. (Millwood)* 9(2): 185–192, 1990.
22. Eckholm, E. Health benefits found to deter job switching. *New York Times.* September 26, 1991, pp. 1, 12.
23. Friedman, E. Insurers under fire. *Health Manage. Q.* 13(3): 23–27, 1991.
24. Committee on Labor and Human Resources. *The American Health Care Crisis: A View from Four Communities.* Government Printing Office, Washington, D.C., 1990.
25. Office of Technology Assessment. *Medical Testing and Health Insurance.* Government Printing Office, Washington, D.C., 1988.
26. Levit, K. R., et al. National health care spending, 1989. *Health Aff. (Millwood)* 10(1): 117–130, 1991.
27. Bastani, R., Marcus, A. C., and Hollatz-Brown, A. Screening mammography rates and barriers to use: A Los Angeles County survey. *Prev. Med.* 20: 350–363, 1991.
28. Zapka, J. G., et al. Interval adherence to mammography screening guidelines. *Med. Care* 29: 697–707, 1991.
29. Department of Health and Human Services. *Health United States 1990.* DHHS publication No. (PHS) 91-1232. Hyattsville, Md., 1991.
30. Rosenthal, E. Measles resurges, and with far deadlier effects. *New York Times.* April 24, 1991, pp. 1, C23.
31. Shulman, N. B., et al. Financial cost as an obstacle to hypertension therapy. *Am. J. Public Health* 76: 1105–1108, 1986.
32. Lohr, K. N., et al. Use of medical care in the Rand Health Insurance Experiment: Diagnosis- and service-specific analyses in a randomized controlled trial. *Med. Care* 24(Suppl.): S1–S87, 1986.
33. Keeler, E. B., et al. How free care reduced hypertension in the Health Insurance Experiment. *JAMA* 254: 1926–1931, 1985.

34. Lurie, N., et al. Preventive care: do we practice what we preach? *Am. J. Public Health* 77: 801–804, 1987.
35. Hayward, R. A., et al. Inequities in health services among insured Americans: Do working-age adults have less access to medical care than the elderly? *N. Engl. J. Med.* 318: 1507–1512, 1988.
36. Brook, R. H., et al. Does free care improve adults' health? Results from a randomized controlled trial. *N. Engl. J. Med.* 309: 1426–1434, 1983.
37. Garrison, J. Health care crisis: firms are dumping sick people. *San Francisco Examiner.* April 5, 1992, pp. A1, A20.
38. Hadley, J., Steinberg, E. P., and Feder, J. Comparison of uninsured and privately insured hospital patients: Condition on admission, resource use, and outcome. *JAMA* 265: 374–379, 1991.
39. Lurie, N., et al. Termination from Medi-Cal—Does it affect health? *N. Engl. J. Med.* 311: 480–484, 1984.
40. Fihn, S. D., and Wicher, J. B. Withdrawing routine outpatient medical services: Effects on access and health. *J. Gen. Intern. Med.* 3: 356–362, 1988.
41. Cantor, J. C. Expanding health insurance coverage: Who will pay? *J. Health Polit. Policy Law* 15: 755–778, 1990.
42. Reinhardt, U. E. What Can Americans Learn from Europeans? *Health Care Financ. Rev.* Suppl., 1989, pp. 97–104.
43. Evans, R. G., and Barer, M. L. What can Europeans learn from Americans? *Health Care Financ. Rev.* Suppl., 1989, pp. 72–77.
44. Glaser, W. A. *Health Insurance in Practice: International Variations in Financing, Benefits, and Problems.* Jossey-Bass, San Francisco, 1991.
45. Enterline, P. E., et al. The distribution of medical services before and after "free" medical care—The Quebec experience. *N. Engl. J. Med.* 289: 1174–1178, 1973.
46. Wennberg, J. E. Outcomes research, cost containment, and the fear of health care rationing. *N. Engl. J. Med.* 323: 1202–1204, 1990.

CHAPTER 9

Canada's National Health Program

David U. Himmelstein and Steffie Woolhandler

MINIMUM STANDARDS FOR CANADA'S PROVINCIAL PROGRAMS (Figure 1)

Canada's provincial programs must meet four minimum criteria in order to quality for federal block grants. First, they must enroll virtually everyone in the province, and eliminate essentially all out-of-pocket costs for covered services. Second, benefits must be portable from province to province—that is, if you are from Ontario and get sick in Quebec you must be covered. Third, the provincial program must cover all medically necessary services. The federal government has not defined this requirement further, but all of the provincial programs have enacted comprehensive acute care coverage. There is variability among the provinces in coverage of long-term care, dental services, prescription drugs, and eye glasses. Fourth, the program must be administered through a public, nonprofit agency. This requirement is based on substantial evidence that public administration is far cheaper and more efficient than private insurance administration.

---

1. UNIVERSAL COVERAGE THAT DOES NOT IMPEDE, EITHER DIRECTLY OR INDIRECTLY, WHETHER BY CHARGES OR OTHERWISE, REASONABLE ACCESS
2. PORTABILITY OF BENEFITS FROM PROVINCE TO PROVINCE
3. COVERAGE FOR ALL MEDICALLY NECESSARY SERVICES
4. PUBLICLY ADMINISTERED, NONPROFIT PROGRAM

Figure 1.

Published in the *National Health Program Chartbook,* 1992, pp. 64–72.

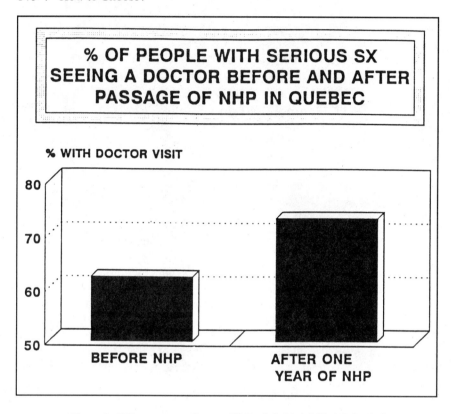

Figure 2. SX, symptoms. Source: *N. Engl. J. Med.* 289: 1174, 1973.

PERCENT OF PEOPLE WITH SERIOUS SYMPTOMS
SEEING A DOCTOR BEFORE AND AFTER PASSAGE
OF THE NHP IN QUEBEC (Figure 2)

Surveys in Quebec found that within one year of the implementation of the national health program (NHP), the proportion of residents with serious symptoms (such as chest pain, persistent cough, or hematemesis) who actually saw a physician increased substantially. A variety of other measures confirm that the national health program greatly improved access to care in Canada.

PERCENT OF AMERICANS AND CANADIANS
UNABLE TO GET NEEDED CARE (Figure 3)

A Harris poll asked Canadians and Americans whether they had experienced difficulties in getting needed medical care. Ten times as many Americans as

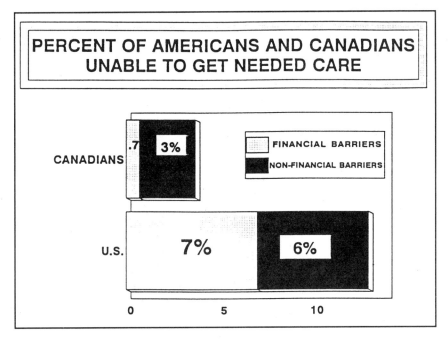

Figure 3. Source: Blendon, *Health Manage. Q.* 1: 1, 1989.

Canadians reported financial barriers to care, a difference that is not surprising since all Canadians are covered by their provincial health insurance program. More surprising is the finding that twice as many Americans as Canadians (6 percent versus 3 percent) reported non-financial barriers to care (e.g., queues for services, unavailability of technology, geographic inaccessibility). These data contradict the impression conveyed by the insurance industry and the American Medical Association (AMA) that medical care is often unavailable or that queues are an important problem in Canada.

AMERICANS AND CANADIANS RATE THEIR HEALTH SYSTEMS (Figure 4)

A Harris poll asked a random sample of Canadians and Americans to evaluate the health system in their own nation. Ninety percent of Americans said that their system needs basic changes or complete rebuilding. Only 10 percent thought that the system works pretty well. In contrast, 56 percent of Canadians said that their system works pretty well.

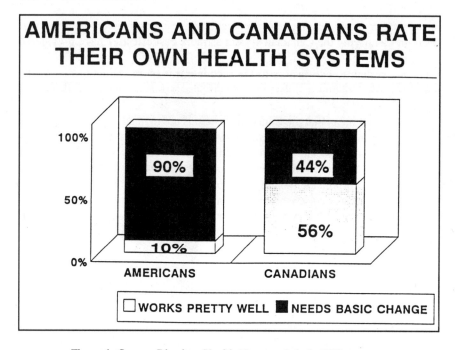

Figure 4. Source: Blendon, *Health Manage. Q.* 1: 1, 1989.

QUANTITY OF PHYSICIAN SERVICES PER CAPITA: UNITED STATES VERSUS CANADA (Figure 5)

The insurance industry and other opponents of a national health program have sought to convey the impression that Canadians' access to care is often restricted. To the contrary, Canadians have substantially more physician visits per capita than do Americans. Moreover, Canadians can go to any doctor or hospital of their choice, while most Americans now have insurance policies that restrict their choice of provider.

HOSPITAL ADMISSIONS OF ELDERLY FOR CARDIAC DISEASE: UNITED STATES VERSUS CANADA, 1985 (Figure 6)

For virtually all cardiac-related diagnoses and interventions, Canadians receive as much care as *insured* Americans. This study compared elderly Americans covered by Medicare with elderly Canadians. Hospital admission rates for both medical and surgical care were comparable, with the single exception of coronary artery bypass graft surgery. This procedure is almost certainly overused in the United States.

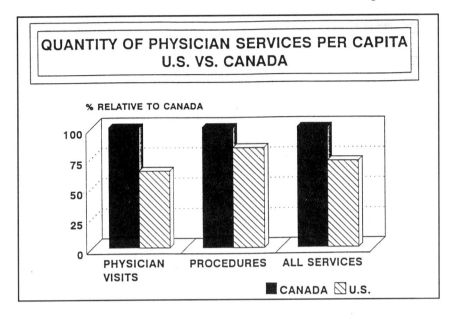

Figure 5. Source: Fuchs, *N. Engl. J. Med.* 323: 884, 1990.

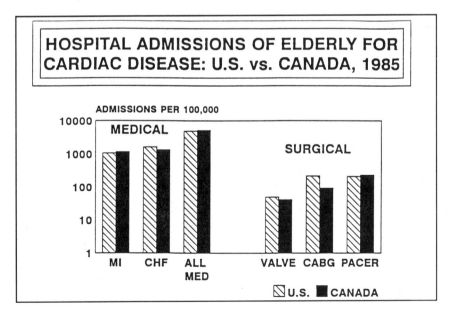

Figure 6. Source: *N. Engl. J. Med.* 321: 1443, 1989. Abbreviations: MI, myocardial infarction (heart attack); CHF, congestive heart failure; All Med, all medical admissions for cardiac conditions; Valve, heart valve surgery; CABG, coronary artery bypass graft surgery; Pacer, placement of a cardiac pacemaker.

Queues for coronary artery surgery developed in some provinces in Canada during the mid and late 1980s, largely because many Canadian coronary care nurses and bypass pump technicians were attracted by bonuses offered by U.S. hospitals expanding their programs. In some areas, patients waited on long queues for a particular surgeon, while other surgeons across town (or even in the same hospital) had little or no queue. The queues, which never affected access to emergency surgery, have now been reduced in most areas of Canada through expanded funding by the provincial single-payer programs, and improved coordination of referral networks.

TRANSPLANTS, UNITED STATES AND CANADA, 1988 (Figure 7)

Opponents of a single-payer system have publicized the false notion that high-technology care is unavailable in Canada. In fact, compared to Americans, Canadians have higher rates of heart and/or lung transplants, and liver transplants; slightly higher rates of bone marrow transplants; and comparable rates of kidney transplants.

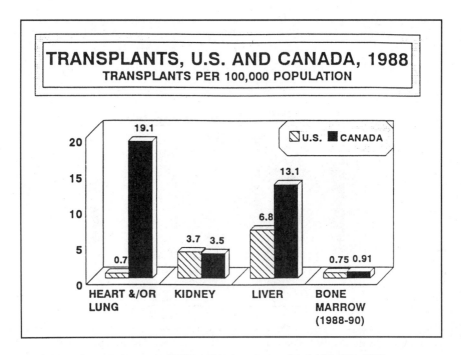

Figure 7. Sources: OECD 1991; *Ann. Intern. Med.* 116: 507, 1992.

Canada has regionalized most of these services. A relatively small number of centers each perform a large number of procedures. Such regionalization improves the quality of care since high-volume centers are better able to maintain competence, and minimizes cost by avoiding the unnecessary duplication of expensive facilities.

PHYSICIAN VISITS PER CAPITA, 1987 (Figure 8)

Americans have slightly fewer physician visits per capita than the British or Canadians, and only half as many physician visits as Italians, Germans, or Japanese. Yet all of these nations have much lower health care costs than the United States.

AVERAGE LENGTH OF STAY IN HOSPITAL (Figure 9)

Many U.S. health policy leaders blame rising health costs on the American people for using too much health care, and base their cost containment strategies

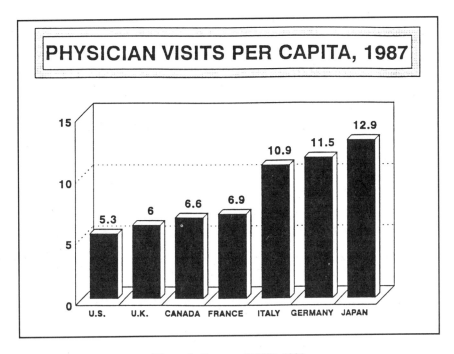

Figure 8. Sources: OECD, 1991.

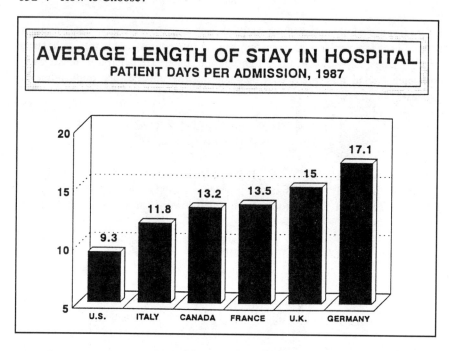

Figure 9. Sources: OECD, 1991.

on limiting the delivery of services through detailed utilization review and managed care bureaucracies. However, for most types of services Americans get less health care than people in many other nations with lower health expenditures. For instance, the average length of stay in hospital is 20 to 40 percent shorter in the United States than in most other developed nations.

CHAPTER 10

Waiting Your Turn:
Hospital Waiting Lists in Canada[1]

Cynthia Ramsay and Michael Walker

There were more televised news stories in Canada on health care than there were on the economy in 1992. Last year [1993], while the media focus returned to the economy, the funding and management of health care remained a major source of public anxiety, which should not be allowed to disappear from the media agenda. With continuing large government deficits and the escalating cost of health care, Canadians will have to make important decisions in the near future about the quality of health care delivery under our universal system. Preserving a universal health care system through rationing is now a topic openly discussed by health administrators (see, for example, 1), as is the need to restrict the amount of new technology provided to hospitals in order to keep hospital costs down.

One manifestation of the rationing of health sector resources in Canada is the existence of waiting lists for medical procedures and treatments. To the extent that nonprice rationing of hospital capacity is occurring, monetary and non-monetary costs may be borne by Canadians even though these costs are not explicitly recognized. These unrecognized costs may include, for example, lost work time, decreased productivity associated with physical impairment and anxiety, and physical and psychological pain and suffering.

A working person incapacitated by an illness bears the costs of the loss of work. These costs are not included in those associated with running the health care system. Cancer patients needing radiation therapy who must drive long distances either to regional health centers or to the United States bear costs in terms of lost time that are not included in health costs nor in any way compensated by the health care system. A woman with a lump in her breast who is told

---

[1] This is the fourth edition of *Waiting Your Turn*, which draws extensively from previous editions.

Published in the Fraser Institute's *Fraser Forum, Critical Issues Bulletin,* 1994.

she must wait four weeks for a biopsy to determine whether the lump is cancerous finds little comfort in the advice from her physician that epidemiological research shows that it doesn't matter to the outcome if the biopsy is delayed that long. The woman's anxiety and tangible psychological pain are not included in the costs of operating the health care system.[2]

In each of these cases, the savings to the government's budget are real and are matched by real though uncounted costs to Canadian health care consumers. While it is difficult or impossible to measure these costs, it is possible to measure the extent of queuing or the length of waiting lists to approximate the extent to which these costs may be mounting.

A number of health sector administrators are skeptical about the meaning and usefulness of waiting lists. They are skeptical both of the relevance of waiting lists as an indicator of the performance of the health care sector and of the reliability of such data as a measure of the extent of rationing of health care services (2). An earlier [1990] Fraser Institute publication evaluated various theoretical issues related to hospital waiting lists, including their relevance as measures of "excess demand" (3). The discussion defended the proposition that waiting lists are a potentially important barometer of performance in the health care sector. It also provided estimates of waiting lists for a set of hospital proce-dures in British Columbia. That study was followed in 1991 by a five-province study similar to the initial British Columbia study. In 1992, all ten provinces in Canada were surveyed.

This report builds upon our earlier studies by updating waiting list estimates for all of the provinces. In the next section, we briefly review the relevant theoretical issues before turning to the 1994 survey results.

WAITING LISTS AS
MEASURES OF EXCESS DEMAND

One interpretation of hospital waiting lists is that they are indices of excess demand for medical treatments performed in hospitals and that they represent the substitution of "nonprice" rationing of scarce resources for rationing by price. The rationing, in this case, takes place through enforced waiting for the available capacity to perform a given treatment or procedure. That waiting is a form of rationing and not simply the "postponement" of a service can be seen in the fact that there are costs involved for those who are forced to wait. If the people waiting had their choice, they probably would not wait in most cases. To the extent that this is true, the wait amounts to a denial of service, and that means rationing. (It is, of course, difficult to know exactly the extent to which people are

[2] All of the foregoing represent actual cases in recent Canadian health care experience. Details are available from the authors on request.

happy to wait. However, it can be presumed that those who are in physical pain or who are unable to work would prefer not to wait. Recently published data by Statistics Canada indicate that 45 percent of those who are waiting for health care in Canada describe themselves as being "in pain" (4).)

A recent [1993] study by the Institute for Clinical Evaluative Studies at the University of Toronto categorized all patients waiting for hip transplants according to their level of pain (5). The study found that in Ontario 40 percent of those who were experiencing severe disability and 40 percent of those who had severe pain were waiting 13 months or more for hip surgery. A further 40 percent of those who were in severe pain waited 7 to 12 months while only 14 percent of those in severe pain waited less than four months. While some of these patients might have been postponing their surgeries for their own reasons, the fact that they were experiencing severe pain probably means that most were being denied prompt access to treatment.

To put the issue somewhat differently, war-time rationing of refrigerators or automobiles could be reinterpreted as simply waiting. Those who wanted "fridges" in 1940 but didn't get them until 1946 were not denied the fridges, they only had to wait. Obviously, the issue of time is an important one in the matter of goods provision. It is also important—in some cases crucial—in the case of waiting for medical services.

Economists generally believe that nonprice rationing of scarce resources is less efficient than rationing through the price system. In particular, prices are efficient mechanisms for signaling the relative scarcity of any good or service, thereby encouraging both producers and consumers to modify their behavior accordingly. A rise in price occasioned by an increase in the demand for a particular medical procedure does cause some health care users to be deterred—effectively rationing the existing supply. The price rise also sends out the signal that not enough health care is being supplied. Assuming that the price rise makes additional profits possible, there will be an increase in the supply of health care as suppliers change their behavior to take advantage of the new profit possibility. This supply response does not necessarily occur if waiting is the system of rationing employed.

Nonprice rationing is also inefficient because it obscures differences in intensities of demand across different sets of consumers. To the extent that some consumers desire a given product more than other consumers, strict nonprice rationing might result in those consumers who desire the product less actually obtaining it. All other things being constant, efficiency is promoted when those consumers who most value a product obtain it. For example, while a nonworking husband and his wife may be equally rationed by a system of waiting lists, the working wife might be willing to pay a little more to be able to get back to work. This would be quite rational behavior on her part even if she and her husband were suffering the same disability. The reason is that she is suffering the additional costs of lost wages, which are not included in the cost of health care and which are not compensated by the universal health care system. With identical illnesses, the wife and husband do not have the same intensity of cost, nor the same need for the medical service that they are both being denied by waiting.

At least two prominent qualifications can be raised about the social inefficiencies of rationing by waiting. One is the claim that many procedures and treatments are performed where the social costs outweigh the social benefits. In these cases, it would be more desirable to discourage the consumption of a given amount of medical services by price rationing rather than by nonprice rationing. In other words, let the working wife pay the increased costs of earlier treatment so that she can get back to work and let her husband wait for an opening on the "elective" surgical waiting list. That is the appropriate approach unless one is prepared to argue that patients will pay any price to receive specific treatments and that government bureaucrats are better able to determine whether treatment is warranted at any cost of providing it.

A second qualification is that nonprice rationing of a vital product such as medical services is fair and is perceived to be fair by society. To the extent that fairness is an objective, one might argue that nonprice rationing provides collective benefits that outweigh the inefficiencies identified above. However, depending upon how the nonprice rationing occurs, the resulting distribution of benefits may not be any improvement upon the price-rationing outcome. If, for example, in a rationing circumstance, personal acquaintance with the head of surgery leads to less waiting, then rationing by waiting simply becomes a cover for a system of personal privilege. Even if the probability of knowing the chief of surgery were *not* related to income, the replacement of rationing by price with rationing by acquaintance will only create a different form of inequity.

The fairness argument can be further qualified if we recognize the potential for providing direct cash transfers to poorer people to enable them to compete in the marketplace for any specific good or service. The argument against direct subsidies is that it is easier to target subsidies-in-kind to appropriate recipients. In the context of health management, this would mean that one would subsidize lower-income people needing specific health care services. However, given the unexpected nature of many illnesses or accidents, it will be difficult to identify these people before the fact. Furthermore, given the potential for catastrophic illness and the associated high costs of treatment, some amount of direct subsidization might have to be extended to a large portion of the population and not just to low-income groups. In this case, the deadweight efficiency losses associated with a system that provides direct cash transfers to poorer people may not be significantly different from those associated with transferring income in-kind through nonprice rationing.

To take the analysis a step further, the government might consider subsidizing purchases of private health care insurance by lower-income individuals and families, thereby indirectly "targeting" health care assistance. The subsidy could be geared to a family's ability to pay so that it could approximate the full cost of the insurance premium for some buyers. At the same time, prices would be relied upon to "clear" the market for medical services.

To be sure, there are many arguments that have been made both for and against private medical insurance systems (6). For the purposes of this report, we accept that the public provision of and payment for health care services is an institutionalized feature of Canadian society for the foreseeable future and that extensive use of market pricing mechanisms to ration scarce capacity is unlikely. Under these circumstances, the extent of any excess demand, as well as how that excess demand is rationed, are relevant public policy issues, since the social costs associated with nonprice rationing should be set against whatever benefits are seen to be associated with it.

NONPRICE RATIONING
AND METHODS OF ADAPTING

There are several ways in which nonprice rationing can take place under the current health care system and many ways by which individuals adapt to rationing. One form of nonprice rationing is a system of triage—the three-way classification system developed by Florence Nightingale for sorting the wounded on the battlefield in wartime. Under such a system, the physician sorts the patients into three groups: those who are beyond help, those who need and will benefit from immediate care, and those who can wait for care.

In peacetime, there may also be a shortage of resources, which requires physicians to employ the triage system to make choices about the order in which people should be treated. In such a selection process, physicians effectively ration access by implicitly or explicitly rejecting candidates for medical treatment whom they would otherwise treat. In the absence of well-defined criteria, doctors might be expected to reject those candidates least likely to suffer morbid consequences from nontreatment and those whose life expectancy would be least improved by treatment. The British experience suggests that some doctors use a foregone present value of earnings criterion for selecting patients for early treatment, thereby giving lower priority to critically ill patients (7). The experience of Canada's largest cancer treatment center suggests that doctors are giving priority for radiation treatment to people whose cancers may be curable, as opposed to using the radiation machines to provide palliative care or limited extensions to life expectancy (8).

It is unlikely that medical practitioners would acknowledge that they are, in effect, rejecting (as opposed to queuing) specific patients who in their medical judgment do need treatment, so it would be difficult to identify this behavior if it were occurring. Patients who have a lower priority or who are not destined to get the care they need simply find that their turn never comes as others take their place in the queue. In this regard, there is no persuasive evidence that mortality rates in Canada are increasing significantly owing to a failure to provide medical services. However, if one regards the elimination of pain and suffering as the objective of medical care, then any additional pain suffered by patients because of delays is medical treatment denied.

Canadians may be adapting to nonprice rationing by substituting private medical services for unavailable public services, specifically by going outside the country for health care. Provincial health care plans cover emergency medical services and other services only available outside Canada. Possibly as a reflection of the increasing prevalence of waiting in the health care system, a Winnipeg-based company began to market an insurance product that provides private insurance for nonemergency treatment outside of Canada (9). Our survey of specialists (reported later in this chapter), found that 2 percent of noncardiovascular patients inquired about treatment in another country. On the other hand, it has been a fairly common practice for many Canadians to buy short-term travelers' health insurance for trips made to the United States. These insurance packages have increased in price, perhaps indicating that Canadians are using this type of insurance more than they did at one time and, perhaps, for medical procedures that have waiting lists in Canada.

REAL SOCIAL COSTS OF RATIONING HEALTH CARE

Observers who argue that hospital waiting lists are not a particularly important social issue believe that waiting lists tend to be inaccurate estimates of rationing and/or that there is little social cost associated with enforced waiting.

One frequently expressed concern is that doctors encourage a greater demand for medical care than is socially optimal. As a result, waiting lists exist for specific treatments. However, there may be no significant social costs associated with rationing since many (perhaps most) individuals on waiting lists are not in "legitimate" need of medical treatment. In a related version of this argument, doctors are suspected of placing a substantial number of patients on hospital waiting lists simply to exacerbate the public's perception of a health care crisis so as to increase public funding of the medical system.

The available evidence on the magnitude of supplier-induced demand for medical services is, at best, ambiguous. The view that this is a modest problem is supported by the fundamental economic argument that competition among physicians will promote a concordance between the physician's interests and those of the patient. General practitioners usually stand as agents for patients in need of specialists. Specialists carry out the bulk of hospital procedures. General practitioners who can mitigate medical problems while sparing patients the pain and discomfort of hospital treatments are more likely to be perceived as doing a good job than those who encourage short-term or long-term hospitalization as a cure. This suggests that general practitioners have an incentive to direct patients to specialists who will not "overprescribe" painful and time-consuming hospital treatments.

Placing excessive numbers of patients on hospital waiting lists may also have direct costs for opportunistic specialists. For example, the latter may come to be seen as using a disproportionate share of hospital resources. This may make it more difficult for them to provide quick access to those resources for patients who are in more obvious (to themselves and to their general practitioners) need of hospital treatment. Similarly, patients facing the prospect of a relatively long waiting list may be tempted to search out other doctors with better connections to hospital facilities.

As an additional consideration, there is no concrete reason for any single physician or group of physicians to believe that an individual physician's waiting lists will significantly affect government funding policies or that they will be net beneficiaries of any increased funding that does occur. In the face of obvious incentives to "free-ride" on the strategic behavior of other physicians, there may be no significant bias for physicians to inflate hospital waiting lists or even to overreport the number of patients they have waiting for admission to hospital.

An often-mentioned concern about measuring waiting is that hospital waiting lists are biased upward by a failure of reporting authorities to identify individual patients listed by more than one doctor and by a failure to prune waiting lists of individuals who have either already received the requested treatment or who, for some reason, are no longer likely to require treatment. Our survey results indicate that doctors generally do not believe that their patients have been booked on waiting lists by other physicians.

In summary, while there are hypothetical reasons to expect that hospital waiting list parameters will overstate true excess demand for hospital treatments, the magnitude of any resulting bias is unclear and is probably relatively small, given countervailing factors that may reduce measured amounts of waiting.

HOSPITAL WAITING LIST SURVEY

In order to develop a more detailed understanding of the magnitude and nature of hospital waiting lists in Canada, we conducted a survey of specialist physicians. Specialists were surveyed rather than hospital administrators because a substantial number of hospitals either do not collect waiting list data in a systematic manner or do not make such data publicly available. In those instances where hospital-based data are available they have been used to corroborate the evidence from the survey data.

As in 1992, the survey was conducted in all ten Canadian provinces. Mailing lists for the specialists polled were provided by Southam Business Lists. The specialists on these lists were drawn from the Canadian Medical Association membership lists. Specialists were offered a chance to win a $2,000 prize as an inducement to respond (without regard to their response). Though answering physicians were undoubtedly motivated in part by the lottery, the large percentage of answering specialists indicates concern about waiting lists for surgical procedures in Canada. Quite clearly, the medical profession has a collective interest in promoting an increased flow of financial and other resources to the health care sector. Nevertheless, it should not be assumed that the survey results are, therefore, unreliable. In particular, it should not be assumed (for reasons suggested earlier) that individual physicians responding to the survey have a strong incentive to skew their responses in a particular direction since physicians were not preselected as to their views about the adequacy of current funding or their views about current health care arrangements. There is a wide dispersion of views among physicians about the desirability of greater ease of access and there is no reason to believe that those who want to create the impression of longer lists are either more likely to distort their responses or more likely to respond to the survey than those who do not.

We chose to survey specialists rather than general practitioners because the former have primary responsibility for health care management of surgical candidates. Survey questionnaires were prepared for 12 different medical specialties: plastic surgery, gynecology, ophthalmology, otolaryngology, general surgery, neurosurgery, orthopedics, cardiology, urology, radiation oncology, medical oncology, and internal medicine. For the 1990 survey, the questionnaires were pretested on a sample of individual member specialists serving on the relevant British Columbia Medical Association specialty committee. In each subsequent use, suggestions for improvement have been made by responding physicians and these modifications have been made to the questionnaires. Adhering to the questionnaire format of the ten specialties originally surveyed, radiation oncology and medical oncology were added to the current survey. The final versions of the questionnaires, comparable to those used in 1990, were mailed to physicians in each specialty. The survey data were collected in December 1993.

For the most part, the survey was sent to all specialists in a category. In the case of internal medicine, ophthalmology, orthopedics, and general surgery in Ontario, 200 names were randomly selected from these categories by Southam Business Lists. As well, in the case of internal medicine in British Columbia, and internal medicine and general surgery in Quebec, 200 names were chosen randomly by Southam Business Lists. The response rate of 30 percent overall was considered quite high for a mailed survey. The response rate in the five provinces initially surveyed (British Columbia, Manitoba, New Brunswick, Newfoundland, Nova Scotia) was 20 percent. Over the last two years [1992, 1993] the response rate for those same provinces has increased dramatically to 33 percent. In this survey the response rates for the Atlantic provinces were: 50 percent in Prince Edward Island, 38 percent in Newfoundland, 35 percent in New Brunswick, and 32 percent in Nova Scotia.

METHODOLOGY

The treatments identified in all of the specialist tables represent a cross-section of common procedures carried out in each specialty. They were suggested by the British Columbia Medical Association specialty boards in 1990, with some procedures being added since then (at the suggestion of survey participants). (All tables appear at the end of the chapter.)

Table 1 (p. 176) provides an overall summary of responses. The major findings from the survey are summarized in Tables 2 through 43. Table 2 (p. 179) reports the average time a patient waits for an appointment with a specialist. This period is measured from the time a general practitioner refers the patient to the specialist. The average wait for an appointment with a specialist is calculated as the average of the weeks indicated by responding specialists. These appointment averages are then weighted by the ratio of the number of specialists surveyed in each specialty in a province, divided by the total number of specialists surveyed in the province, to obtain the weighted average reported on the last line of Table 2.

Table 3 through 14 (pp. 180–186) report the average time a patient must wait for treatment after having seen a specialist where the average waiting time per patient is calculated from the survey responses. The weighted averages reported in the last line of each table are calculated by summing the products of the average wait for each operation, and the ratio of the number of persons undergoing each operation and the total number of operations performed in each specialty by province.

Tables 15 through 26 (pp. 187–193) report the estimated number of patients waiting for surgery. The 1990 estimates of the number of people waiting for treatment in British Columbia were extrapolated from the physicians' responses to a query concerning the number of patients they had waiting. There were problems with this methodology: while the variance in the responses concerning waiting times was fairly low, the variance in responses concerning the length of the queue was high. This would indicate that physicians' access to surgical facilities is positively related to the number of patients that they have waiting, since patients of specialists with longer queues receive their treatment within approximately the same number of weeks as patients of specialists with shorter queues. Hence, the time it takes to process patients is comparable across all specialists in any given province. In this situation, the reported average time waited would appear to be fairly reliable, whereas concerns exist about the reliability of estimating the total number waiting in the province from an average number of patients waiting per specialist.

The estimation method used this year [1993] and last avoids these problems. The 1993 estimates are derived using the average weeks waited and Statistics Canada's Health Report No. 82-217, "Surgical Procedures and Treatments 1990-91." This report provides a count of the total number of surgical procedures performed annually by each province. To estimate the number of individuals waiting for surgery at any given point, we divided the average weeks waiting for a given operation by 52 and then multiplied this number by the total number of persons undergoing this operation annually. Thus a waiting period of, say, one month implies that, on average, patients are waiting one-twelfth of a year's total capacity to get their surgery. The next person added to the list would find one-twelfth of a year's patients ahead of him or her in the queue. The main assumption underlying this estimate is that the number of surgeries performed will neither increase nor decrease annually in response to waiting lists.

We encountered a number of minor problems while matching Statistics Canada's operation categories to the ones reported in our survey. In several instances, an operation such as rhinoplasty was listed for more than one specialist. In these cases, average waiting times were identified with the classification of the responding specialist. Hence, the flow or number of patients annually undergoing this type of operation is divided between specialties according to the proportion of overall surgery performed in each specialty. In other instances, the orthopedic operation polled in our study, "removal of pins and other hardware," had no match in the Statistics Canada report, nor did the urology operation, "ureteral reimplantation for reflux." Accordingly, we made no estimate of the number of patients waiting for these operations.

Tables 27a and 27b (pp. 194–195) offer a comparison of average waiting times and the estimated number of patients waiting across specialties and provinces. Of course, our calculation of the estimated number of patients waiting in each specialty includes only those patients waiting for the operations surveyed. The 52 operations we surveyed represent between 50 and 65 percent of nonemergency surgery performed in all of the provinces studied.

The final row of Table 27a is a weighted average of the 12 specialties listed above. These weighted averages are calculated by summing the products of average waiting and the proportion of polled surgery. To estimate the number of people waiting at any time for nonemergency surgeries that were *not* included in our survey, we found the residual operations for each province. The estimate of residual waiting is the product of the residual number of operations in each province and the provincial weighted averages divided by 52 (weeks). The estimate of total residual waiting is reported in Table 27b, as is the estimate of total patients waiting in each province at any given time.

Tables 31 through 43 (pp. 202–209) report what specialists consider to be clinically reasonable amounts of time to wait for treatments, on average. The methodology of these tables is comparable to that of Tables 3 through 14.

DATA VERIFICATION WITH GOVERNMENT SOURCES

All of the data were sent to provincial ministries of health across Canada. Replies were received from British Columbia, Alberta, Saskatchewan, Manitoba, and New Brunswick. The Ministry of Health and the Ministry Responsible for

Seniors in British Columbia confirmed our finding that approximately 1,832 patients are waiting for hip or knee surgery in the province and that over 200 patients are waiting to receive cancer treatment. Alberta Health could not comment on the results in general as waiting time information is collected and maintained independently by health care institutions throughout the province. The Department of Health in Saskatchewan found our data on average waits for treatment to be consistent with the data they had collected. There were discrepancies between the numbers of people waiting for treatment, but their data showed the same trends, with ophthalmology and orthopedics having the longer waiting lists. The Department of Health and Community Services in New Brunswick felt that the total numbers of patients waiting indicated by our survey results were reasonable, but could make no further comments as they do not maintain a central waiting list registry for the province.

DATA VERIFICATION WITH OTHER
WAITING LIST STUDIES

In 1967, a survey of British Columbia hospitals was done by the British Columbia Hospital Insurance Service, the forerunner to MSA (10). This study was undertaken primarily to project bed needs in the future. Thus, its data were for individual hospitals and regions and do not allow for direct comparison with our study. However, some general comments can be made. In 1967, reported waiting times ranged from 2 to 300 days with an average time of about 5 weeks, though this figure varied substantially among hospitals. Our survey results show that waiting times in British Columbia range from 3 to 214 days, with an average waiting time of about 9 weeks. Another difference between patients waiting today and those in 1967 is that today's patient is more likely to be classified as urgent. The 1967 study found that 93 percent of patients in their sample population were waiting for elective surgery, 7 percent for urgent, and 0.5 percent for emergency. In contrast, figures made available to us by Vancouver General Hospital for 1988 suggest that 76 percent of the patients waiting are classified as elective and 24 percent are classified as urgent. The final major difference between the 1967 survey and today's [1993] is the number of patients waiting. The Hospital Insurance study estimated that in 1967 the total number of people on hospital waiting lists in British Columbia exceeded 12,000—0.6 percent of the population in British Columbia that year. Our estimate of 28,209 people waiting for surgery in British Columbia, although a decrease of 1,828 from our 1992 revised estimate, represents 0.9 percent of the population in 1993. This is a large increase over two decades.

In 1982, the Ontario Medical Association undertook a survey of its members in seven surgical specialties (11). The results were based on the responses of 836 specialists from a total of 2,100 specialists surveyed. Given the differences in wording between the Ontario survey and our own, differences in the precise treatments identified, and so forth, comparisons between the two surveys are problematic. We did identify 22 treatments for which average waiting times in the two surveys could be compared. Despite the ten-year difference between these two surveys, the Ontario waiting times are remarkably similar. In 1993, 12 treatments had average waiting times that exceeded the 1982 waiting times by less than one week and, of these, four had average waiting times that were slightly less than the 1982 waiting times. Seven operations, however, had waiting times that differed by more than a month; the largest increases being for cataract surgery, which is 11.2 weeks longer, and hip replacement surgery, which is 13.6 weeks longer.

A brief survey of Ontario hospitals undertaken in October 1990 for the General Accounting Office of the United States Government (12) suggests that patients waiting for elective orthopedic surgery were waiting from 8.5 weeks to 51 weeks, that elective cardiovascular patients were waiting 1 to 25 weeks, and that elective ophthalmology patients were waiting 4.3 to 51 weeks. Limited as this survey was, its results are consistent with ours.

A study on waiting times for radiotherapy in Ontario (13) found that the median waiting times between diagnosis and initiation of radiotherapy for carcinoma of the larynx, carcinoma of the cervix, non-small cell lung cancer, and carcinoma of the prostate were 30.3 days, 27.2 days, 27.3 days, and 93.3 days, respectively. While our survey looked at radiotherapy as a whole without specifying the types of cancer being treated, our average waiting time of 32.9 days (from referral, to meeting with a specialist, to treatment) is consistent with these results.

FOCUS ON CARDIOVASCULAR SURGERY

More people in Canada will die this year of cardiovascular disease than of any other single cause. Because cardiovascular disease is a degenerative process and the decay of the cardiac surgery candidate is gradual, under a system of rationed supply some cardiovascular surgery candidates tend to be bumped by patients with other conditions that require immediate care. This is not a direct process but rather a reflection of the fact that budgets for hospitals are set separately for "conventional illness" and for other, high-cost interventions such as cardiac bypass. Only a certain number of the latter are included in a hospital's overall annual budget. Complicating matters is the ongoing debate about whether cardiac bypass surgery actually extends life. If it *only* improves the quality of life there will be no statistics that point to a decay of health care in the population and, hence, no basis for increased funding.

The result has been lengthy waiting lists, often as long as a year or more, followed by public outcry, which in turn has prompted short-term funding. For instance, two years ago [1992] we reported that Newfoundland's waiting list for coronary bypass surgery was a year long. Last year, the hospital performing open heart surgery received a special temporary grant to deal with its waiting lists. U.S.

hospitals have also provided a convenient short-term solution to excessive waiting lists for cardiac surgery. The British Columbia government contracted Washington state hospitals to perform some 200 operations in 1989 following a public outcry over the six-month waiting list for cardiac bypass surgery in that province. Wealthy individuals are sometimes choosing to avoid the waiting lists by having their heart surgery performed in the United States. In fact, a California heart surgery center has advertised its services in a Vancouver newspaper. Our survey suggests that over 5 percent of British Columbians with heart disease inquire about the possibility of treatment outside Canada and about 2 percent actually have their surgery performed outside the country. For Canada as a whole, about 2 percent of cardiac patients inquire about surgery outside Canada while 0.7 percent actually have their heart surgery performed outside the country.

Excess demand and limited supply have led to the development of a fairly stringent system for setting priorities in some hospitals. In some provinces, patients scheduled for cardiovascular surgery are classified by the urgency of their medical conditions. In these cases, the amount of time they wait for surgery will depend on their classifications. Priorities are usually set based on the amount of pain or angina that patients are experiencing, the amount of blood flow through their arteries (usually determined by an angiogram test), and the "shape" their hearts are in.

Reporting average waiting times as we have done in previous years fails to take into account the importance of these systems for prioritizing patients. More importantly, the false impression may be given that the medical community is not sensitive to an individual's medical needs. On the contrary, an individual needing immediate cardiac surgery will not end up at the end of a waiting list. In fact, if the patient's medical needs warrant it, he or she will be admitted for surgery immediately in most parts of the country.

For the past two years, the cardiovascular survey questionnaire has distinguished among emergent, urgent, and elective patients: the traditional classification by which patients are prioritized. However, in discussing the situation with physicians and by talking with hospital administrators, it has become clear that these classifications are not standardized across provinces. British Columbia and Ontario use a nine-level prioritization system developed in Ontario. Other provinces have a four-level system, with two urgent classifications. Decisions as to where to group patients was thus left to answering physicians and heart centers. Direct comparisons among provinces should, therefore, be made tentatively while recognizing that this survey provides the only comparative data available on the topic.

Efforts were made in this survey to verify the cardiovascular survey results specifically with hospital statistics and with data from provincial health ministries. The ministries of health in British Columbia and Quebec provided us with the actual number of patients on their waiting lists, while the Department of Health in Saskatchewan provided us with the number of patients waiting for surgery as well as the average amount of time that these patients are waiting. Hospital officials in Alberta, Nova Scotia, Newfoundland, and New Brunswick provided us with provincial data. Hospital officials in Manitoba wanted to provide us with data but are in the midst of implementing a province-wide cardiac surgery database and requested that we not release any cardiac data for Manitoba until the system is in place.

Estimates of the length of waiting lists were either taken directly from hospital information or were extrapolated in the same manner as other estimates from the average wait times. The numbers presented for Nova Scotia, Newfoundland, and New Brunswick are not estimates but are the actual numbers of people waiting. These numbers were provided by the hospitals from central registries. The numbers presented for Alberta, Saskatchewan, and Quebec are the actual numbers of people waiting for bypasses and valve operations, but they are estimates of the number of people waiting for pacemaker operations. The estimated numbers of people waiting for heart surgery in all other provinces were derived using the average waiting time for urgent patients. The reason the urgent average waiting time was used rather than the emergent or elective average wait times was that it provided a convenient median measure. In provinces where the length of the waiting list was provided by the hospitals, it became clear that the average wait for elective surgery overestimated the length of the line while the emergent average waiting time underestimated it. For example, in British Columbia, the Ministry recorded 351 patients waiting for cardiac surgery. From this number, an average waiting time of 6.4 weeks can be calculated which exactly corresponds to our estimate of the average weeks waited for urgent cardiac surgery reported in Table 27a.

In a 1991 paper, an Ontario panel of 16 cardiovascular surgeons attempted to outline explicit criteria for prioritizing patients (14). They also suggested time frames considered safe waiting times for coronary surgery candidates. For comparative purposes, it was necessary to collapse their nine priority categories down to the three used in this study. Having done this, we found that they suggest that emergent patients should be operated on within three days (or 0.43 of a week). The majority of average emergent wait times fall outside this range. However, physicians in these provinces may define emergent to include patients that might be considered urgent in other provinces. Urgent surgeries should, according to the Ontario surgeons, be performed within six weeks. The average waits for urgent coronary surgery in British Columbia and Alberta fall outside this range. The Ontario panel suggests that elective surgeries be performed within a period of six months. All provinces except Alberta and Newfoundland fall within this time frame. Unfortunately, hospital officials in Alberta could not separate their data for average waiting times by the type of operation, thus we could not use the data that they provided. The average wait for bypass and valve operations combined, according to Alberta hospital officials, was 5.7 weeks for urgent surgery and 17.1 weeks for elective, both of which fall within the Ontario panel's guidelines. With regard to Quebec, the number of people indicated as waiting for bypass surgery (Table 22) does not include the 84 people who have been registered for surgery for more than a year. Hospital officials felt that these were people who had been scheduled for surgery that had been canceled for various personal or clinical reasons but who wanted to be kept on the waiting list or were people whose conditions required surgery in the future but who were not yet ready for it.

SURVEY RESULTS:
ESTIMATED WAITING IN CANADA

Waiting for an Appointment with a Specialist

Table 2 (p. 179) indicates the average number of weeks that patients wait for initial appointments with specialists after referral from their general practitioners or from other specialists. Most waits for specialists' appointments are between one and two months. However, the longest wait is 20 weeks to see a neuro-surgeon in Manitoba, followed closely by a 19.9-week wait to see an ophthal-mologist in New Brunswick. The weighted averages, depicted in Figure 1, sug-gest that Saskatchewan and Newfoundland have the shortest waits in the country for appointments with specialists, while New Brunswick has the longest.

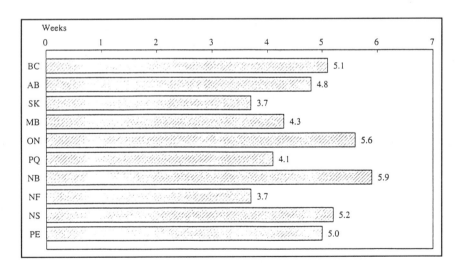

Figure 1. Waiting times by province in 1993: Weeks waited from general practitioner's referral to appointment with specialist. Source: The Fraser Institute's annual waiting list survey, 1994. Abbreviations used in all figures and tables: BC, British Columbia; AB, Alberta; SK, Saskatchewan; MB, Manitoba; ON, Ontario; PQ, Quebec; NB New Brunswick; NF, Newfoundland; NS, Nova Scotia; PE, Prince Edward Island.

Waiting for Treatment

Several general observations can be made about Tables 3 through 14 and Tables 31 through 41. Residents of all provinces surveyed are waiting significant periods of time for hospital treatments. While some treatments have short waits, most procedures require waits of at least a month. For many procedures, the waiting time is at least two months. Eighty-five percent of the actual average waiting times were greater than what specialists considered to be reasonable average waiting times. The average wait for a hip replacement in Manitoba (arthroplasty of the hip) is more than a year. A clinically reasonable amount of time to wait for this procedure in Manitoba, according to specialists, is about three months.

Ranking the provinces according to the weighted averages reported in Table 27a indicates that the longest average wait for surgery occurs in New Brunswick and the shortest in Ontario. Prince Edward Island had the second longest weighted average and Quebec had the second shortest average wait.

Waits were generally longer for most procedures in the Maritimes and shorter in Ontario than in other parts of the country. Overall, there was about a five-week difference between the shortest and the longest weighted averages. Graphically, the average waits for treatment by province can be seen in Figure 2.

Table 29 (p. 200) presents a frequency distribution of the average waits for polled surgery by province and by region. In all provinces, the majority of polled operations have waiting lists of less than three months. However, in New

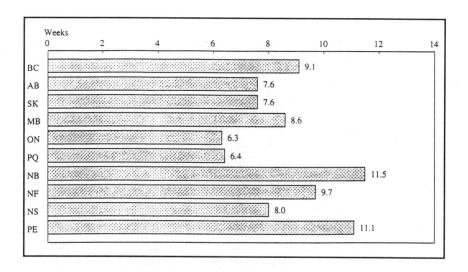

Figure 2. Waiting times by province in 1993: Weeks waited from appointment with specialist to treatment. Source: The Fraser Institute's annual waiting list survey, 1994.

Brunswick, only 54 percent of the polled waiting lists have average waits of less than three months and in Prince Edward Island those lists with less than three-month waits are down to just 51 percent. In fact, the Maritime provinces collectively have the greatest proportion of average waiting times over six months and the lowest proportion under three. In contrast, 96 percent of Quebec's average waits and 95 percent of Ontario's average waits are under three months long and none are over six months.

Comparison with Last Year's Results

As this is the second consecutive year this survey has been undertaken across Canada, a comparison ccccan be made between this year's results and last year's, although last year's results reported here are not exactly the same as those published in last year's publication, "Waiting Your Turn: Hospital Waiting Lists in Canada" [1992 results, published in 1993]. In order to compare the estimates of the number of patients waiting in 1993 with those in 1992, the 1992 estimates were updated using the 1990-91 Statistics Canada count of operations done in that year, as opposed to the 1989-90 counts that were the only ones available when the previous study was written up. The results are compared in Tables 28a and 28b (pp. 196–199). Some of the variation in waiting times and in the number of people waiting for treatment over the last two years in provinces such as Prince Edward Island and Newfoundland is the result of the small sample sizes being studied. In such cases, the presence of a specialist whose patients must wait an especially long time will skew the specialty average upwards. If such a specialist responds to the survey one year and not the next, the difference between years will be large but will not necessarily be an indication of an actual change in the average waiting times for a province.

Our study shows an overall reduction in the waiting times for all provinces except Alberta, Saskatchewan, and Ontario. Quebec and Prince Edward Island showed the greatest improvement in waiting. The waiting list situation, albeit improving overall, worsened in a number of specialties. Generally, waiting for plastic surgery, neurosurgery, elective cardiology, urology, and internal medicine increased across Canada.

There was an increase in the number of patients waiting in Alberta, Saskatchewan, and Ontario. The increase in the number of people waiting in Ontario was generally attributed to the effect of "Rae Days." The other seven provinces showed a general decrease in waiting. The decrease in waiting was most notable in Prince Edward Island where, over the last year, the number of people waiting has decreased by just over 22 percent. The decrease in the number of people waiting for surgery in Canada from 189,218 in 1992 (revised estimate) to 183,528 in 1993 is partially attributable to an increase in the amount of same-day surgery performed, shorter hospital stays, and an increase in the number of private clinics in Canada.

Clinically Reasonable Waiting Times

In almost every instance, the responding specialists felt that waiting times for treatment were excessive. When asked to indicate a clinically reasonable waiting time for the various procedures, specialists generally indicated a period of time substantially shorter than that given for the average number of weeks patients were actually waiting for treatment. Table 42 (p. 207) summarizes the weighted averages for the specialties surveyed. These weighted averages were calculated in the same manner as those given in Table 27a. The variability among the provincial weighted averages is much less than it was in Table 27a. Whereas the actual waiting times among provinces varied by as much as 5 weeks, the number of weeks that specialists felt was reasonable to wait varied by less than 2 weeks among provinces.

Figure 3 compares the actual average number of weeks patients are waiting for treatment after having seen a specialist with the average number of weeks specialists feel are reasonable to have patients wait. The largest difference in these two periods is for ophthalmology where the actual waiting time is 8.4 weeks (or more than 2 months) longer than what is considered to be reasonable by specialists. The smallest divergence is in medical oncology, yet the actual waiting time is still the longer of the two.

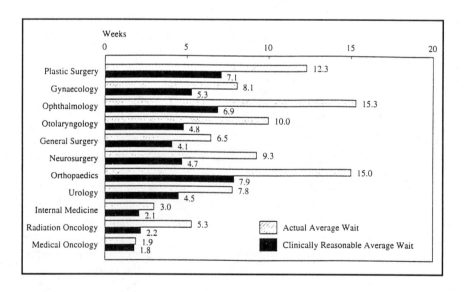

Figure 3. Actual versus reasonable waiting times by specialty for Canada: Time waited from appointment with specialist to treatment in 1993. Source: The Fraser Institute's annual waiting list survey, 1994.

Estimated Total Waiting in Canada

While waiting times for surgery convey a mixed impression about the apparent extent of rationing of health care, there is much less ambiguity when the overall wait for health care is considered. This overall wait, which records the time between the referral by a general practitioner to the time that the required surgery is performed, includes an additional wait for the appointment to see the specialist. Table 30 (p. 201) and Figure 4 present the combined waiting times. They indicate that, on average, patients wait over two months for relief of their ailments, from a weighted average of 10.5 weeks in Quebec to 17.4 weeks in New Brunswick.

Across Canada, the longest waits for treatment tend to be for two specialties: orthopedics and ophthalmology. The average waits for these specialties exceed 20 weeks. As is indicated in Figure 5, the average wait for orthopedic surgery in Canada is 25 weeks, or over 6 months, and the average wait for ophthalmic surgery is 22.4 weeks. The shortest wait in Canada is for cancer patients being treated with chemotherapy. These patients must wait 3.5 weeks, on average, to receive their treatments.

HEALTH EXPENDITURES AND WAITING TIMES

Last year, Ontario performed better than the other provinces with regard to hospital waiting lists. This year, although Ontario's waiting lists increased,

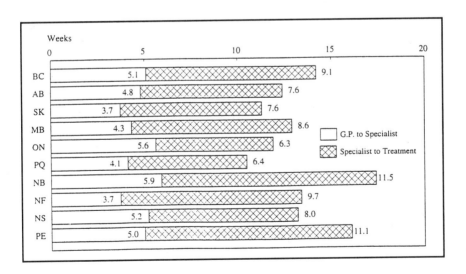

Figure 4. Total waiting times by Province: Weeks waited from general practitioner's referral to treatment in 1993. Source: The Fraser Institute's annual waiting list survey, 1994.

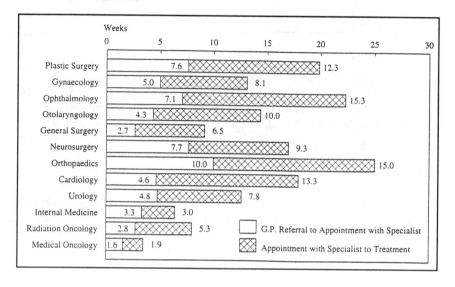

Figure 5. Total waiting times by specialty for Canada: Time waited from general practitioner's referral to treatment in 1993. Source: The Fraser Institute's annual waiting list survey, 1994.

Ontario is still the province with the shortest waiting list. The model of waiting lists that underlies our analysis (which has been sketched out in this study) is that waiting is a manifestation of rationing. It would, therefore, seem to follow that one possible explanation for the result in Ontario is that the province is simply engaging in less rationing than are the other provinces. Rationing is not, of course, a necessary consequence of the way in which the health care system is organized, but merely a possible consequence of that organization if the budgetary allocations to the health care sector are insufficient to keep up with the demand. Budget constraint leads to constraints on the supply of health care services, to an excess of demand over available supply, and thus to the observed rationing by waiting.

It follows from this that one possible explanation for Ontario's superior performance is that Ontario simply spent more money on health care than did the other provinces and that this enabled it to respond more fully to the demands of patients than was possible in other provinces.

In order to examine the truth of this explanation, we calculated a crude measure of expenditures on health care in the form of adjusted per capita expenditure on health care in each province by the public and private sectors. (The per capita figures were adjusted by weighting the number of people in each age group by the percentage of total cost incurred by people in that age group. The reason for using this method of weighting is that if a population in a particular province has more people in age cohorts that are more in need of health care, the same dollar amount per capita spent on health care in that province would yield a less effective supply effort than it would in a province with fewer elderly citizens.) This is shown in Figure 6, which displays the differences from the national average in weighted per capita expenditures for all provinces and the differences from the national average waiting time, by province. (Waiting time is measured from patients' appointments with their general practitioner to the time when they actually receive treatment.) As the figure clearly shows, those provinces with costs at or above the average have waiting times at or below the average wait. As well, those provinces that spent less than the national average generally have waiting times above the national average. The only two exceptions are British Columbia and Nova Scotia, which have, respectively, above average costs and waits, and below average costs and waits. Another anomaly is Quebec, which has costs at about the average level but an average waiting time that is three weeks less than the national average. A statistical test reveals that variation in health care spending explain about half of the total variation among the provinces in the average time waited for treatment.

Evidently there are many factors that influence the waiting times in the provinces and that operate in conjunction with the supply of resources, for example: the age of the population and, therefore, the underlying demand for health care (for which we have tried to make adjustments); the management of resources, including the extent of effort to decrease the number of patients on specific

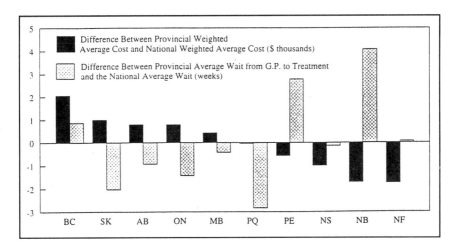

Figure 6. Comparison between weighted average costs and average waiting times (divergence from the Canadian averages). Sources: Average wait for treatment data from The Fraser Institute's annual waiting list survey, 1994. Population data from Statistics Canada, 1991. Expenditure data for 1991 from the Centre for Health Services and Policy Research, University of British Columbia, 1993.

doctors' waiting lists; the extent of same-day surgery; the average length of hospital stays; and the extent of reliance on private clinics. It is also possible that Quebec's superior performance is due to yet other factors. For example, Dr. Naylor of the Institute for Clinical Evaluative Studies (14) notes that the rate of hip replacement in Quebec is only one-third the rate of that in the other provinces. This, Naylor remarks, is due to the fact that the Quebec government has a policy limiting the extent of joint replacement. The effect of such a policy is to produce lower apparent waiting times since patients in need of this operation in Quebec are simply denied it and, hence, do not appear on a waiting list. If there are other such policies in Quebec or elsewhere, they would affect the comparative length of waiting times without leaving any trace in our survey.

A NOTE ON TECHNOLOGY

The wait to see a specialist and the wait to receive treatment are not the only waits that patients face. Our study also looked at the wait for various diagnostic tests. Table 44 (p. 210) shows the average number of weeks patients must wait for access to a computerized axial tomography (CT) scanner, a magnetic resonance imager (MRI), and an ultrasound machine. The average wait for an MRI in Canada (9 weeks) is twice that for a CT scan (4.2 weeks) and is probably an underestimate of the actual waiting time since specialists who do not prescribe MRI tests because of the lengthy waits for access to a machine are not included in the calculation of the average. The longest wait for an MRI is in Alberta (11.4 weeks). MRIs are not available in Prince Edward Island and New Brunswick, and there is only one MRI in Newfoundland. Ultrasound tests are quite common and many specialists have their own machines, which resulted in an average wait for ultrasound in Canada of only 1.7 weeks.

CONCLUSION

While the 1994 "Waiting Your Turn" survey indicates that the waiting list situation has improved for the most part, waiting for health services in Canada is a reality—an indicator that rationing is taking place. On average, in all specialties, less than 10 percent of patients were on waiting lists because they requested a delay or postponement of their treatment. Conversely, the average percentage of patients who would have their surgeries the next day if there were an operating room available was greater than 50 percent in all specialties. These two figures are especially noteworthy given that the survey was conducted in December and that most people would prefer one or two weeks to prepare for a hospital stay.

As well, even if one debates the reliability of waiting list data, our survey reveals that specialists feel that their patients are waiting too long to receive treatment, up to four and a half times longer than is considered to be reasonable.

REFERENCES

1. Who calls the shots, if rationing becomes routine? *Globe and Mail,* April 30, 1992, p. A12.
2. Amoko, D. H. A., Modrow, R. E., and Tan, J. K. H. Surgical waiting lists II: Current practices & future directions. Using the province of British Columbia as a test study. *Healthcare Management FORUM,* 5(4): 34-39, 1992.
3. Globerman, S., and Hoye, L. Waiting your turn: Hospital waiting lists in Canada. *Fraser Forum,* May 1990.
4. Statistics Canada. *General Social Survey—Health.* Public Use Microdata File. Ottawa, Ont., 1991.
5. Williams, J. I. and Naylor, C. D. *Patterns of Healthcare in Ontario #5: Hip and Knee Replacement in Ontario.* Institute for Clinical Evaluative Studies in Ontario, October 18, 1993.
6. Blomqvist, A. *The Health Care Business.* The Fraser Institute, 1979.
7. Aaron, H. J., and Schwartz, W. B. *The Painful Prescription: Rationing Hospital Care.* The Brookings Institution, Washington, D.C., 1984.
8. Cancer patients face wait for treatment. *Globe and Mail,* September 13, 1989, p. A1.
9. Insurance plan skirts lineups. *Province,* Vancouver, April 6, 1993, p. A19.
10. Pallan, P. *A Study of Hospital Waiting Lists.* Research Division, British Columbia Hospital Insurance Service, Department of Health Services and Hospital Insurance.
11. O'Keefe, G. Survey of waiting for elective surgery. *Ontario Med. Rev.,* November 1982.
12. General Accounting Office, Human Resources Division. *Canadian Health Insurance: Lessons for the U.S., 91-90.* Report to the Chairman of the Committee of Government Operations, House of Representatives, June 1991.
13. Mackillop, W. J., et al. *Waiting for Radiotherapy in Ontario.* The Radiation Research Unit, Queen's University, Kingston Regional Cancer Centre and Kingston General Hospital, 1993.
14. Naylor, C. D., et al. Assigning priority to patients requiring coronary revascularization: Consensus principles from a panel of cardiologists and cardiac surgeons. *Can. J. Cardiol. Med.* 7(5): 207–213, 1991.

Table 1

Summary of responses, 1993[a]

Specialty	Number of questionnaires mailed out										
	BC	AB	SK	MB	ON	PQ	NB	NF	NS	PE	Total
Plastic surgery	50	31	10	10	143	114	12	2	6	2	380
Gynecology	146	115	35	53	581	384	25	19	44	6	1,408
Ophthalmology	152	72	18	27	250	253	16	11	35	2	836
Otolaryngology	72	32	13	15	195	186	9	4	19	3	548
General surgery	161	128	56	65	311	254	31	21	59	9	1,095
Neurosurgery	26	18	7	4	64	54	5	2	7	0	187
Orthopedics	137	81	20	30	234	279	18	15	22	3	839
Urology	59	34	14	19	201	140	19	7	22	2	517
Internal medicine	213	193	73	124	207	274	34	33	88	7	1,246
Radiation oncology	30	21	2	0	96	62	5	2	8	1	227
Medical oncology	13	8	4	2	56	22	2	0	1	1	109
Cardiology	34	16	7	5	69	56	3	2	4	0	196
Total	1,093	749	259	354	2,407	2,078	179	118	315	36	7,588

Number of responses

Specialty	BC	AB	SK	MB	ON	PQ	NB	NF	NS	PE	Total
Plastic surgery	23	11	5	3	48	34	4	1	2	1	132
Gynecology	51	38	11	20	164	98	10	6	17	3	418
Ophthalmology	67	34	7	11	83	85	6	5	13	1	312
Otolaryngology	25	14	4	5	62	56	4	4	7	2	183
General surgery	46	38	19	18	104	50	7	8	16	4	310
Neurosurgery	13	6	3	1	21	16	3	1	3	—	67
Orthopedics	54	29	5	7	67	59	6	5	7	2	241
Urology	19	12	4	5	61	32	9	6	7	1	156
Internal medicine	55	42	18	25	42	63	10	7	24	2	288
Radiation oncology	10	10	1	—	27	11	1	1	3	1	65
Medical oncology	6	6	1	1	19	5	1	—	1	1	41
Cardiology	12	4	3	—	21	11	1	1	1	—	54
Total	381	244	81	96	719	520	62	45	101	18	2,267

177

Table 1

(Cont'd.)

Specialty	Response rate percent										
	BC	AB	SK	MB	ON	PQ	NB	NF	NS	PE	Average
Plastic surgery	46%	35%	50%	30%	34%	30%	33%	50%	33%	50%	35%
Gynecology	35	33	31	38	28	26	40	32	39	50	30
Ophthalmology	44	47	39	41	33	34	38	45	37	50	37
Otolaryngology	35	44	31	33	32	30	44	100	37	67	33
General surgery	29	30	34	28	33	20	23	38	27	44	28
Neurosurgery	50	33	43	25	33	30	60	50	43	—	36
Orthopedics	39	36	25	23	29	21	33	33	32	67	29
Urology	32	35	29	26	30	23	47	86	32	50	30
Internal medicine	26	22	25	20	28	23	29	21	27	29	23
Radiation oncology	33	48	50	—	28	18	20	50	38	100	29
Medical oncology	46	75	25	50	34	23	50	—	100	100	37
Cardiology	35	25[b]	100[c]	—	30	20[b]	100[c]	100[c]	100[c]	—	27
Average	35	33	31	27	30	25	35	38	32	50	30

[a] Abbreviations for all tables as in Figure 1, p. 167.
[b] These data were supplemented with hospital data.
[c] These data were provided by the province's health registry or by the province's Ministry of Health.

178

Table 2

Average 1993 patient wait to see a specialist after referral from a general practitioner, in weeks

Specialty	BC	AB	SK	MB	ON	PQ	NB	NF	NS	PE
Plastic surgery	8.8	9.4	6.1	10.0	7.2	4.5	11.3	12.0	8.0	1.5
Gynecology	3.9	6.2	4.7	3.3	5.5	3.9	6.0	2.6	5.6	7.0
Ophthalmology	3.7	2.9	9.1	9.9	7.1	5.4	19.9	3.9	8.6	16.0
Otolaryngology	2.5	6.5	2.0	3.8	4.9	3.7	2.6	2.3	7.0	6.0
General surgery	2.7	3.0	1.8	2.5	2.5	2.4	2.3	4.3	3.8	1.8
Neurosurgery	7.1	6.8	4.8	20.0	9.0	5.6	5.8	6.0	6.2	—
Orthopedics	10.4	7.3	6.8	9.9	13.2	6.1	5.1	3.5	9.9	3.5
Cardiology	7.5	3.6	4.5	—	4.2	3.8	2.5	3.5	4.0	—
Urology	5.3	5.2	2.4	4.5	5.3	4.1	4.1	6.2	3.8	18.0
Internal medicine	5.1	4.2	2.9	2.5	2.7	3.3	4.0	3.0	3.7	3.0
Radiation oncology	4.4	2.6	2.0	—	2.0	1.5	1.0	1.0	1.2	1.0
Medical oncology	1.3	1.6	1.0	2.0	1.6	1.8	1.0	—	2.0	0.5
Weighted average	5.1	4.8	3.7	4.3	5.6	4.1	5.9	3.7	5.2	5.0

Table 3

Plastic surgery (1993): Average patient wait for treatment after appointment with specialist, in weeks

Treatment	BC	AB	SK	MB	ON	PQ	NB	NF	NS	PE
Mammoplasty	19.7	11.0	18.8	14.0	11.3	9.4	35.7	364.0	100.0	24.0
Neurolysis	7.7	7.6	5.8	7.3	7.2	6.2	11.3	7.0	20.0	—
Blepharoplasty	9.9	10.3	7.7	9.0	6.6	5.2	29.5	8.0	50.0	—
Rhinoplasty	11.5	10.4	17.8	12.0	8.1	6.5	31.7	8.0	31.0	—
Scar revision	9.9	12.2	21.3	12.0	8.2	8.9	23.8	8.0	31.0	1.0
Hand surgery	12.1	9.6	9.8	7.3	8.2	6.7	22.3	6.5	15.5	4.0
Weighted average	11.5	9.8	12.9	10.4	8.4	7.3	26.5	19.9	32.5	7.6

Table 4

Gynecology (1993): Average patient wait for treatment after appointment with specialist, in weeks

Treatment	BC	AB	SK	MB	ON	PQ	NB	NF	NS	PE
Dilation and curettage (D&C)	4.2	5.9	3.2	4.3	3.5	3.6	12.9	2.1	4.6	4.5
Tubal ligation	8.0	7.6	4.5	9.5	5.3	5.9	24.0	1.6	9.4	11.7
Hysterectomy	8.6	10.1	7.0	6.1	6.1	5.7	22.0	3.3	10.0	9.7
Vaginal repair	10.3	10.5	7.5	6.3	6.0	5.7	24.4	2.9	10.2	11.5
Tuboplasty	10.3	10.9	6.8	4.6	8.0	7.5	23.2	8.5	6.9	10.0
Laparoscopy	5.9	7.3	4.5	5.9	5.3	5.3	20.6	1.4	6.1	7.7
Weighted average	8.2	8.9	5.4	6.4	5.9	5.4	21.2	2.9	9.0	10.1

Table 5

Ophthalmology (1993): Average patient wait for treatment after appointment with specialist, in weeks

Treatment	BC	AB	SK	MB	ON	PQ	NB	NF	NS	PE
Cataract removal	13.3	11.8	29.8	22.6	17.9	11.1	15.4	4.2	15.6	23.0
Lacrimal duct	10.4	9.5	26.0	4.5	9.8	8.7	12.8	2.5	4.3	—
Strabismus	10.3	9.7	11.0	6.0	13.2	7.9	11.8	5.5	4.8	—
Operations on eyelids	9.8	8.7	20.0	6.0	9.2	6.4	12.8	4.8	5.3	—
Weighted average	12.4	11.5	27.0	20.2	17.1	10.8	15.2	4.2	14.5	23.0

Table 6

Otolaryngology (1993): Average patient wait for treatment after appointment with specialist, in weeks

Treatment	BC	AB	SK	MB	ON	PQ	NB	NF	NS	PE
Myringotomy/ tonsillectomy/ adenoidectomy	8.8	10.6	6.0	8.7	7.2	6.5	5.1	28.0	16.6	3.0
Tympanoplasty	10.5	9.1	10.7	5.7	9.0	6.5	8.5	—	14.5	24.5
Rhinoplasty/septal surgery	12.4	10.0	12.7	4.8	9.6	6.6	10.5	24.0	25.6	24.5
Nasal polyps	10.2	10.0	12.7	5.8	8.4	5.3	4.7	7.0	18.2	21.5
Weighted average	9.5	10.4	7.3	7.9	7.6	6.4	5.7	23.7	17.8	7.9

Table 7

General surgery (1993): Average patient wait for treatment after appointment with specialist, in weeks

Treatment	BC	AB	SK	MB	ON	PQ	NB	NF	NS	PE
Hernia repair	9.8	8.0	5.7	5.0	4.3	6.4	7.6	14.1	4.7	19.5
Cholecystectomy	9.2	6.7	5.5	4.8	4.2	5.8	11.2	25.3	4.5	21.3
Breast biopsy	2.1	1.8	1.6	2.1	2.0	2.2	1.6	1.7	2.0	3.1
Mastectomy	1.8	1.5	1.3	1.5	1.7	1.5	1.5	1.0	1.7	2.4
Hemorrhoidectomy	11.0	8.4	5.2	6.4	4.7	8.1	14.8	30.4	3.9	21.5
Colonoscopy	4.0	3.6	3.4	2.3	3.5	3.4	5.5	2.8	4.1	4.5
Varicose vein	13.9	9.7	4.3	6.0	5.1	8.4	19.0	35.8	5.3	26.0
Weighted average	8.1	6.3	4.4	4.4	3.8	5.4	8.8	18.0	4.1	15.2

Table 8

Neurosurgery (1993): Average patient wait for treatment after appointment with specialist, in weeks

Treatment	BC	AB	SK	MB	ON	PQ	NB	NF	NS	PE
Neurolysis (peripheral nerve)	4.4	5.2	5.3	8.0	6.8	9.3	6.7	4.0	6.0	—
Intervertebral disc surgery	9.3	6.2	7.3	14.0	9.7	14.6	6.7	4.0	6.0	—
Elective cranial bone flap	6.5	5.7	6.0	6.0	6.7	8.8	6.7	—	3.3	—
Weighted average	8.5	6.0	6.8	11.0	8.7	12.4	6.7	4.0	5.3	—

Table 9

Orthopedic surgery (1993): Average patient wait for treatment after appointment with specialist, in weeks

Treatment	BC	AB	SK	MB	ON	PQ	NB	NF	NS	PE
Meniscectomy	8.9	6.7	11.0	11.8	10.1	7.2	8.3	6.1	7.6	16.0
Removal of pins	10.5	7.0	13.0	11.7	11.8	8.6	25.8	5.9	9.1	13.5
Arthroplasty (Hips)	30.5	19.7	21.8	61.6	19.8	19.7	16.7	7.6	19.1	21.5
Arthroplasty (interphalangeal)	11.1	7.9	12.0	13.5	8.1	8.5	6.3	6.0	12.8	21.5
Digital neuroma	7.9	5.6	8.0	13.5	6.4	6.4	—	6.7	8.8	20.0
Rotator cuff repair	12.5	6.1	15.5	17.3	10.1	8.4	10.5	6.0	8.9	12.0
Osteotomy	15.5	9.9	14.3	15.7	11.4	8.4	13.6	7.2	10.5	19.0
Hallux valgus/hammer toe	11.8	10.7	15.4	13.6	10.0	10.4	28.8	8.0	10.4	16.0
Weighted average	19.0	11.4	15.4	29.8	13.1	11.0	13.2	6.8	14.5	20.1

Table 10

Cardiovascular surgery (1993): Average patient wait for treatment after appointment with specialist, in weeks

Treatment	BC	AB	SK[a]	MB	ON	PQ	NB[b]	NF[b]	NS[b]	PE
Emergency										
Coronary artery bypass	4.4	0.1	1.0	—	1.5	—	0.0	0.1	1.0	—
Operations on valves and septa of heart	6.4	0.2	1.0	—	1.7	—	0.0	—	—	—
Implantation, removal, or replacement of pacemaker	0.0	1.0	0.5	—	0.1	—	—	0.0	—	—
Urgent										
Coronary artery bypass	6.1	12.2	3.2	—	1.9	1.4	6.0	2.5	5.0	—
Operations on valves and septa of heart	7.6	10.8	2.8	—	1.5	1.1	6.0	—	5.0	—
Implantation, removal, or replacement of pacemaker	2.1	2.5	—	—	0.6	0.8	—	—	2.0	—
Elective										
Coronary artery bypass	13.0	25.5	7.9	—	9.8	9.8	12.0	28.0	14.0	—
Operations on valves and septa of heart	14.6	25.0	8.5	—	8.7	5.8	12.0	28.0	14.0	—
Implantation, removal, or replacement of pacemaker	5.8	4.0	—	—	2.2	1.3	—	—	—	—

[a]Department of Health and survery data for the province.
[b]Hospital data for the province.

Table 11

Urology (1993): Average patient wait for treatment after appointment with specialist, in weeks

Treatment	BC	AB	SK	MB	ON	PQ	NB	NF	NS	PE
Prostatectomy	14.9	4.1	20.0	4.0	4.7	6.5	15.7	3.1	8.6	16.0
TUR bladder	4.7	3.8	4.0	1.8	3.4	2.9	5.5	2.1	4.0	7.0
Cystoscopy	8.2	4.0	2.4	2.8	4.2	5.9	15.6	5.1	8.4	7.0
Hernia/hydrocele	12.8	5.1	5.0	5.0	5.6	10.5	15.4	11.5	14.0	—
Bladder fulguration	5.3	2.8	3.0	2.5	2.8	4.3	7.8	3.6	3.5	7.0
Ureteral reimplantation	14.3	3.9	1.5	3.0	3.6	4.2	18.2	7.4	20.0	—
Weighted average	11.4	4.0	9.7	3.7	4.5	7.1	13.8	4.9	8.4	11.2

Table 12

Internal medicine (1993): Average patient wait for treatment after appointment with specialist, in weeks

Treatment	BC	AB	SK	MB	ON	PQ	NB	NF	NS	PE
Colonoscopy	1.7	3.1	2.1	2.5	2.1	1.9	3.0	4.6	3.1	2.0
Angiography	3.3	4.4	0.9	7.9	4.5	4.7	6.0	3.6	4.4	—
Gastroscopy	1.5	2.8	2.2	2.4	1.7	1.9	1.8	2.9	2.5	4.5
Weighted average	2.5	3.6	1.7	4.6	2.9	2.9	2.0	3.5	3.5	4.0

Table 13

Radiation oncology (1993): Average patient wait for treatment after appointment with specialist, in weeks

Treatment	BC	AB	SK	MB	ON	PQ	NB	NF	NS	PE
Radiotherapy	9.6	4.2	1.5	—	2.7	3.5	4.0	1.0	1.3	1.0
Treatment of side effects	0.6	0.3	0.0	—	0.4	0.4	0.0	1.0	0.0	—
Weighted average	9.6	4.2	1.5	—	2.7	3.5	4.0	1.0	1.3	1.0

Table 14

Medical oncology (1993): Average patient wait for treatment after appointment with specialist, in weeks

Treatment	BC	AB	SK	MB	ON	PQ	NB	NF	NS	PE
Chemotherapy	1.3	2.4	0.0	1.0	2.3	0.5	1.2	—	1.0	2.0
Treatment of side effects	0.4	0.0	0.0	0.0	0.2	0.0	0.0	—	0.0	—
Weighted average	1.3	2.4	0.0	1.0	2.3	0.5	1.2	—	1.0	2.0

Table 15

Plastic surgery (1993): Estimated number of patients waiting for treatment after appointment with specialist

Treatment	BC	AB	SK	MB	ON	PQ	NB	NF	NS	PE
Mammoplasty	140	75	28	21	300	274	86	72	60	6
Neurolysis	84	108	54	27	301	175	34	10	45	—
Blepharoplasty	25	20	11	4	46	21	14	1	10	—
Rhinoplasty	201	81	140	59	351	290	185	19	66	—
Scar revision	114	101	85	32	220	114	43	11	65	1
Hand surgery	61	46	28	13	145	56	21	2	9	1
Total	625	431	346	156	1,363	930	383	115	255	8

Table 16

Gynecology (1993): Estimated number of patients waiting for treatment after appointment with specialist

Treatment	BC	AB	SK	MB	ON	PQ	NB	NF	NS	PE
D & C	89	229	86	45	345	330	92	37	28	10
Tubal ligation	126	212	60	164	188	340	126	7	41	107
Hysterectomy	1,191	1,011	214	214	2,490	1,525	862	96	466	50
Vaginal repair	69	64	31	10	130	107	48	4	31	5
Tuboplasty	259	252	66	42	686	229	90	22	30	8
Laparoscopy	71	88	20	26	210	202	63	3	33	5
Total	1,805	1,856	477	501	4,049	2,733	1,281	169	629	185

Table 17

Ophthalmology (1993): Estimated number of patients waiting for treatment after appointment with specialist

Treatment	BC	AB	SK	MB	ON	PQ	NB	NF	NS	PE
Cataract removal	554	693	665	441	4,662	3,250	501	26	590	80
Lacrimal duct	40	20	55	6	114	86	7	4	7	—
Strabismus	57	20	29	3	127	89	11	6	7	—
Operations on eyelids	74	40	50	8	111	59	8	4	6	—
Total	725	773	799	458	5,014	3,484	527	40	610	80

Table 18

Otolaryngology (1993): Estimated number of patients waiting for treatment after appointment with specialist

Treatment	BC	AB	SK	MB	ON	PQ	NB	NF	NS	PE
Myringotomy/ tonsillectomy/ adenoidectomy	1,069	1,317	376	350	3,391	864	207	863	609	18
Tympanoplasty	121	78	43	18	259	150	20	—	39	10
Rhinoplasty/ septal surgery	312	80	130	35	567	480	46	142	172	25
Nasal polyps	128	100	33	7	231	124	11	13	49	9
Total	1,630	1,575	582	410	4,448	1,618	284	1,018	869	62

188

Table 19

General surgery (1993): Estimated number of patients waiting for treatment after appointment with specialist

Treatment	BC	AB	SK	MB	ON	PQ	NB	NF	NS	PE
Hernia repair	1,017	706	244	197	1,284	1,461	197	211	164	95
Cholecystectomy	1,132	721	238	211	1,810	1,692	433	679	229	117
Breast biopsy	48	51	13	20	115	143	10	4	12	3
Mastectomy	86	46	34	21	272	165	13	7	24	5
Hemorrhoidectomy	268	215	44	52	321	515	92	82	27	20
Colonoscopy	48	39	31	8	258	139	42	11	24	11
Varicose vein	237	157	21	33	358	574	70	74	22	10
Total	2,836	1,935	625	542	4,418	4,689	857	1,068	502	261

Table 20

Neurosurgery (1993): Estimated number of patients waiting for treatment after appointment with specialist

Treatment	BC	AB	SK	MB	ON	PQ	NB	NF	NS	PE
Neurolysis (peripheral nerve)	25	43	34	12	127	125	8	6	16	—
Intervertebral disc surgery	905	347	229	188	2,027	1,461	92	69	114	—
Elective cranial bone flap	163	116	49	44	600	419	38	—	26	—
Total	1,093	506	312	244	2,754	2,005	138	75	156	—

Table 21

Orthopedic surgery (1993): Estimated number of patients waiting for treatment after appointment with specialist

Treatment	BC	AB	SK	MB	ON	PQ	NB	NF	NS	PE
Meniscectomy	148	113	88	59	380	119	33	17	8	7
Arthroplasty (Hips)	1,832	707	418	866	3,371	1,284	207	39	316	54
Arthoplasty (interphalangeal)	259	185	117	89	836	621	36	24	72	11
Digital neuroma	109	70	45	74	185	131	—	16	19	4
Rotator cuff repair	45	22	36	16	120	127	7	3	9	1
Osteotomy	588	291	176	163	1,544	633	131	32	105	19
Hallux valgus/hammer toe	49	6	2	2	95	47	23	1	6	1
Total	3,030	1,394	882	1,269	6,531	2,962	437	132	535	97

Table 22

Cardiovascular surgery (1993): Estimated number of patients waiting for treatment after appointment with specialist

Treatment	BC[a]	AB[b]	SK[c]	MB	ON	PQ[c]	NB[c]	NF[c]	NS[c]	PE
Coronary artery bypass	334	264	247	—	372	548	24	87	95	—
Operations on valves and septa of heart	114	106	190	—	62	25	14	27	13	—
Implantation, removal, or replacement of pacemaker	72	44	—	—	44	30	—	0	5	—
Total	520	386	437	—	478	603	38	114	113	—

[a]Confirmed with Ministry data.
[b]Hospital and survey data for the province. Twenty-eight patients are waiting for both bypass and valve surgery in Alberta. This is reflected in the provincial total.
[c]Hospital or Ministry data for the province. For Quebec, the pacemaker data are derived from the survey data.

Table 23

Urology (1993): Estimated number of patients waiting for treatment after appointment with specialist

Treatment	BC	AB	SK	MB	ON	PQ	NB	NF	NS	PE
Prostatectomy	1,797	228	664	111	1,487	1,013	407	38	186	63
TUR bladder	157	56	41	9	322	123	44	9	29	6
Cystoscopy	259	115	47	19	633	290	268	30	152	15
Hernia/hydrocele	487	120	54	58	1,165	1,322	245	61	182	—
Bladder fulguration	130	63	39	15	172	140	54	10	33	11
Total	2,830	582	845	212	3,779	2,888	1,018	148	582	95

Table 24

Internal medicine (1993): Estimated number of patients waiting for treatment after appointment with specialist

Treatment	BC	AB	SK	MB	ON	PQ	NB	NF	NS	PE
Colonoscopy	27	50	25	16	103	84	25	27	27	4
Angiography	294	300	26	132	994	452	—	67	188	—
Gastroscopy	92	158	72	45	482	269	63	48	82	37
Total	413	508	123	193	1,579	805	88	142	297	41

Table 25

Radiation oncology (1993): Estimated number of patients waiting for treatment after appointment with specialist

Treatment	BC	AB	SK	MB	ON	PQ	NB	NF	NS	PE
Radiotherapy	151	75	11	—	129	83	2	3	12	0

Table 26

Medical oncology (1993): Estimated number of patients waiting for treatment after appointment with specialist

Treatment	BC	AB	SK	MB	ON	PQ	NB	NF	NS	PE
Chemotherapy	94	57	0	8	328	45	10	—	20	2

Table 27a

Average wait to receive treatment by selected specialties in 1993, in weeks

Treatment	BC	AB	SK	MB	ON	PQ	NB	NF	NS	PE
Plastic surgery	11.5	9.8	12.9	10.4	8.4	7.3	26.5	19.9	32.5	7.6
Gynecology	8.2	8.9	5.4	6.4	5.9	5.4	21.2	2.9	9.0	10.1
Ophthalmology	12.4	11.5	27.0	20.2	17.1	10.8	15.2	4.2	14.5	23.0
Otolaryngology	9.5	10.4	7.3	7.9	7.6	6.4	5.7	23.7	17.8	7.9
General surgery	8.1	6.3	4.4	4.4	3.8	5.4	8.8	18.0	4.1	15.2
Neurosurgery	8.5	6.0	6.8	11.0	8.7	12.4	6.7	4.0	5.3	—
Orthopedics	19.0	11.4	15.4	29.8	13.1	11.0	13.2	6.8	14.5	20.1
Cardiology (elective)[a]	13.3	25.4	8.0	—	9.6	9.4	12.0	28.0	14.0	—
Cardiology (urgent)[a]	6.4	12.0	3.1	—	1.8	1.4	6.0	2.5	5.0	—
Urology	11.4	4.0	9.7	3.7	4.5	7.1	13.8	4.9	8.4	11.2
Internal medicine	2.5	3.6	1.7	4.6	2.9	2.9	2.0	3.5	3.5	4.0
Radiation oncology	9.6	4.2	1.5	—	2.7	3.5	4.0	1.0	1.3	1.0
Medical oncology	1.3	2.4	0.0	1.0	2.3	0.5	1.2	—	1.0	2.0
Weighted average	9.1	7.6	7.6	8.6	6.3	6.4	11.5	9.7	8.0	11.1

[a]Weighted averages do not include pacemaker waits.

194

Table 27b

Estimated number of patients waiting by specialty in 1993

Treatment	BC	AB	SK	MB	ON	PQ	NB	NF	NS	PE
Plastic surgery	625	431	346	156	1,363	930	383	115	255	8
Gynecology	1,805	1,856	477	501	4,049	2,733	1,281	169	629	185
Ophthalmology	725	773	799	458	5,014	3,484	527	40	610	80
Otolaryngology	1,630	1,575	582	410	4,448	1,618	284	1,018	869	62
General surgery	2,836	1,935	625	542	4,418	4,689	857	1,068	502	261
Neurosurgery	1,093	506	312	244	2,754	2,005	138	75	156	—
Orthopedics	3,030	1,394	882	1,269	6,531	2,962	437	132	535	97
Cardiology	520	386	437	—	478	603	38	114	113	—
Urology	2,830	582	845	212	3,779	2,888	1,018	148	582	95
Internal medicine	413	508	123	193	1,579	805	88	142	297	41
Radiation oncology	151	75	11	—	129	83	2	3	12	0
Medical oncology	94	57	0	8	328	45	10	—	20	2
Residual	12,457	8,082	3,417	3,677	24,352	15,590	3,277	2,155	3,482	564
Total	28,209	18,160	8,856	7,670	59,222	38,435	8,340	5,179	8,062	1,395
Proportion of population	0.9%	0.7%	0.9%	0.7%	0.6%	0.6%	1.1%	0.9%	0.9%	1.1%

Canada totals   183,528 (0.67% of population)

195

Table 28a

Comparison of average weeks waited to receive treatment by selected specialties (Δ = change), 1992 and 1993

Treatment	BC '93	BC '92	BC Δ	AB '93	AB '92	AB Δ	SK '93	SK '92	SK Δ	MB '93	MB '92	MB Δ	ON '93	ON '92	ON Δ
Plastic surgery	11.5	11.2	3%	9.8	9.3	5%	12.9	14.1	-9%	10.4	11.0	-5%	8.4	6.9	22%
Gynecology	8.2	9.3	-12	8.9	7.6	17	5.4	9.7	-44	6.4	14.8	-57	5.9	5.5	7
Ophthalmology	12.4	13.7	-9	11.5	8.5	35	27.0	23.1	17	20.2	20.4	-1	17.1	12.9	33
Otolaryngology	9.5	7.5	27	10.4	11.1	-6	7.3	4.1	78	7.9	7.4	7	7.6	5.7	33
General surgery	8.1	8.3	-2	6.3	4.6	37	4.4	6.9	-36	4.4	6.5	-32	3.8	3.9	-3
Neurosurgery	8.5	7.1	20	6.0	7.4	-19	6.8	3.6	89	11.0	7.3	51	8.7	6.6	32
Orthopedics	19.0	18.6	2	11.4	12.8	-11	15.4	13.5	14	29.8	30.5	-2	13.1	12.0	9
Cardiology (elective)[a]	13.3	13.0	2	25.4	18.6	37	8.0	16.2	-51	—	9.5	—	9.6	9.4	2
Cardiology (urgent)[a]	6.4	6.1	5	12.0	7.9	52	3.1	6.0	-48	—	2.0	—	1.8	2.6	-31
Urology	11.4	12.8	-11	4.0	3.6	11	9.7	6.0	62	3.7	3.2	16	4.5	3.6	25
Internal medicine	2.5	3.6	-31	3.6	2.9	24	1.7	2.2	-23	4.6	3.1	48	2.9	1.6	81
Weighted average[b]	9.1	9.7	6	7.6	7.0	9	7.6	7.6	0	8.6	10.4	-17	6.3	5.5	15

Treatment	PQ '93	PQ '92	PQ Δ	NB '93	NB '92	NB Δ	NF '93	NF '92	NF Δ	NS '93	NS '92	NS Δ	PE '93	PE '92	PE Δ
Plastic surgery	7.3	9.2	−21%	26.5	17.9	48%	19.9	75.5	−74%	32.5	13.3	144%	7.6	—	—
Gynecology	5.4	5.0	8	21.2	26.4	−20	2.9	4.7	−38	9.0	9.4	−4	10.1	25.7	−61%
Ophthalmology	10.8	14.9	−28	15.2	20.7	−27	4.2	4.3	−2	14.5	19.1	−24	23.0	27.5	−16
Otolaryngology	6.4	7.1	−10	5.7	8.6	−34	23.7	25.1	−6	17.8	17.7	1	7.9	8.4	−6
General surgery	5.4	5.8	−7	8.8	5.7	54	18.0	14.4	25	4.1	5.5	−25	15.2	10.0	52
Neurosurgery	12.4	28.3	−56	6.7	2.0	235	4.0	—	—	5.3	7.3	−27	—	—	—
Orthopedics	11.0	12.9	−15	13.2	17.9	−26	6.8	12.7	−46	14.5	20.0	−28	20.1	31.2	−36
Cardiology (elective)[a]	9.4	48.5	−81	12.0	20.0	−40	28.0	24.0	17	14.0	14.0	0	—	—	—
Cardiology (urgent)[a]	1.4	5.2	−73	6.0	4.0	50	2.5	3.5	−29	5.0	6.3	−21	—	—	—
Urology	7.1	4.8	48	13.8	10.2	35	4.9	14.3	−66	8.4	4.9	71	11.2	7.6	47
Internal medicine	2.9	2.7	7	2.0	3.5	−43	3.5	2.4	46	3.5	3.1	13	4.0	3.0	33
Weighted average[b]	6.4	8.0	−20	11.5	11.9	−3	10.2	12.5	−18	8.0	8.9	−10	11.3	14.8	−24

[a]Weighted averages do not include pacemaker waits.
[b]The overall weighted average includes only those specialties which are comparable over both years of the study.

197

Table 28b

Comparison of estimated numbers of patients waiting for treatment by selected specialties (Δ = change), 1992 and 1993

Treatment	BC			AB			SK			MB			ON		
	'93	'92	Δ	'93	'92	Δ	'93	'92	Δ	'93	'92	Δ	'93	'92	Δ
Plastic surgery	625	665	-6.0%	431	415	3.9%	346	371	-6.7%	156	159	-1.9%	1,363	1,019	33.8%
Gynecology	1,805	2,041	-11.6	1,856	1,590	16.7	477	859	-44.5	501	1,156	-56.7	4,049	3,798	6.6
Ophthalmology	725	785	-7.6	773	572	35.1	799	686	16.5	458	463	-1.1	5,014	3,801	31.9
Otolaryngology	1,630	1,296	25.8	1,575	1,682	-6.4	582	326	78.5	410	389	5.4	4,448	3,353	32.7
General surgery	2,836	2,783	1.9	1,935	1,401	38.1	625	977	-36.0	542	795	-31.8	4,418	4,915	-10.1
Neurosurgery	1,093	905	20.8	506	623	-18.8	312	165	89.1	244	163	49.7	2,754	2,102	31.0
Orthopedics	3,030	2,906	4.3	1,394	1,566	-11.0	882	778	13.4	1,269	1,301	-2.5	6,531	6,031	8.3
Cardiology	520	522	-0.4	386	435	-11.3	437	—	—	—	55	—	478	746	-35.9
Urology	2,830	3,395	-16.6	582	530	9.8	845	529	59.7	212	188	12.8	3,779	2,701	39.9
Internal medicine	413	604	-31.6	508	403	26.1	123	158	-22.2	193	130	48.5	1,579	865	82.5
Total[a]	15,507	15,902	-2.5	9,946	9,217	7.9	4,991	4,849	2.9	3,985	4,744	-16.0	34,413	29,331	17.3

Treatment	PQ '93	PQ '92	PQ Δ	NB '93	NB '92	NB Δ	NF '93	NF '92	NF Δ	NS '93	NS '92	NS Δ	PE '93	PE '92	PE Δ
Plastic surgery	930	895	3.9%	383	243	57.6%	115	392	−70.7%	255	119	114.3%	8	—	—
Gynecology	2,733	2,511	8.8	1,281	1,597	−19.8	169	268	−36.9	629	755	−16.7	185	472	−60.8%
Ophthalmology	3,484	4,839	−28.0	527	718	−26.6	40	42	−4.8	610	801	−23.8	80	94	−14.9
Otolaryngology	1,618	1,821	−11.1	284	431	−34.1	1,018	1,063	−4.2	869	859	1.2	62	64	−3.1
General surgery	4,689	5,635	−16.8	857	572	49.8	1,068	877	21.8	502	664	−24.4	261	168	55.4
Neurosurgery	2,005	4,676	−57.1	138	41	236.6	75	—	—	156	201	−22.4	—	—	—
Orthopedics	2,962	3,512	−15.7	437	618	−29.3	132	247	−46.6	535	733	−27.0	97	152	−36.2
Cardiology	603	896	−32.7	38	48	−20.8	114	94	21.3	113	88	28.4	—	—	—
Urology	2,888	1,570	83.9	1,018	733	38.9	148	432	−65.7	582	343	69.7	95	73	30.1
Internal medicine	805	731	10.1	88	148	−40.5	142	97	46.4	297	265	12.1	41	33	24.2
Total[a]	22,717	27,086	−16.1	5,051	5,149	−1.9	2,946	3,512	−16.1	4,548	4,828	−5.8	821	1,056	−22.3

[a]Total includes only those specialties which are comparable over both years of the study.

Table 29

Frequency distribution of waiting times (specialist to treatment) by province and by region in 1993:
Proportion of average waiting times that fall in the specified ranges[a]

Range	BC	AB	SK	MB	ON	PQ	NB	NF	NS	PE
0–3.9 wks	14.0%	22.8%	31.6%	22.4%	29.8%	22.2%	16.1%	35.3%	21.4%	18.9%
4–7.9 wks	22.8	31.6	31.6	42.9	31.6	46.3	25.0	37.3	30.4	21.6
8–11.9 wks	40.4	36.8	10.5	12.2	33.3	27.8	12.5	9.8	17.9	10.8
12–23.9 wks	21.1	5.3	22.8	20.4	5.3	3.7	33.9	2.0	21.4	37.8
24–51.9 wks	1.8	3.5	3.5	—	—	—	12.5	13.7	7.1	10.8
1 yr+	—	—	—	2.0	—	—	—	2.0	1.8	—

	BC	Prairies	ON	PQ	Atlantic
0–3.9 wks	14.0%	25.8%	29.8%	22.2%	23.0%
4–7.9 wks	22.8	35.0	31.6	46.3	29.0
8–11.9 wks	40.4	20.2	33.3	27.8	13.0
12–23.9 wks	21.1	16.0	5.3	3.7	23.0
24–51.9 wks	1.8	2.5	—	—	11.0
1 yr+	—	0.6	—	—	1.0

[a]Average waits for pacemaker implantation, removal, or replacement are not included. Also not included are those operations for which no data were obtained.

Table 30

Total expected waiting time from general practitioner referral to treatment in 1993, in weeks

Treatment	BC	AB	SK	MB	ON	PQ	NB	NF	NS	PE
Plastic surgery	20.3	19.2	19.0	20.4	15.6	11.8	37.8	31.9	40.5	9.1
Gynecology	12.1	15.1	10.1	9.7	11.4	9.3	27.2	5.5	14.6	17.1
Ophthalmology	16.1	14.4	36.1	30.1	24.2	16.2	35.1	8.1	23.1	39.0
Otolaryngology	12.0	16.9	9.3	11.7	12.5	10.1	8.3	26.0	24.8	13.9
General surgery	10.8	9.3	6.2	6.9	6.3	7.8	11.1	22.3	7.9	17.0
Neurosurgery	15.6	12.8	11.6	31.0	17.7	18.0	12.5	10.0	11.5	—
Orthopedics	29.4	18.7	22.2	39.7	26.3	17.1	18.3	10.3	24.4	23.6
Cardiology (elective)[a]	20.8	29.0	12.5	—	13.8	13.2	14.5	31.5	18.0	—
Urology	16.7	9.2	12.1	8.2	9.8	11.2	17.9	11.1	12.2	29.2
Internal medicine	7.6	7.8	4.6	7.1	5.6	6.2	6.0	6.5	7.2	7.0
Radiation oncology	14.0	6.8	3.5	—	4.7	5.0	5.0	2.0	2.5	2.0
Medical oncology	2.6	4.0	1.0	3.0	3.9	2.3	2.2	—	3.0	2.5
Weighted average	14.2	12.4	11.3	12.9	11.9	10.5	17.4	13.4	13.2	16.1

[a]Weighted average does not include pacemaker waits.

Table 31

Plastic surgery (1993): Average reasonable patient wait for treatment after appointment with specialist, in weeks

Treatment	BC	AB	SK	MB	ON	PQ	NB	NF	NS	PE
Mammoplasty	8.6	8.2	17.3	8.0	8.3	8.6	8.0	—	12.0	—
Neurolysis	4.3	7.0	5.5	4.0	4.3	4.6	5.0	—	3.5	—
Blepharoplasty	7.1	8.2	9.5	8.0	6.6	5.7	10.0	—	12.0	—
Rhinoplasty	7.0	8.5	15.0	8.0	6.9	6.2	8.0	—	12.0	—
Scar revision	7.0	8.4	15.0	8.0	7.5	6.6	10.0	—	12.0	—
Hand surgery	6.1	5.8	7.5	4.0	4.6	4.8	8.0	—	11.0	—
Weighted average	6.6	7.6	10.8	6.5	6.3	6.3	7.7	—	9.5	—

Table 32

Gynecology (1993): Average reasonable patient wait for treatment after appointment with specialist, in weeks

Treatment	BC	AB	SK	MB	ON	PQ	NB	NF	NS	PE
D & C	3.0	4.4	3.1	2.7	2.7	3.1	4.1	3.7	4.0	5.0
Tubal ligation	5.8	7.5	4.7	6.3	5.0	5.9	5.3	7.3	7.1	5.0
Hysterectomy	5.4	7.4	5.2	5.1	4.6	4.9	6.7	7.0	5.9	5.0
Vaginal repair	6.2	7.7	6.0	5.9	5.2	5.2	9.0	8.0	7.6	5.0
Tuboplasty	7.2	8.8	9.2	6.2	6.6	7.3	—	6.0	7.5	—
Laparoscopy	3.9	5.4	4.2	5.0	3.8	3.9	7.5	6.3	5.8	5.0
Weighted average	5.3	6.9	4.9	5.2	4.6	4.8	6.4	6.0	6.0	5.0

Table 33

Ophthalmology (1993): Average reasonable patient wait for treatment after appointment with specialist, in weeks

Treatment	BC	AB	SK	MB	ON	PQ	NB	NF	NS	PE
Cataract removal	7.8	7.0	8.2	8.6	6.6	5.8	13.0	5.2	9.5	6.0
Lacrimal duct	6.2	7.3	6.7	7.0	4.8	5.9	10.0	3.0	5.0	—
Strabismus	7.2	7.7	7.0	7.0	5.5	4.9	10.0	3.0	4.6	4.0
Operations on eyelids	7.1	8.6	6.7	5.0	4.7	5.1	10.0	5.0	6.0	—
Weighted average	7.5	7.1	7.9	8.3	6.4	5.8	12.8	4.6	9.1	5.9

Table 34

Otolaryngology (1993): Average reasonable patient wait for treatment after appointment with specialist, in weeks

Treatment	BC	AB	SK	MB	ON	PQ	NB	NF	NS	PE
Myringotomy/ tonsillectomy/ adenoidectomy	5.0	5.2	4.5	3.0	3.9	3.9	4.0	—	4.9	—
Tympanoplasty	6.8	6.3	9.0	3.8	5.7	5.0	6.0	—	5.5	—
Rhinoplasty/ septal surgery	8.6	7.0	9.3	5.0	6.3	5.5	6.3	—	8.4	—
Nasal polyps	5.5	4.9	8.0	4.2	4.3	4.2	5.0	—	3.3	—
Weighted average	5.7	5.5	5.5	3.4	4.2	4.5	4.3	—	5.3	—

203

Table 35

General surgery (1993): Average reasonable patient wait for treatment after appointment with specialist, in weeks

Treatment	BC	AB	SK	MB	ON	PQ	NB	NF	NS	PE
Hernia repair	6.9	5.7	5.5	4.9	4.4	4.1	5.2	3.5	4.8	7.3
Cholecystectomy	4.8	4.6	5.0	4.4	3.9	3.4	3.7	3.8	3.5	7.3
Breast biopsy	1.6	1.6	1.7	2.0	1.8	1.6	1.1	1.5	2.2	1.3
Mastectomy	1.5	1.4	1.5	1.6	1.6	1.5	1.1	0.8	2.1	1.3
Hemorrhoidectomy	8.2	7.1	6.0	4.9	4.1	5.0	6.2	3.6	3.9	11.7
Colonoscopy	2.9	3.0	2.4	2.1	2.6	2.5	3.0	2.1	3.4	2.0
Varicose vein	12.0	7.5	6.4	7.3	5.7	8.5	14.2	7.0	7.2	13.5
Weighted average	5.3	4.6	4.3	4.2	3.6	3.7	4.2	3.3	3.8	5.9

Table 36

Neurosurgery (1993): Average reasonable patient wait for treatment after appointment with specialist, in weeks

Treatment	BC	AB	SK	MB	ON	PQ	NB	NF	NS	PE
Neurolysis (peripheral nerve)	4.1	3.8	5.7	8.0	4.5	5.0	—	—	4.0	—
Intervertebral disc surgery	4.5	3.4	7.0	8.0	4.1	5.6	—	—	3.3	—
Elective cranial bone flap	4.2	4.2	5.0	8.0	5.6	3.1	—	—	7.0	—
Weighted average	4.4	3.6	6.5	8.0	4.5	4.8	—	—	4.3	—

Table 37

Orthopedic surgery (1993): Average reasonable patient wait for treatment after appointment with specialist, in weeks

Treatment	BC	AB	SK	MB	ON	PQ	NB	NF	NS	PE
Meniscectomy	5.1	4.4	5.3	8.0	4.2	3.5	3.6	5.0	3.0	—
Removal of pins	7.5	7.2	7.5	11.0	7.3	6.3	14.8	5.0	6.0	—
Arthroplasty (hips)	11.0	10.3	11.5	11.3	10.0	6.9	8.7	5.0	9.0	—
Arthoplasty (interphalangeal)	8.6	7.5	12.0	8.3	7.6	5.9	8.0	5.0	9.8	—
Digital neuroma	7.0	5.3	5.3	9.3	5.7	4.1	9.0	—	3.5	—
Rotator cuff repair	7.4	6.0	9.0	—	5.4	4.0	6.8	—	5.3	—
Osteotomy	9.4	7.1	9.3	12.5	7.6	5.3	7.7	5.0	7.7	—
Hallux valgus/hammer toe	8.7	7.8	9.8	10.7	7.2	6.2	9.7	5.0	7.8	—
Weighted average	9.2	7.5	9.5	10.5	8.0	5.6	7.7	5.0	8.2	—

Table 38

Urology (1993): Average reasonable patient wait for treatment after appointment with specialist, in weeks

Treatment	BC	AB	SK	MB	ON	PQ	NB	NF	NS	PE
Prostatectomy	6.6	4.6	4.9	4.5	4.4	4.0	5.6	4.0	10.8	—
TUR bladder	2.5	2.3	2.5	2.5	2.4	2.1	2.6	1.0	2.8	—
Cystoscopy	4.2	3.2	1.2	2.9	3.1	3.1	4.8	4.0	5.2	—
Hernia/hydrocele	8.7	6.2	3.5	5.8	5.2	5.3	5.1	—	8.0	—
Bladder fulguration	3.0	3.0	2.0	3.7	2.4	2.5	2.4	—	2.9	—
Ureteral reimplantation	6.1	3.8	1.5	5.0	3.4	2.5	7.1	—	11.2	—
Weighted average	5.7	4.1	3.0	4.4	3.9	3.9	4.8	3.4	7.2	—

Table 39

Internal medicine (1993): Average reasonable patient wait for treatment after appointment with specialist, in weeks

Treatment	BC	AB	SK	MB	ON	PQ	NB	NF	NS	PE
Colonoscopy	1.5	2.1	2.1	2.0	2.1	2.0	2.2	2.0	2.4	1.0
Angiography	2.0	2.5	1.5	1.4	2.9	2.5	6.0	2.3	3.2	—
Gastroscopy	1.2	1.7	1.8	2.1	1.7	1.8	1.9	1.8	2.5	2.0
Weighted average	1.7	2.1	1.7	1.8	2.2	2.1	2.0	2.1	2.8	1.8

Table 40

Radiation oncology (1993): Average reasonable patient wait for treatment after appointment with specialist, in weeks

Treatment	BC	AB	SK	MB	ON	PQ	NB	NF	NS	PE
Radiotherapy	2.1	2.5	2.0	—	1.9	2.5	4.0	2.0	—	2.0
Treatment of side effects	0.4	0.1	—	—	0.7	0.7	0.0	2.0	0.0	—
Weighted average	2.1	2.5	2.0	—	1.9	2.5	4.0	2.0	—	2.0

Table 41

Medical oncology (1993): Average reasonable patient wait for treatment after appointment with specialist, in weeks

Treatment	BC	AB	SK	MB	ON	PQ	NB	NF	NS	PE
Chemotherapy	1.2	1.5	2.0	—	2.3	0.6	—	—	0.0	2.0
Treatment of side effects	0.2	0.1	0.0	0.0	0.3	0.0	—	—	0.0	0.0
Weighted average	1.2	1.5	2.0	—	2.3	0.6	—	—	0.0	2.0

Table 42

Reasonable number of weeks to wait to receive treatment by selected specialists in 1993

Treatment	BC	AB	SK	MB	ON	PQ	NB	NF	NS	PE
Plastic surgery	6.6	7.6	10.8	6.5	6.3	6.3	7.7	—	9.5	—
Gynecology	5.3	6.9	4.9	5.2	4.6	4.8	6.4	6.0	6.0	5.0
Ophthalmology	7.5	7.1	7.9	8.3	6.4	5.8	12.8	4.6	9.1	5.9
Otolaryngology	5.7	5.5	5.5	3.4	4.2	4.5	4.3	—	5.3	—
General surgery	5.3	4.6	4.3	4.2	3.6	3.7	4.2	3.3	3.8	5.9
Neurosurgery	4.4	3.6	6.5	8.0	4.5	4.8	—	—	4.3	—
Orthopedics	9.2	7.5	9.5	10.5	8.0	5.6	7.7	5.0	8.2	—
Urology	5.7	4.1	3.0	4.4	3.9	3.9	4.8	3.4	7.2	—
Internal medicine	1.7	2.1	1.7	1.8	2.2	2.1	2.0	2.1	2.8	1.8
Radiation oncology	2.1	2.5	2.0	—	1.9	2.5	4.0	2.0	—	2.0
Medical oncology	1.2	1.5	2.0	—	2.3	0.6	—	—	0.0	2.0
Weighted average	5.3	5.1	5.1	5.1	4.4	4.2	5.5	3.8	5.2	4.6

Table 43

Comparison between actual (A) average number of weeks waited to receive treatment and the reasonable (R) average number of weeks to wait for treatment in 1993 (D = difference)

Treatment	BC			AB			SK			MB			ON		
	A	R	D	A	R	D	A	R	D	A	R	D	A	R	D
Plastic surgery	11.5	6.6	74.2%	9.8	7.6	28.9%	12.9	10.8	19.4%	10.4	6.5	60.0%	8.4	6.3	3.3%
Gynecology	8.2	5.3	54.7	8.9	6.9	29.0	5.4	4.9	10.2	6.4	5.2	23.1	5.9	4.6	28.3
Ophthalmology	12.4	7.5	65.3	11.5	7.1	62.0	27.0	7.9	241.8	20.2	8.3	143.4	17.1	6.4	167.2
Otolaryngology	9.5	5.7	66.7	10.4	5.5	89.1	7.3	5.5	32.7	7.9	3.4	132.4	7.6	4.2	81.0
General surgery	8.1	5.3	52.8	6.3	4.6	37.0	4.4	4.3	2.3	4.4	4.2	4.8	3.8	3.6	5.6
Neurosurgery	8.5	4.4	93.2	6.0	3.6	66.7	6.8	6.5	4.6	11.0	8.0	37.5	8.7	4.5	93.3
Orthopedics	19.0	9.2	106.5	11.4	7.5	52.0	15.4	9.5	62.1	29.8	10.5	183.8	13.1	8.0	63.8
Urology	11.4	5.7	100.0	4.0	4.1	-2.4	9.7	3.0	223.3	3.7	4.4	-15.9	4.5	3.9	15.4
Internal medicine	2.5	1.7	47.1	3.6	2.1	71.4	1.7	1.7	0.0	4.6	1.8	155.6	2.9	2.2	31.8
Radiation oncology	9.6	2.1	357.1	4.2	2.5	68.0	1.5	2.0	-25.0	—	—	—	2.7	1.9	42.1
Medical oncology	1.3	1.2	8.3	2.4	1.5	60.0	0.0	2.0	-100.0	1.0	—	—	2.3	2.3	0.0
Weighted average	9.3	5.3	75.5	7.4	5.1	45.1	7.7	5.1	51.0	8.7	5.1	70.6	6.5	4.4	47.7

Treatment	PQ			NB			NF			NS			PE		
	A	R	D	A	R	D	A	R	D	A	R	D	A	R	D
Plastic surgery	7.3	6.3	15.9%	26.5	7.7	244.2%	19.9	—	—	32.5	9.5	242.1%	7.6	—	—
Gynecology	5.4	4.8	12.5	21.2	6.4	231.3	2.9	6.0	-51.7%	9.0	6.0	50.0	10.1	5.0	102.0%
Ophthalmology	10.8	5.8	86.2	15.2	12.8	18.7	4.2	4.6	-8.7	14.5	9.1	59.3	23.0	5.9	289.8
Otolaryngology	6.4	4.5	42.2	5.7	4.3	32.6	23.7	—	—	17.8	5.3	235.8	7.9	—	—
General surgery	5.4	3.7	45.9	8.8	4.2	109.5	18.0	3.3	445.5	4.1	3.8	7.9	15.2	5.9	157.6
Neurosurgery	12.4	4.8	158.3	6.7	—	—	4.0	—	—	5.3	4.3	23.3	—	—	—
Orthopedics	11.0	5.6	96.4	13.2	7.7	71.4	6.8	5.0	36.0	14.5	8.2	76.8	20.1	—	—
Urology	7.1	3.9	82.1	13.8	4.8	187.5	4.9	3.4	44.1	8.4	7.2	16.7	11.2	—	—
Internal medicine	2.9	2.1	38.1	2.0	2.0	0.0	3.5	2.1	66.7	3.5	2.8	25.0	4.0	1.8	122.2
Radiation oncology	3.5	2.5	40.0	4.0	4.0	0.0	1.0	2.0	-50.0	1.3	—	—	1.0	2.0	-50.0
Medical oncology	0.5	0.6	-16.7	1.2	—	—	—	—	—	1.0	0.0	100.0	2.0	2.0	0.0
Weighted average	6.7	4.2	59.5	12.0	5.5	118.2	3.7	3.8	-2.6	8.4	5.2	61.5	11.2	4.6	143.5

[a]The overall weighted average includes only those specialties which contained data for actual average waiting times and clinically reasonable waiting times.

Table 44

Waiting for technology: Average number of weeks waited to receive
selected diagnostic tests in 1993

Province	CT	MRI	Ultrasound
BC	4.3	10.7	1.7
AR	2.9	11.4	1.3
SK	5.4	5.5	1.4
MB	4.7	6.7	2.5
ON	4.6	10.6	1.3
PQ	3.9	7.5	2.3
NB	3.2	—	2.2
NF	6.0	5.9	2.8
NS	2.4	4.9	1.9
PE	5.1	—	3.9
Weighted average	4.2	9.0	1.7

CHAPTER 11

Patient Access to
Magnetic Resonance Imaging Centers
in Orange County, California

Beverly C. Morgan

It is becoming increasingly common for physicians to invest in free-standing health care businesses to which they refer their patients but at which they do not practice. These arrangements, known as joint ventures, include a wide variety of diagnostic and therapeutic services; a salient example is centers offering magnetic resonance imaging (MRI). Discussion of the appropriateness and ethics of these arrangements has been widespread. Opponents of this practice say that referring physicians have a direct conflict of interest when they are owners of businesses to which patients are referred. The main argument of proponents is that investment by physicians enhances patients' access to care.

Orange County, California, has 2.4 million residents, 798 square miles, and 41 MRI centers (1). By comparison, Canada has 27 million residents, 4 million square miles, and 22 MRI centers (2). In Orange County, nine MRI centers are based at six hospitals (one hospital has three units, and another has two). Fourteen centers are mobile. Seventeen MRI units are "free-standing," some directly adjacent to hospitals. These free-standing units are all independently owned; physicians are investors in almost all of them.

To test the hypothesis that free-standing MRI centers in Orange County increase patients' access, I conducted the following survey. Over a three-month period, I randomly called all 17 free-standing centers, posing as three persons. First, I called as a patient with a minor orthopedic problem, referred by my physician for an MRI. When asked about insurance, I identified my own plan (Prudential High Option Health Care). I was offered an appointment at any time;

Reprinted by permission of *The New England Journal of Medicine* from 328(12), pp. 884–885, 1993.
Copyright 1993, Massachusetts Medical Society.

48 hours was the longest delay I encountered. Virtually every unit offered next-day service.

I made the next two series of calls posing as a patient referred by my physician with the diagnosis of a possible brain tumor and the recommendation that I undergo MRI as soon as possible. When questioned about my insurance status in the second series of calls, I stated that Medi-Cal (Medicaid) was my payer. Representatives of 6 of the 17 centers said that they could schedule such a study within two to three weeks if my physician would be willing to complete the extensive paperwork necessary to obtain special authorization from Medi-Cal. Representatives of the other 11 units stated that they did not accept Medi-Cal coverage under any circumstances.

In the third series of calls, I stated that I was uninsured and had no funds immediately available to pay for the MRI. None of the 17 centers would accept a patient without funds; under the most satisfactory arrangement I was offered, I would have to pay $500 cash before the procedure and show "evidence of ability to pay the remainder of the $500 to $700 due promptly."

As both the patient with Medi-Cal coverage and the patient without funds, I asked for an alternative way to obtain the test. Most of the representatives said they were unaware of any; the only suggestion I received was to try "UCI"—the University of California, Irvine, Medical Center, the not-for-profit hospital in which I work. The MRI unit at the medical center is owned by American Medical International, a for-profit organization, and provides services for the large number of Medicaid and uninsured patients cared for at the institution. The full use of this unit precludes acceptance of referrals of patients financially screened out at other MRI centers in the county.

Despite the plethora of MRI centers in Orange County, access is severely limited for both Medicaid patients and patients who lack health insurance. These findings cast serious doubt on the argument that joint ventures in MRI improve access to care. I suspect that the situation in Orange County is not unique. The Clinton administration and state governments should consider legislation to prohibit such joint ventures and to ensure that when medically indicated, sophisticated forms of technology such as MRI are available to patients regardless of their insurance status.

REFERENCES

1. Community radiologists and industry representatives, personal communication.
2. Canadian Coordinating Office for Health Care Technology Assessment. *Technology Brief,* Issue 5.1. Ottawa, Ont., October 1992.

CHAPTER 12

Postsurgical Mortality in Manitoba and New England

Leslie L. Roos, Elliott S. Fisher, Sandra M. Sharp,
Joseph P. Newhouse, Geoffrey Anderson,
and Thomas A. Bubolz

On a per capita basis, the United States spends from 25 to 50 percent more on hospitals than Canada (1, 2). Such differences cannot be attributed to higher rates of hospital admission in the United States; rather, "patients at U.S. hospitals appear to use either more inputs or more highly paid inputs (or both) than do patients at Canadian hospitals" (1). Are the greater hospital expenditures per patient stay in the United States associated with better outcomes?

To address this question, we used insurance databases to examine differences between Manitoba and New England in postsurgical mortality among patients 65 years of age and older. Both short-term (30-day) and long-term (6-month) mortality were examined. Because surgical procedures are clearly defined in administrative data systems and have narrower clinical indications than most medical hospitalizations, comparing outcomes of surgical care reduces the problems of case-mix measurement (3). Specific procedures were chosen on the basis of their frequency and cost.

Although data from Manitoba and New England were used because of their availability, Manitoba is generally representative of Canada in terms of average earnings, hospital expenditures per capita, and the rates for a number of common surgical procedures (4-6). Manitoba had 202 physicians (including interns and residents) and 590 hospital beds (acute and extended treatment) per 100,000 population in 1985 (7). Manitoba has a multiethnic population of mostly European origin, with about 5.4 percent Treaty Indians and about 0.5 percent

Published in the *Journal of the American Medical Association,* 263(18), pp. 2453–2458, 1990.
Copyright 1990, American Medical Association.

black. Besides using global budgeting to control hospital costs, the Canadian health care system differs from the American along several dimensions. Manitoba, in particular, has a well-coordinated system of home health care and personal care homes that provide universal access to the elderly with minimal user fees. In addition, the pressures for hospital discharge after surgery may be less in Manitoba than under Medicare; lengths of stay, controlling for diagnosis related group, are about 95 percent longer in Canada (1).

The New England population is relatively affluent and generally white, with just 4.6 percent nonwhite in 1988. New England is well supplied with physicians and hospital beds, having 242 physicians (including residents and fellows) and 598 hospital beds per 100,000 population in 1986 (8). New England expenditures are approximately 15 percent higher ($783 per capita) than the U.S. average of $680 per capita in 1985 (1).

Health care in Manitoba does have some features in common with that of the United States. Physicians are paid on a fee-for-service basis, moving freely between hospital and community practice. Anderson and colleagues (3) have noted the similarities between two Canadian provinces (Manitoba and Ontario) and the United States, both in overall mortality rates for ischemic heart disease and in the recent decreases in mortality rates (9, 10).

METHODS

Data Sources

Both Medicare and the Manitoba Health Services Commission databases contain computerized information on hospital discharges and patient enrollment in the respective insurance systems. The hospital files include patient and hospital identifiers, admission and discharge dates, and data on diagnoses and procedures (using codes from the *International Classification of Diseases, Ninth Revision, Clinical Modification*). The enrollment files include individual identifiers and specify a date of death, regardless of whether that death occurred inside or outside a hospital.

In Manitoba, all hospital and medical care, with a few minor exceptions (such as private room, cosmetic surgery, and some out-of-province care), is without user fees or limitations on use. The Manitoba health insurance database contains information on all individuals registered in the province (11, 12). New England Medicare data were based on the hospital claims file (Medicare Part A) and the enrollment file maintained by the Health Care Financing Administration (13).

Both the Manitoba and New England data sets are population based, containing information on almost all elderly residents, regardless of where their care was received. This study includes the 1.5 percent of Manitoba elderly residents and 2 percent of the New England Medicare patients 65 years of age and over who had their procedures performed outside their own areas. A very few Manitobans might have had out-of-province surgery without authorization for reimbursement by the provincial Health Services Commission. From 3 to 4 percent of New England Medicare patients have their surgery in Department of Veterans Affairs hospitals; this is not recorded in the Medicare database. About 8 percent of elderly New England residents were members of health maintenance organizations during at least part of the period from 1984 to 1986. They are included in the study, but some of their inpatient claims may not have been filed.

Small numbers of hospital claims either could not be assigned an operation date or noted two operations that we studied as occurring during the same hospital stay. In total, 0.5 percent of both Manitoba and New England claims were so excluded. Very few individuals became unavailable for follow-up during the 6 months after surgery (0.2 percent in Manitoba and essentially none in New England). Date of surgery was added to the Manitoba hospital claims through linkage to physicians billing information. For 3 percent of the Manitoba procedures, date of operation was assigned on the basis of the specific operation's average presurgical length of stay; this general approach to missing data has been adopted from Daley and colleagues (14).

Study Population

The study population consists of individuals 65 years of age and older in New England and Manitoba. Except as noted below, the primary procedure on the discharge abstract was used to define the operations. To minimize potential case-mix differences, an effort was made to select relatively homogeneous groups of surgical patients. Patients who received concurrent bypass and valve replacement were analyzed separately. Both diagnostic codes and procedure codes were used to construct the groups for total hip replacement (no hip fracture diagnosis) and for hip fracture repair procedures (hip fracture diagnosis and "surgery for repair" performed). Although diagnosing, coding, and treating malignancies may differ between the two regions, the percentage of transurethral prostatectomies with diagnoses of cancer of the bladder or prostate was similar (23 to 24 percent of the total) in both settings. Twelve percent of the open prostatectomies were excluded because of cancer of the bladder or prostate; similarly, 1.5 percent of the cholecystectomies were eliminated from consideration because of cancer of the gallbladder.

Definition of Variables

Age and gender are verified, and mortality ascertained, by linkage of hospital claims with the enrollment files. Covariates used in the analysis of mortality were age, sex, the absence or presence of high-risk diagnoses that independently predict mortality (15, 16), and type of operation—"emergency," "scheduled," or "delayed." The covariates are represented categorically, with groupings for age

(65 to 69, 70 to 74, and ≥ 75 years of age) based on previous work (17, 18). The high-risk diagnoses were malignant neoplasm, old myocardial infarction, peripheral vascular disease, chronic obstructive pulmonary disease, diabetes, dementia, moderate or severe chronic liver disease, renal failure, and ulcers. Emergency, scheduled, and delayed operations were defined on the basis of the number of days between admission and surgery (19). Emergency operations were defined as those that occurred on the date of admission. Scheduled operations are generally performed within 2 days of admission. Patients hospitalized 3 or more days prior to surgery were classified as having delayed operations; these may be high-risk cases that require further diagnostic procedures or sicker patients whose condition must be stabilized before surgery (20). Length of stay before trans-urethral prostatectomy differed to such an extent between Manitoba and New England that the "type of operation" variable was not included for this procedure. Because of inconsistency in the coding of hospital transfers in the New England data, we did not include this variable to control for case mix.

The covariates were selected after extensive Manitoba analyses that combined retrospectively collected administrative data (from the surgical hospitalization and from any hospitalizations in the previous 6 months) with the widely used patient's physical status score (as prospectively judged by the attending anes-thesiologist) (15, 16, 21). Among possible covariates relevant across a range of different procedures, those applied herein explained a substantial portion of the total variation in individual postsurgical mortality that was predictable from the administrative and clinical data described above.

Statistical Methods

Because of the small numbers of certain types of procedures performed in Manitoba, we also grouped procedures into three categories according to mortality in the 6 months following surgery: low (mortality rates <6 percent), moderate (6 to 15 percent), and high (>15 percent). To generate adequate statistical power, more years of data are used for Manitoba. Manitoba postsurgical mortality from 1980 to 1986 is compared with New England mortality from 1984 and 1985. Power calculations show that for the low and moderate categories we can detect a 20 percent mortality difference (significant at the $P < .05$ level) between countries with 90 percent certainty; for high-rate procedures, we can detect a 15 percent difference with equivalent power and significance. Analyses using Manitoba data from 1983 to 1986 (the 4 years closest to 1984 and 1985) generated similar findings for the low- and moderate-mortality procedures (but with wider confidence intervals for the odds ratios). As discussed later, survival following hip fracture repair (a high-mortality procedure) improved somewhat between the periods 1980 to 1982 and 1983 to 1986 in Manitoba.

We calculated odds ratios and adjusted for patient characteristics, using a multiple logistic regression model to estimate the independent effects of location

(Manitoba compared with New England) on postsurgical mortality (22). Only 7 of 124 possible interactions between location and each of the covariates were statistically significant at the .05 level; this was close to the number expected by chance. Inclusion of the significant interactions did not substantially alter our findings. Other statistical analyses that tested models adjusted for only age and sex and models adjusted for only age, sex, and comorbidity led to few changes in the odds ratios.

RESULTS

Surgical Rates in Manitoba and New England

New England showed markedly higher rates of coronary artery bypass surgery, valve replacement surgery, and carotid endarterectomy among the elderly. Manitoba rates of prostatectomy and cholecystectomy (from 1980 to 1986) were substantially higher, while the two regions were quite similar in rates of total hip replacement and repair of hip fracture (Table 1). When Manitoba rates from 1983 to 1986 are used for a closer comparison with the New England data, the Manitoba rates increased substantially for coronary artery bypass surgery (10.4 per 10,000 elderly for 1983 to 1986) and heart valve replacement (2.8 per 10,000).

Individual procedures varied in the characteristics of patients who underwent surgery, but differences between Manitoba and New England were relatively small. Except for open heart procedures, Manitoba patients appeared to have somewhat fewer high-risk diagnoses. Although these high-risk diagnoses should be coded on hospital discharge abstracts in both regions, some differences may result from the financial incentives for American hospitals to code their Medicare cases more thoroughly (23).

Mortality Comparisons

Analyses of individual procedures show relatively small differences in risk of death and unadjusted mortality ratios between Manitoba and New England (Table 2). The unadjusted odds ratios for procedures with low and moderate postsurgical mortality suggest better outcomes in Manitoba; two of the four comparisons (for 30-day and 6-month mortality) were statistically significant. On the other hand, the two conditions with high postsurgical mortality, repair of hip fracture and concurrent valve replacement/bypass surgery, showed greater mortality in Manitoba.

Controlling for case mix has little effect on the short- and long-term mortality data (Table 3). Six months after surgery, outcomes for both low- and moderate-mortality procedures favored Manitoba, while for the two high-mortality procedures, both 30-day and 6-month outcomes indicated a lower risk of death in the

Table 1

Rates of surgery and characteristics of elderly surgical patients in Manitoba and New England[a]

Procedure	Manitoba (1980–1986)				New England (1984–1985)			
	Surgical Rate[b]	Mean age, yr	High-risk diagnoses, %	No. of operations	Surgical rate[b]	Mean age, yr	High-risk diagnoses, %	No. of operations
Procedures with low mortality								
Total hip replacement	17.1	73.3[c]	11.9[c]	1,569	16.1	73.9	15.3	5,163
Simple cholecystectomy	32.3	72.1[c]	15.4[c]	2,961	28.1	73.6	22.6	9,041
Open prostatectomy	10.9	74.5	12.8[c]	1,004	3.8	73.9	20.8	1,235
Carotid endarterectomy	5.1	71.2[c]	26.9	465	11.8	72.5	30.9	3,802
Transurethral prostatectomy	124.6	74.7	19.1[c]	4,932	122.2	74.5	24.5	15,078
All low-mortality procedures	—	73.6[c]	16.8[c]	10,931	—	73.9	23.2	34,319
Procedures with moderate mortality								
Cholecystectomy with exploration of the common bile duct	8.7	75.4	17.8[c]	794	7.3	76.1	23.3	2,346
Coronary artery bypass graft surgery	8.0	70.0[c]	24.8	734	16.0	70.5	24.4	5,151
Transurethral prostatectomy with malignancy	40.1	77.0	100.0	1,589	37.1	76.6	100.0	4,583
Heart valve replacement	2.3	71.1	16.0	212	3.8	72.0	16.0	1,231
All moderate-mortality procedures	—	74.7[c]	58.5[c]	3,329	—	73.7	49.4	13,311
Procedures with high mortality								
Repair of hip fracture	50.0	81.6	22.9[c]	4,584	50.5	81.9	25.0	16,235
Concurrent valve replacement/bypass surgery	1.1	71.4	25.7	101	1.4	72.6	20.9	435
All high-mortality procedures	—	81.4	23.0[c]	4,685	—	81.6	24.9	16,670

[a]Sources: Population and rate data for New England (1984–1985 operations) are from Medicare discharge abstracts from the Health Care Financing Administration. Data for Manitoba (1980–1986 operations, 1984 population) are from Manitoba Health Services Commission hospital admission/discharge abstracts and enrollment file.
[b]Each rate is expressed as the number of discharges per 10,000 population 65 years of age and older.
[c]Manitoba–New England differences were significant at $P < .01$.

Table 2

Risk of death (per 100) according to type of operations among patients 65 years of age and older

Procedure	30-Day mortality			6-Month mortality		
	Manitoba	New England	Unadjusted odds ratio: Manitoba–New England	Manitoba	New England	Unadjusted odds ratio: Manitoba–New England
Procedures with low mortality						
Total hip replacement	1.3	1.0	1.32	2.1	2.3	0.92
Simple cholecystectomy	1.5	2.4	0.64[a]	2.8	5.3	0.53[a]
Open prostatectomy	1.1	1.1	1.04	3.2	2.3	1.36
Carotid endarterectomy	1.9	2.3	0.86	4.7	5.8	0.82
Transurethral prostatectomy	1.3	1.0	1.22	5.3	5.2	1.02
All low-mortality procedures	1.3	1.5	0.89	3.9	4.7	0.83[a]
Procedures with moderate mortality						
Cholecystectomy with exploration of the common bile duct	3.4	4.2	0.81	7.1	7.5	0.95
Coronary artery bypass graft surgery	5.3	5.6	0.95	7.2	8.7	0.83
Transurethral prostatectomy with malignancy	1.4	1.8	0.80	9.0	9.4	0.96
Heart valve replacement	6.6	7.9	0.84	10.8	14.1	0.77
All moderate-mortality procedures	3.1	4.3	0.73[a]	8.3	9.2	0.90
Procedures with high mortality						
Repair of hip fracture	8.1	5.6	1.44	18.8	16.0	1.18[a]
Concurrent valve replacement/bypass surgery	20.8	12.2	1.71[a]	21.0	17.9	1.17
All high-mortality procedures	8.4	5.8	1.45[a]	18.9	16.1	1.18[a]

[a]Manitoba–New England differences were significant at $P < .05$.

219

Table 3

Adjusted comparisons for mortality in the 30 days and 6 months after surgery

Procedure	30-Day mortality			6-Month mortality		
	Adjusted odds ratio: Manitoba–New England[a]	P	No. of deaths	Adjusted odds ratio: Manitoba–New England[a]	P	No. of deaths
Procedures with low mortality						
Total hip replacement	1.19 (0.70–2.03)	.52	70	0.79 (0.53–1.18)	.25	152
Simple cholecystectomy	0.77 (0.55–1.07)	.12	260	0.60 (0.47–0.77)	<.01	568
Open prostatectomy	—[b]	—	—	1.26 (0.74–2.15)	.39	61
Carotid endarterectomy	0.91 (0.45–1.82)	.78	95	0.84 (0.54–1.33)	.46	241
Transurethral prostatectomy	1.27 (0.94–1.71)	.11	218	1.08 (0.93–1.25)	.30	1,038
All low-mortality procedures	0.93 (0.77–1.12)	.43	667	0.79 (0.71–0.89)	<.01	2,058
Procedures with moderate mortality						
Cholecystectomy with exploration of the common bile duct	0.83 (0.54–1.29)	.41	126	0.96 (0.70–1.32)	.80	231
Coronary artery bypass graft surgery	0.87 (0.61–1.23)	.42	326	0.75 (0.56–1.02)	.07	501
Transurethral prostatectomy with malignancy	0.78 (0.49–1.24)	.29	106	0.95 (0.78–1.16)	.60	573
Heart valve replacement	0.87 (0.48–1.57)	.65	111	0.72 (0.45–1.16)	.18	196
All moderate-mortality procedures	0.83 (0.66–1.03)	.09	669	0.82 (0.71–0.94)	<.01	1,501
Procedures with high mortality						
Repair of hip fracture	1.38 (1.21–1.57)	<.01	1,279	1.14 (1.04–1.25)	<.01	3,460
Concurrent valve replacement/bypass surgery	1.93 (1.06–3.51)	.03	74	1.26 (0.71–2.23)	.43	99
All high-mortality procedures	1.40 (1.24–1.59)	<.01	1,353	1.14 (1.05–1.25)	<.01	3,559

[a]Values in parentheses are 95% confidence intervals.
[b]Insufficient number of deaths for statistical adjustment.

United States. Among individual procedures studied, mortality after simple cholecystectomy (but not after cholecystectomy with common duct exploration) was significantly lower in Manitoba at 6 months. Patients who underwent concurrent valve replacement and coronary bypass in New England had significantly lower mortality at 30 days, but not at 6 months. This finding is based on relatively small numbers and does not hold for the other cardiovascular surgical procedures.

The rate of hip fracture, the age of the patients, and the presence of other high-risk diagnoses were nearly identical in Manitoba and New England (Table 1). Depending on the procedure used, short-term mortality after repair of hip fracture was from 34 to 70 percent higher in Manitoba. Statistically significant differences in mortality after repair of hip fracture both 30 days and 6 months after surgery were found when Manitoba data from 1980 to 1986 were used for the comparison. Differences in mortality had diminished by 6 months after surgery.

Using Manitoba hip fracture data from 1983 to 1986 weakened the comparisons with New England data from 1984 and 1985. Manitoba 30-day mortality dropped from 8.8 percent in 1980 to 1982 to 7.4 percent in 1983 to 1986; similar improvements were noted for 6-month mortality. This change led to a decline in the Manitoba–New England odds ratios for mortality after repair of hip fracture; for 30-day mortality the adjusted odds ratios dropped from 1.38 (for Manitoba data from 1980 to 1986) to 1.25 (significant at the .01 level) and, for 6-month mortality, from 1.14 to 1.03 (not significant at the .05 level). Similar recalculations using Manitoba data from 1983 to 1986 produced no changes in Table 3, except that the confidence intervals for adjusted 6-month mortality of "all high-mortality procedures" then included 1.0 (not significant, $P = .55$).

Hospital Volume

Each hospital was categorized as having "relatively high" or "relatively low" surgical volume on each procedure according to the number of operations performed on the elderly; hospitals were specified as above or below the median value generated by pooling Manitoba and New England data for each procedure. The mean annual hospital volumes for prostatectomy and total hip replacement were significantly greater in Manitoba, while the mean annual volume for cholecystectomy was higher in New England. Volumes for the open heart procedures, carotid endarterectomy, and repair of hip fracture were roughly similar.

When surgical volume was incorporated into the regression equations, high-volume hospitals showed lower mortality in four of five statistically significant comparisons. With five different procedures involved, there appeared to be no special pattern to the results. The Manitoba–New England odds ratios changed very little with the addition of this volume variable; thus, differences between New England and Manitoba in each hospital's experience with each procedure do not markedly affect the comparisons between countries.

Using Manitoba data from 1980 to 1986 and pooling across all procedures, the odds ratios for 30-day mortality slightly favor New England (1.12 to 1.22, depending on the statistical model); these ratios are close to 1.00 (0.90 to 0.99) when repair of hip fracture (which has the largest number of cases) is not included. Considering 6-month mortality for all procedures, the odds ratios are again close to 1.00 (0.94 to 1.05); if repair of hip fracture is left out, the ratios slightly favor Manitoba (0.79 to 0.92). Adjusted odds ratios do show higher postsurgical mortality rates in New England in 6 of 10 comparisons at 30 days and 7 of 11 comparisons at 6 months (Table 3). In 8 of 10 cases, long-term mortality comparisons were more favorable to Manitoba than were short-term comparisons.

COMMENT

To determine whether higher health care expenditures in the United States than in Canada are associated with improved health outcomes, we used health insurance databases to compare mortality rates in Manitoba and New England after 11 surgical procedures. Short-term mortality favored New England after hip fracture repair and concurrent valve replacement/coronary bypass grafting. For other procedures, no significant differences in short-term mortality were found. By 6 months after surgery, mortality rates had shifted toward favoring Manitoba for low- and moderate-risk procedures.

While controlling for case mix using observational data, whether administrative or otherwise, is contentious (24), randomization among hospitals or countries is impractical. Observational studies provide the only plausible source of insight. Moreover, administrative data have been shown to do nearly as well for risk adjustment as data that rely on physiological measures and physician judgment of health status (15, 21). Given current interest in reducing U.S. health care expenditures, studying the outcomes of treatment in Canada and the United States in more detail seems especially timely. Our data offer this opportunity.

It is also important to distinguish between the factors that may influence operative mortality (30-day mortality) and 6-month mortality. The former is strongly associated with the severity of the illness and such institutional effects as volume (25) or intensity of care (26). Differences in hospital expenditures would have their greatest effect on short-term mortality. Long-term mortality may be more strongly influenced by the underlying health status of the population.

The lack of significant differences in short-term mortality for the low- and moderate-risk procedures suggests that the increased hospital expenditures within the United States may not lead to substantially improved outcomes for these procedures. That concurrent valve replacement/coronary bypass surgery is associated with lower mortality in New England, while no differences were detected for valve replacement and coronary artery bypass graft when performed separately, is difficult to interpret. While different selection criteria operating in each health care system might lead to unmeasured case-mix differences, the inconsistency of the findings for these three cardiovascular procedures argues against substantial differences in the quality of care between Manitoba and New England. Similarly, the lack of a difference that favors New England for the remainder of the low- and moderate-risk procedures argues against major differences favoring New England.

We need to explore possible reasons both for the short-term mortality differences observed in patients with hip fractures and for the improvement in Manitoba survival between the periods 1980 to 1982 and 1983 to 1986. Case mix seems unlikely to explain the short-term mortality differences observed for patients with hip fractures. First, hip fracture represents a condition for which hospitalization and surgical treatment are unavoidable; differential selection is unlikely to be a cause of unmeasured confounding by case mix. Both the incidence of hip fracture and hip fracture survival are strongly related to age, gender, and underlying health status (27), while the incidence rates for hip fracture are similar in the two regions. Even though we find somewhat higher rates of hip fracture repair among Manitobans in the 85- to 89-year and 90+-year age ranges, the Manitoba–New England odds ratios dropped only slightly (0.01 or 0.02) when six, rather than three, age groups were used in the analysis. Second, the available evidence suggests that the underlying health status of the population is better in Manitoba than in New England. Mortality rates for men and women aged 65, 75, and 85 years favor Manitoba by from 2 to 19 percent. This bias would thus be in favor of Manitoba, while our results demonstrated improved outcomes in New England.

Short-term mortality differences may also be influenced both by the geographic distribution of patients and hospitals in Manitoba (with the subsequent delays in treatment) and by differences among hospitals associated with surgical volume. Twenty-four percent of Manitoba patients are transferred prior to hip fracture repair, compared with about 5 percent for New England. From 1980 to 1986, short-term mortality after hip fracture repair was 7.3 percent for metropolitan Winnipeg residents, but 9.2 percent for other Manitobans. Such 30-day mortality averaged 9.5 percent for Manitoba patients who had their hip fractures repaired at 13 low-volume hospitals (annual volume, <54 operations among the elderly), while patients at 5 high-volume hospitals averaged 7.7 percent. More detailed study of the causes of these observed differences might be particularly valuable.

The trends toward lower long-term mortality rates in Manitoba (compared with New England) are more difficult to interpret. The lower risk may simply be a consequence of the overall lower age-specific risk of death in Manitoba. Differences in access to outpatient and long-term care in Manitoba may influence not only postsurgical mortality, but also overall mortality in the population. However, our data can provide no evidence for either of these hypotheses.

Our study suggests that operative mortality in New England is similar to that in Manitoba for most of the conditions examined. That mortality following hip fracture repair is significantly higher in Manitoba is cause for concern, and further investigation has been initiated. Because mortality is only one of many important outcomes, our analyses represent just a first step in investigating similarities and differences between the U.S. and Canadian health care systems. As with studies of small-area variations that have pointed out the need to determine "which rate is right" (28), our findings should be used primarily to identify fruitful areas for additional research. Careful study of the processes of care in each system and their association with a broad range of outcomes will contribute to improved health care effectiveness for both Canadians and Americans.

REFERENCES

1. Newhouse, J.P., Anderson, G. M., and Roos, L. L. Hospital spending in the United States and Canada: A comparison. *Health Aff.* 7(5): 6–16, 1988.
2. Evans, R. G. Perspectives: Canada. *Health Aff.* 7(5): 17–24, 1988.
3. Anderson, G. M., Newhouse, J. P., and Roos, L. L. Hospital care for elderly patients with diseases of the circulatory system: A comparison of hospital use in the United States and Canada. *N. Engl. J. Med.* 321: 1443–1448, 1989.
4. Minister of Supply and Services, Canada. *Canada Yearbook 1988.* Ottawa, Ontario, Publication Division, Statistics Canada, 1988.
5. Mindell, W. E., Vayda, E., and Cardillo, B. Ten-year trends in Canada for selected operations. *Can. Med. Assoc. J.* 127: 23–27, 1982.
6. Health Economics and Statistics Branch. *National Health Expenditures, 1975–1985 (Provincial).* Health and Welfare Canada, Ottawa, 1987.
7. Minister of Supply and Services Canada. *Health Personnel in Canada 1987.* Minister of National Health and Welfare, Ottawa, 1988.
8. American Medical Association. *Physician Characteristics and Distribution in the United States.* Chicago, Ill., 1987.
9. Nicholls, E. S., Jung, J., and Davies, J. W. Cardiovascular disease mortality in Canada. *Can. Med. Assoc. J.* 125: 981–992, 1981.
10. Higgins, M. W. and Luepker, R. V. *Trends in Coronary Heart Disease Mortality: The Influence of Medical Care.* Oxford University Press, New York, 1988.
11. Roos, L. L., Sharp, S. M., and Wajda, A. Assessing data quality: A Computerized approach. *Soc. Sci. Med.* 28: 175–182, 1989.
12. Wajda, A. and Roos, L. L. Simplifying record linkage: Software and strategy. *Comput. Biol. Med.* 17: 239–248, 1987.
13. Lave, J., Dobson, A., and Walton, C. The potential use of Health Care Financing Administration data sets for health care services research. *Health Care Financ. Rev.* 5: 93–98, 1983.
14. Daley, J., et al. Predicting hospital-associated mortality for Medicare patients: A method for patients with stroke, pneumonia, acute myocardial infarction, and congestive heart failure. *JAMA* 260: 3617–3624, 1988.
15. Charlson, M. E., et al. A new method of classifying prognostic comorbidity in longitudinal studies: Development and validation. *J. Chronic Dis.* 40: 373–383, 1987.

16. Pompei, P., Charlson, M. E., and Douglas, R. G. Clinical assessments as predictors of one-year survival after hospitalization: Implication for prognostic stratification. *J. Clin. Epidemiol.* 41: 275–284, 1988.
17. Roos, L. L., Sharp, S. M., and Cohen, M. M. Risk adjustment in claims-based research: The search for efficient approaches. *J. Clin. Epidemiol.* 42: 1193–1206, 1989.
18. Roos, N. P., et al. Mortality and reoperation after prostatic hyperplasia. *N. Engl. J. Med.* 320: 1120–1124, 1989.
19. Showstack, J. A., et al. Association of volume with outcome of coronary artery bypass graft surgery: Scheduled vs nonscheduled operations. *JAMA* 257: 785–789, 1987.
20. Kenzora, J. E., et al. Hip fracture mortality: Relation to age, treatment, preoperative illness, time of surgery and complications. *Clin. Orthop.* 186: 45–56, 1984.
21. Flood, A. B. and Scott, W. R. *Hospital Structure and Performance.* The Johns Hopkins University Press, Baltimore, Md., 1987.
22. Harrell, F. E. The LOGIST procedure. In *SUGI Supplemental Library User's Guide, Version 5 Edition,* edited by R. P. Hastings, et al., pp. 269–293. SAS Institute, Cary, N.C., 1986.
23. Ginsberg, P. M. and Carter, G. M. Medicare case-mix index increase. *Health Care Financ. Rev.* 4: 51–65, 1986.
24. Byar, D. P. Why databases should not replace randomized clinical trials. *Biometrics.* 36: 337–342, 1980.
25. Lubitz, J., Riley, G. and Newton, M. Outcomes of surgery among the Medicare aged: Mortality after surgery. *Health Care Financ. Rev.* 6: 103–115, 1985.
26. Garber, A. M., Fuchs, V. R., and Silverman, J. F. Case mix, costs, and outcomes—differences between faculty and community services in a university hospital. *N. Engl. J. Med.* 310: 1231–1237, 1984.
27. Robbins, J. A. Hip fractures. *Med. Rounds* 2: 99–115, 1989.
28. Wennberg, J. E. Which rate is right? *N. Engl. J. Med.* 314: 310–311, 1986.

CHAPTER 13

Use of Coronary Artery Bypass Surgery in the United States and Canada: Influence of Age and Income

Geoffrey M. Anderson, Kevin Grumbach, Harold S. Luft, Leslie L. Roos, Cameron Mustard, and Robert Brook

The continuing debate over health care reform in the United States has led to growing interest in alternative forms of health care financing and organization. The Canadian health care system is one of the most frequently mentioned alternatives. This interest stems in large part from the ability of the single-payer Canadian system to provide universal coverage at a lower per capita cost than the United States, while having lower infant mortality rates and longer life expectancy. However, these apparent advantages in terms of aggregate measures of cost and outcome may obscure some important differences in terms of specific aspects of access and quality of care. Coronary artery bypass surgery (CABS) has often been cited as a specific procedure that may highlight some of the important differences in quality and access to care in the two countries.

Critics of the Canadian system point to waiting lists for CABS as a visible indication of the restrictions placed on high-technology procedures and of poor access to needed services that result from government regulation of health care (1). On the other hand, studies in the United States that indicate differences in use of CABS by race (2), income (3), and insurance status (4) can be taken as an indication of the continuing inequities in access found in a health care system that relies more on market forces than on regulation.

Published in the *Journal of the American Medical Association*, 269(13), pp. 1661–1666, 1993. Copyright 1993, American Medical Association.

Our study used comprehensive hospital discharge databases from the Canadian provinces of Ontario, Manitoba, and British Columbia and from the states of California and New York to estimate the CABS rates in these jurisdictions. The study also examined differences in access to CABS by age group and by income class.

In Canada, both the number of hospitals performing CABS and the number of procedures performed are controlled by provincial governments. In New York, the number of hospitals performing CABS, but not the number of procedures, is controlled. Essentially, California has no controls over either the number of hospitals offering CABS or the number of procedures performed. Analysis of overall and age-specific rates of CABS use will help clarify the impact of the control of supply on utilization. Analysis by income class will shed light on the differences in access between the Canadian universal health insurance system and the system in the United States, where a large proportion of the nonelderly population is underinsured or uninsured.

METHODS

Sources of Data on CABS

This population-based study used comprehensive hospital discharge data collected in New York, California, Ontario, Manitoba, and British Columbia. Nonfederal hospitals in each jurisdiction are required to submit an abstract for each discharge to a central agency. Each abstract contains information on procedures performed on the patient, as well as information on the age and place of residence of the patient. California, New York, and Manitoba code procedures using the *International Classification of Diseases, Ninth Revision, Clinical Modification.* In these jurisdictions, CABS cases were defined as codes 36.1, 36.10 through 36.16, and 36.19. Ontario and British Columbia code procedures using the *Canadian Classification of Diagnostic, Therapeutic, and Surgical Procedures.* In these two jurisdictions, CABS cases were defined as codes 48.11 through 48.19. In all jurisdictions, cases were identified if a CABS procedure was listed as any one of the procedures contained on the abstract. Therefore, the identified cases included CABS performed with other procedures, including surgery on the valves of the heart. The cases used in the study were limited to procedures performed in hospitals in the jurisdiction on residents of that jurisdiction. In the American jurisdictions, cases were identified by calendar year. In the Canadian jurisdictions, cases were identified by fiscal year (April 1 to March 31).

Calculation of Overall and Age-Specific Use Rates

The CABS cases identified from the discharge abstracts were used as the numerators in the calculation of rates. Data on the population distributions in the various jurisdictions obtained from federal or provincial authorities were used as denominators in overall or age-specific rates. The adult population was defined as residents aged 20 years and older in the Canadian jurisdictions and 21 years and older in the American jurisdiction. Age-adjusted rates were calculated using the direct method, with California as the standard population and the age-specific rates in each jurisdiction applied to this population distribution.

Calculation of Use Rates by Income Class

Data on the income of individual patients are not available from hospital discharge abstracts in either Canada or the United States. In our study, census data were used to define income categories for geographic areas. Patients were assigned to these areas on the basis of the ZIP or postal code of their residence listed on the discharge abstracts. Because median household income data were not available for all areas in Canada, mean household income was used to measure income status in all geographic areas.

Canadian postal codes consist of six characters. The first three characters of the postal code define a forward sorting area (FSA), and these FSAs were used to define geographic areas. Census data for the population living in or near urban centers are available at the FSA level directly from Statistics Canada. Census data at the FSA level are not available directly from Statistics Canada for those living in rural areas. Census data at the FSA level for these rural areas were constructed by aggregating census data from enumeration areas (the smallest unit of analysis available within the Canadian census) up to the FSA level, using a file that links enumeration areas to postal codes. In the United States, the five-digit ZIP code from discharge abstracts was linked directly to census data using a commercially available data file.

The Canadian income data were drawn from the 1986 census and population figures from 1987 estimates. ZIP code level population and income data for New York and California for 1987 were interpolated from 1980 and 1990 data.

In each jurisdiction, the census population and income data were used to divide FSA or ZIP code areas into population-based income quintiles. This was done by first ranking the areas within each jurisdiction by mean household income. Areas with the lowest incomes were then aggregated until their population accounted for 20 percent of the population of the jurisdiction. These areas were identified as the lowest income quintile areas. This process was repeated to generate each of the succeeding income quintiles in each jurisdiction.

The average adult population of an FSA in the three Canadian jurisdictions was between 14,000 and 15,000 compared with 12,000 for an average ZIP code area in California and 7,000 for the average ZIP code area in New York. Larger populations per ZIP code or FSA area may result in greater heterogeneity of household incomes within an area. However, despite the differences in average ZIP code or FSA population size across the jurisdictions, the distribution and variation in average household income among the five income quintiles were similar.

In Ontario, approximately 5 percent of cases of CABS identified as being performed on residents had missing or invalid postal codes and these cases were excluded from the income analysis. All discharges from British Columbia and Manitoba were linked to census data. In California and New York, approximately 1 percent and 1.5 percent, respectively, of discharges had missing or invalid ZIP codes and were not linked to income categories.

Rates of use by income were calculated by using the census data to define the relevant denominators in each income quintile and the postal or ZIP code information on the discharge abstracts to assign cases to the appropriate numerator. The use by income quintile was calculated for all jurisdictions using only 1987 discharges, the discharge year closest to the year in which the income data were available for Canada.

RESULTS

Figure 1 indicates the rates of CABS performed in each jurisdiction per 100,000 adults. In all five regions, an initial decrease in utilization between 1983 and 1985 was followed by a subsequent increase in utilization. In 1989, the overall rates in California were more than twice those found in Manitoba, and the rate in New York was about 40 percent higher than the rate in Ontario.

Table 1 presents data on age-specific CABS rates in both 1983 and 1989. As shown in Figure 2, each of the jurisdictions has experienced growth in the rates of surgery in the elderly population, with the largest proportional increases occurring in the population aged 75 years and older. During the same time in which rates increased rapidly in the elderly age groups, rates for 20- to 44-year-olds decreased in four of the jurisdictions and rates for 45- to 54-year-olds decreased consistently in all five jurisdictions. Rates for 55- to 64-year-olds remained relatively stable.

In 1989, California had the highest age-specific rates for every age category with the exception of the youngest age group, for which both Ontario and New York had somewhat higher rates than California. The largest proportional differences in age-specific rates between California and the other jurisdictions were found in the oldest age groups. For those aged 75 years and older, California rates were 72 percent higher than those in New York and over three times that of any of the three Canadian jurisdictions. Over time, procedures in the elderly constituted a steadily increasing proportion of CABS performed in each jurisdiction. By 1989, in all jurisdictions other than Ontario, greater than one half of CABS were performed on the elderly (aged 65 years and older).

Table 2 demonstrates the relative importance of age distributions and age-specific CABS rates in explaining the overall difference in CABS rates between California and the other jurisdictions. In 1989, the combined rate for the three

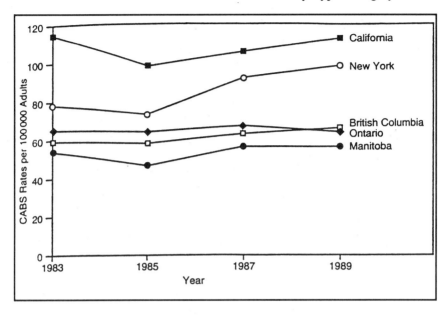

Figure 1. Coronary artery bypass surgery (CABS) rates per 100,000 adults.

Table 1

Age-specific coronary artery bypass surgery rates[a] in 1983 and 1989

Jurisdiction	Age group, yr				
	20–44[b]	45–54	55–64	65–74	≥75
	1983				
California	10.2	144.7	314.4	404.1	153.9
New York	9.2	106.0	214.5	205.6	48.0
British Columbia	7.9	88.1	192.5	202.5	20.5
Ontario	9.7	99.6	185.8	136.9	30.9
Manitoba	3.2	74.3	163.5	150.8	39.4
	1989				
California	6.3	95.1	268.2	478.7	312.2
New York	7.0	85.9	231.4	362.3	181.1
British Columbia	4.0	57.3	158.3	237.5	100.0
Ontario	7.4	88.5	186.9	226.5	50.0
Manitoba	3.4	48.1	152.4	212.8	89.4

[a]Per 100,000.
[b]Ages 21–44 years for New York and California.

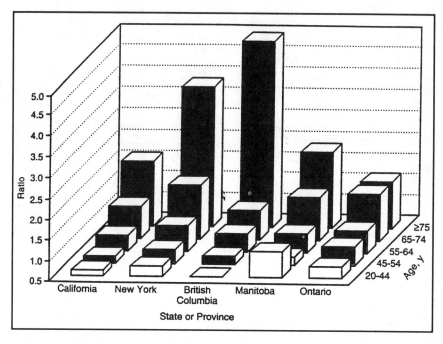

Figure 2. Ratio of 1989 age-specific coronary artery bypass surgery (CABS) rates to 1983 age-specific CABS rates.

Table 2

Effect of age distribution and rates in the elderly on difference in surgical rates[a]

Jurisdiction	1989 crude rate	Absolute difference from California	1989 age-adjusted rate[b]	Absolute difference from California	1989 rate using California rates for elderly	Absolute difference from California
California	112.5	—	112.5	—	112.5	—
New York	97.4	−15.1	88.4	−24.1	107.3	−5.2
British Columbia	63.2	−49.3	57.4	−55.1	90.8	−21.7
Manitoba	53.2	−59.3	49.5	−63.0	89.3	−23.2
Ontario	66.2	−46.3	63.1	−49.4	102.7	−9.8
Three Canadian jurisdictions combined	65.5	−47.0	62.4	−50.1	100.0	−12.5

[a]Per 100,000.
[b]Using direct age adjustments with California as the referent population.

Canadian jurisdictions was 58 percent of the rate in California. The effect of differences in age distribution can be accounted for by calculating age-adjusted rates. Direct age-adjusted rates based on the 1989 California age distribution are presented in column 4 of Table 2. In 1989, the age-adjusted CABS rate in the three Canadian jurisdictions combined was 55 percent of the rate in California.

The impact of differences in use rates among the elderly can be measured by calculating the rates expected in each jurisdiction if that jurisdiction had the same age distribution as California as well as the same age-specific rates among the elderly as California. The differences between age-adjusted rates using California rates for the elderly are much smaller than those for age adjustment only, indicating that use among the elderly plays a major role in explaining the higher overall rates in California. For example, all but 5.2 per 100,000 (22 percent) of the 24.1 per 100,000 difference in age-adjusted rates between New York and California can be accounted for by higher rates of use by the elderly in California. Similarly, all but 12.5 per 100,000 (25 percent) of the difference in rates between California and the three Canadian jurisdictions combined can be accounted for by the higher rates of use in the elderly in California.

Table 3 presents CABS rates in 1987 by the income quintile of residence. In Figure 3, the relationship between these rates and the relative income of the quintile, measured as the ratio of the average income within the quintile to the average income of the entire jurisdiction, is presented. The range of relative incomes across the quintiles is somewhat broader in the U.S. jurisdictions than in

Table 3

1987 Coronary artery bypass surgery rates[a] by average household income of area of residence

Income area	Quintile	Canada[b]	California	New York
		Nonelderly population		
Highest	Q1	43.7	64.4	74.2
	Q2	42.7	60.0	61.2
	Q3	43.5	58.2	59.5
	Q4	44.1	56.3	54.2
Lowest	Q5	48.1	49.7	38.1
		Elderly population		
Highest	Q1	194.6	357.5	302.3
	Q2	168.3	361.6	236.7
	Q3	147.5	364.0	209.8
	Q4	151.5	348.5	188.3
Lowest	Q5	145.2	298.8	159.2

[a]Per 100,000.
[b]British Columbia, Manitoba, and Ontario.

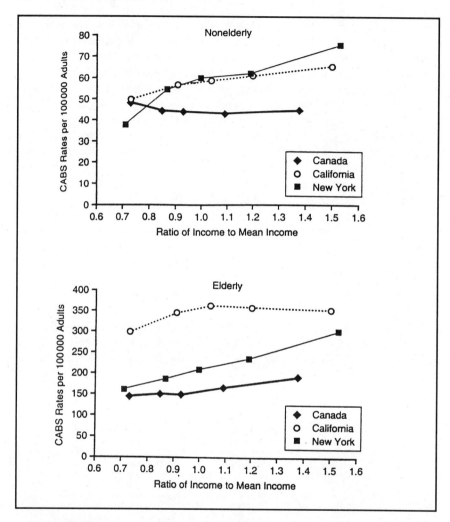

Figure 3. Coronary artery bypass surgery (CABS) rates and relative incomes, 1983 through1989. Note that the scales used on the vertical axes differ between nonelderly (top) and elderly (bottom) data.

Canada, with the lowest quintile in New York having a relative income of 0.71 and the highest quintile having a relative income of 1.53. In Canada, the respective relative rates are 0.73 and 1.38.

In the nonelderly population, CABS rates steadily increased from the lowest to the highest income quintile in California and in New York. In Canada, those living in the lowest income areas had the highest CABS rate, while rates were similar across the four other income groups. The pattern of use for the elderly by income of the area of residence is less straightforward. New York shows a steady gradient with the highest rates for those living in the highest income areas. In California, the rates are similar for those living in the four highest income areas and lowest for those living in the lowest income areas. In Canada, those living in the three lowest income areas have similar rates with higher rates in the two more affluent income areas.

COMMENT

This study draws on administrative data to examine the use of coronary artery bypass surgery in Canada and the United States. Although these data sources contain a great amount of information, our results should be interpreted in light of some important limitations.

One limitation is that our data are drawn from only five jurisdictions and may not be completely representative of national practice. However, the data do cover care provided to about 20 percent of the United States population and over 50 percent of the Canadian population.

Another potential limitation is inaccuracies in the administrative data. Although no systematic validation of all the data sources used in this study was undertaken, there is evidence to support their accuracy. For the Canadian jurisdictions, the overall numbers of procedures identified using the hospital discharge abstracts were very similar to the numbers identified using comprehensive physician billing data. In Manitoba, a separate study showed that 99.3 percent of CABS cases identified from hospital discharge abstracts could be matched with a procedure claim filed by the physician (5). Also, as a follow-up to this study, the hospital discharge abstract data from New York, Ontario, and British Columbia were used to select charts for more detailed analysis of clinical factors associated with CABS. Virtually all cases of CABS identified in the discharge abstracts were verified in chart audits.

Our analysis has been limited to services provided within each jurisdiction for residents of that jurisdiction and, therefore, excludes a detailed examination of out-of-jurisdiction use. Data from 1987 and 1988 indicate that 2 percent of the Medicare population residing in California who received CABS did so outside that state, a figure consistent with overall out-of-state hospital admissions. In New York, almost 13 percent of the Medicare population who had CABS were operated on outside the state, a figure over twice as the high overall proportion of out-of-state admissions. Over half of these out-of-state procedures occurred in southern states. Data from Ontario and British Columbia indicate that in 1989 approximately 5 percent of the CABS billed to the provincial health insurance plans were performed outside these provinces. Also, it should be noted that our analysis excluded procedures performed in federal hospitals. For California and New York, this means that operations performed in Veterans Affairs hospitals were not included in the calculation of rates. Aggregate data provided by the Department of Veterans Affairs indicate that these hospitals accounted for less than 3 percent of total CABS in either jurisdiction in 1989 (6). In Canada, no CABS procedures were performed in federal hospitals.

Our analysis shows declines in CABS rates in each jurisdiction between 1983 and 1985 and then increases between 1985 and 1989. The drop in rates between 1983 and 1985 may reflect changes in the indications for the procedure, changes in the prevalence or severity of coronary artery disease, or the introduction of percutaneous transluminal coronary angioplasty (PTCA) as an alternative form of revascularization. In both countries, uniform coding of PTCA first became standardized in 1987, although PTCA was widely used prior to that date.

In New York, rates of PTCA in the nonelderly grew from 37 per 100,000 in 1987 to 46 per 100,000 in 1989, and rates in the elderly grew from 69 per 100,000 to 110 per 100,000. In California, rates of PTCA in the nonelderly rose from 71 per 100,000 in 1987 to 83 per 100,000 in 1989, and in the elderly from 252 per 100,000 to 361 per 100,000. Accurate age-specific data on PTCA were not available for the Canadian jurisdictions. In 1989, rates for PTCA in the three Canadian jurisdictions reached levels of about 40 to 50 per 100,000 adults.

Between 1983 and 1989, overall CABS rates were consistently highest in California and lowest in the Canadian jurisdictions and the differences were greatest for the oldest age groups. These differences in CABS rates were much greater than the differences in mortality rates for ischemic heart disease (7) or hospital discharge rates for ischemic heart disease (8) between the two countries. This suggests that the differences in CABS rates are not primarily driven by differences in disease prevalence, but rather by differences in treatment practices.

Also between 1983 and 1989, each jurisdiction experienced a shift of CABS utilization, with decreasing rates of use in the younger age groups and increasing rates of use in the elderly. In particular, use rates increased most rapidly in the very elderly—those aged 75 years and older. As a result of these age-specific shifts and (to a much lesser degree) the aging of the population, by 1989, CABS patients in every jurisdiction but Ontario were more likely to be elderly than nonelderly. The increase in CABS volume among the elderly almost completely offset and, in the case of New York, actually exceeded the decrease in volume among the nonelderly.

This redistribution of use by age might be expected in an environment of constrained resources for CABS that makes CABS use a "zero sum game" in which increased access for one group must come at the expense of diminished access for others. However, even open-ended systems such as that in use in California experienced this age-shift in utilization, suggesting that other forces might be behind this shift.

Evidence from both countries suggests that the prevalence of ischemic heart disease has been decreasing for the last two decades (7, 9). The lower rates of CABS in the nonelderly population may be the result of the decreased prevalence of ischemic heart disease in that age group. However, the increased CABS rates in the elderly suggest that there has been a broadening of the indications for use of the procedure in this group.

High rates of CABS in the elderly are not only important in understanding changes in use within jurisdictions, but also in understanding differences across jurisdictions. In particular, the higher overall rates of CABS in California are driven predominantly by the higher rates for the elderly. In 1989, an individual in California aged 75 years and older was 1.7 times more likely than an individual of the same age in New York and over three times more likely than an individual from the same age group in any of the Canadian jurisdictions to undergo CABS. About 75 percent of the difference in the overall rate of CABS between California and the Canadian jurisdictions and between California and New York is the result of higher rates of CABS in those aged 65 years and older in California.

Canadian provincial governments strictly control both the number of hospitals performing CABS and the funding for those procedures, New York controls the number of hospitals performing CABS but does not control the number of procedures performed in those institutions, and California does not limit either the number of institutions or the funding for CABS. Our results suggest that the regulation possible under the centralized control of a Canadian-style, single-payer system is associated with lower levels of use of CABS and particularly lower levels of use among the elderly. This control of use within a jurisdiction may exert pressure on the system that results in public demands for expanded services, as found in Canada, or high levels of out-of-state care, as found in New York.

In terms of the quality of care, the differences in use in these different jurisdictions raise the important question of whether the control of the resources for CABS results in a rationing of care that denies access to needed medical services (particularly for the elderly) or whether a lack of centralized control of resources in a fee-for-service system results in the overuse of CABS. This question can only be addressed with detailed analyses of unmet need, appropriateness (10), and outcomes (11) of care.

We also examined the relationship between income and CABS rates to determine if there might be financial barriers to care in the United States that might not be found under the universal health insurance system in Canada. Because the hospital discharge abstracts used in the analysis do not contain specific information on patient income, this part of the study used data on the average income of families in the area in which patients resided as a proxy for data on the income of individual patients. Although this approach has some limitations, it has been used in previous studies of access to hospital services (3, 12) in both countries and provides an accepted method to study the important issue of equity of access.

In both Canada and the United States, ischemic heart disease is most common in the lowest income groups (12, 13). In Canada, the nonelderly living in the poorest areas had somewhat higher CABS rates than those living in higher income areas. In California and New York, the nonelderly living in the poorest areas had the lowest CABS rates and rates increased with the average income of the area. Although overall CABS rates for the nonelderly were higher in the U.S. jurisdictions, those living in the poorest areas of New York and California had similar or lower rates than those living in the poorest parts of Canada.

The analysis of income and use rates for the elderly is complicated by the fact that our measures of income are not age specific and that wealth, rather than income, may be a better indicator of financial resources for the elderly. Moreover, in both countries, the elderly are covered under universal health insurance programs. Thus, although in each jurisdiction the elderly living in the lowest income areas had the lowest CABS rates, we did not detect the same consistent gradient in CABS rates with respect to income in the United States that we found among nonelderly Americans.

CONCLUSIONS

Our results show that CABS rates in all five jurisdictions have increased rapidly for the elderly and have remained relatively stable or decreased in the nonelderly. This may reflect the replacement of CABS with PTCA as a revascularization technique for a portion of the nonelderly and broadening indications for revascularization by any method for older patients. Whether rates of CABS in the elderly have reached their zenith or will continue to grow and whether this growth is appropriate remain to be determined.

The single-payer system in Canada is associated with lower overall rates of CABS, and in particular lower rates of CABS for the elderly, than found in the United States. Within the United States, CABS rates are lower in regulated New York than in unregulated California. These differences cannot be primarily attributed to differences in the incidence of ischemic heart disease. This suggests differences in the choice of treatment of ischemic heart disease—differences that may be the result of control of the resources required to perform CABS.

Among the nonelderly in both New York and California, CABS rates are lowest for people living in the lowest income areas; in Canada, they are highest for people living in the lowest income areas. This suggests that the Canadian universal health insurance system reduces the influence of income on access to services.

Although the differences in CABS utilization between the two countries are clear, further research is needed to clarify the effects of these differences on the costs and quality of care.

REFERENCES

1. Naylor, C. D. A different view of queues in Ontario. *Health Aff.* 10: 110–128, 1991.
2. Wenneker, M. B., and Epstein, A. M. Racial inequalities in the use of procedures for patients with ischemic heart disease in Massachusetts. *JAMA* 261: 253–257, 1989.

3. Gittelsohn, A. M., Halpern, J., and Sanchez, R. L. Income, race and surgery in Maryland. *Am. J. Public Health* 81: 1435–1440, 1991.
4. Hadley, J., Steinberg, E. P., and Feder, J. Comparison of uninsured and privately insured hospital patients: Condition on admission, resource use, and outcome. *JAMA* 265: 374–379, 1991.
5. Roos, L. L., Sharp, S. M., and Wajda, A. Assessing data quality: A computerized approach. *Soc. Sci. Med.* 28: 175–182, 1989.
6. Hammermeister, K., Veterans Administration Hospital, Denver, Colo. Personal communication, 1992.
7. Nicholls, E., et al. *Cardiovascular Disease in Canada.* Catalogue 82-544. Statistics Canada and Health and Welfare Canada, Ottawa, December 1986.
8. Anderson, G. M., Newhouse, J. P., and Roos, L. L. Hospital care for elderly patients with diseases of the circulatory system: A comparison of hospital use in the United States and Canada. *N. Engl. J. Med.* 321: 1443–1448, 1989.
9. Sempos, C., et al. Divergence of recent trends in coronary mortality for the four major race-sex groups in the United States. *Am. J. Public Health* 78: 1422–1427, 1988.
10. Winslow, C. M., et al. The appropriateness of performing coronary artery bypass surgery. *JAMA* 260: 505–509, 1988.
11. Roos, L. L., et al. Health and surgical outcomes in Canada and the United States. *Health Aff.* 11: 56–72, 1992.
12. Wilkins, R., Adams, O., and Brancker, A. Changes in mortality by income in urban Canada from 1971 to 1986. *Health Rep.* 1: 137–174, 1989.
13. National Center for Health Statistics. *Current Estimates From the National Health Interview Survey, 1989.* Series 10, No. 176, publication PHS 90-1504. U.S. Dept. of Health and Human Services, Washington, D.C., 1990.

CHAPTER 14

Coronary Angiography and Bypass Surgery in Manitoba and the United States: A First Comparison

Leslie L. Roos, Ruth Bond, C. David Naylor,
Mark R. Chassin, and Andrew L. Morris

Comparisons between Canadian and American health care systems are of interest to policymakers and health services researchers on both sides of the border. The high levels of public popularity for Canadian health insurance and the combination of lower costs and greater life expectancy have caught American attention (1–3). At the same time, some practitioners, both American and Canadian, have complained that Canadian restrictions on the availability of expensive advanced technology may make it increasingly difficult to maintain high quality care (4, 5).

Debates over quality of care and cost containment may be informed by comparing the characteristics of patients receiving various diagnostic and therapeutic procedures in the two countries. The use of appropriateness panels is one method to formulate such comparisons; inappropriate procedures subject patients to unnecessary risk and waste resources. Moreover, the percentage of procedures deemed appropriate seems only weakly related to the rates of a given procedure in any region. Therefore, opportunities may exist to improve the level of appropriateness, regardless of whether a procedure is being performed at a high or low rate (6).

This chapter compares the appropriateness of coronary angiography (CA) and coronary artery bypass surgery (CABS) performed during the early 1980s by one Manitoba teaching hospital with the same procedures done in several American hospitals during roughly the same period. Because no explicit Canadian criteria

Reproduced with permission of *Canadian Journal of Cardiology*, 1994, 10(1), pp. 49–56.

for appropriateness were available for the period under review, patterns of practice were compared using standards of appropriateness developed by American clinicians. Past comparisons between British and American panelists' ratings of cardiovascular procedures have shown American standards to be more liberal, rating a higher proportion of cases appropriate for treatment (7, 8). Since country-specific standards for appropriateness are likely to differ, comparisons were made based on clinical presentation and the amount of vessel disease, as well as on terms of appropriateness.

SUBJECTS AND METHODS

Sample Selection

The Manitoba hospital studied performed approximately 70 percent of the CAs and 80 percent of all cardiac surgeries done in the province in the May 1981 to December 1982 period (when the angiography patients were first entered on a waiting list for an earlier study) (9). Manitoba's mean annual rates of CAs (13.3 per 10,000 population aged 65 or over in 1981–82) and bypass surgery (6.6 per 10,000 in the same age group) in the early 1980s were considerably lower than those in the United States (6, 10–12).

Table 1 summarizes the comparison groups. The American angiography patients were 65 years of age or older (the Medicare population); these data were collected in 1981 from three hospitals in three states, representing regions with angiography rates of 50, 23, and 22 per 10,000 elderly. There were only minimal differences between Manitoba angiography patients aged 55 to 64 (200) and

Table 1

Manitoba–American comparison groups

Group	Main comparisons	Patient age	Time period	Sample size
Coronary angiography patients	1 Manitoba hospital	55 or older	1981–82	351
	3 American hospitals	65 or older	1981	628, 514, and 535, respectively
Coronary artery disease patients				
Surgically treated	1 Manitoba hospital	All ages	1981–83	245
	3 Other American hospitals	All ages	1979, 1980, 1982	161, 96, and 129, respectively
Medically treated/ no surgery	1 Manitoba hospital	All ages	1981–83	153

those 65 years of age or older (151) (see Appendix); thus, the Manitoba age qualification was set at 55 years (compared with 65 years in the United States sample) in order to increase the number of Manitoba patients.

The American bypass patients constituted a stratified random sample of all patients undergoing CABS in three other hospitals in a western state in 1979, 1980, and 1982. By tracing Manitoba angiography patients through time, we were able to compare those who were medically treated with those having bypass surgery. The Manitoba bypass patients studied were representative of all those receiving surgery at their hospital but differed somewhat from the bypass patients at the Manitoba hospital performing the remaining 20 percent of these operations. Out-of-province patients (49 cases) and cases who could not be linked with hospital discharge data (11 cases) were not included in the study (Figure 1). For the CA sample, the first angiography was chosen; the bypass group included patients undergoing surgery within 12 months of angiography. Thirteen patients in the "no surgery" group crossed over, having bypass surgery more than a year after angiography (up until March 1987). In the bypass sample, the angiography closest to the date of surgery provided the data used here; only three bypass patients had another angiogram within 1 year before surgery. Patients with prior revascularization, other heart surgery, or valvular heart disease were excluded from both the Manitoba and the American bypass samples (Figure 1).

Appropriateness Rating

The definition of appropriateness used by the expert panel, the way the panel was conducted, and the method for classifying indications as appropriate, equivocal, and inappropriate have been described elsewhere (13). The American panel results were used to organize the data for both countries; previous reports have used these criteria for chart audits of both CA and coronary artery surgery (14, 15). In the present study, those criteria and data were drawn on to make direct comparisons with Canadian procedures.

In both Canada and the United States, trained medical record abstractors used the abstraction form to assign indications to each case. Data elements recorded in the abstraction forms were the basis for assigning one or more indications to each case. For cases with more than one indication, the highest appropriateness rating was designated as the primary indication and used throughout the analysis. Complicated cases (particularly those involving both unstable angina and myocardial infarction) were classified by one of the investigators from a summary of the medical record. Instrument reliability has been described elsewhere (16); in Manitoba, inter-rater reliability in the assessment and coding of 10 duplicate records was greater than 97 percent.

Exercise treadmill results were generally present in the American hospital charts; furthermore, missing information was obtained by going back to American physicians' offices and clinics as necessary. The Manitoba research,

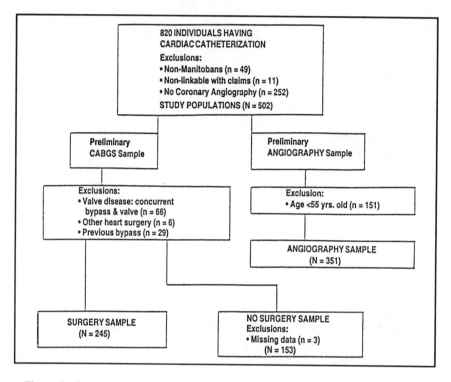

Figure 1. Generating the Manitoba samples. The surgery group includes patients with ICD-9-CM procedure codes 36.10 to 36.14; however, it excludes crossovers: surgery codes within the 36.10 to 36.14 range but occurring more than one year after angiography. The latter are included in the "no surgery" sample.

originally designed to study waiting lists, did not include contact with the referring physician in order to obtain exercise treadmill results. Although 87 percent of the Manitoba angiography patients had exercise tests in the six months before referral, results for such tests were not available in the Manitoba hospital charts. It was felt that almost all Manitoba exercise tests seen were positive. Because exercise test results influence some of the appropriateness judgements, several different assumptions as to the results of these tests were used in the analyses.

RESULTS

Coronary Angiography

The Manitoba angiography sample consisted of 351 individuals, aged 55 years or older, 66 percent of whom were male. Catheterization findings revealed similar proportions of those suffering from one-vessel disease (19 percent) and two-vessel disease (22 percent); three-vessel disease occurred relatively frequently (37 percent) while left main disease was found in 13 percent of the angiography sample.

Table 2 groups the 300 indications for CA into 12 clinical groups according to major presenting complaint (13). Compared with their American counterparts, Manitoba patients present more chronic stable angina and unstable angina, but less valve disease. Fewer Manitobans fell into the "following myocardial infarction" group; however, a number of postmyocardial infarction patients were classified into the "unstable angina" category.

Table 3 summarizes the comparative data in terms of the major categories: appropriate, equivocal, and inappropriate. Most Manitoba patients fell into categories in which treadmill testing was not needed to establish appropriateness. The first two columns in Table 3 assume that 75 and 50 percent, respectively, of the relevant Manitoba patients had positive treadmill tests. If only 25 percent had

Table 2

Clinical presentation of patients undergoing coronary angiography by site

Clinical presentation	Manitoba hospital (n = 351)	American hospital number[a]		
		1 (n = 628)	2 (n = 514)	3 (n = 535)
Chronic stable angina[b]	46%	28%	25%	28%
Unstable angina[c]	30	17	22	20
Valve disease[b]	8	19	19	17
Following myocardial infarction[b,d]	4	10	12	9
Nonspecific chest pain	8	8	4	11
Following unstable angina[e]	<1	5	7	8
Following coronary artery bypass surgery	0	5	2	1
Asymptomatic	0	3	1	2
During an acute myocardial infarction[f]	1	2	2	1
Congestive heart failure	<1	2	33	2
Following survival from sudden cardiac arrest	<1	<1	<1	<1
Other	3	1	1	2

[a]Column percentages may not add up to 100% due to rounding.

[b]Differences between the Manitoba hospital and the individual American hospitals were statistically significant at at least the 0.001 level (by χ^2 tests, $df = 6$).

[c]Coronary angiography was performed during the hospital admission occasioned by unstable angina.

[d]Defined as within six months of a myocardial infarction (but more than six days after its onset).

[e]Defined as within three months of hospital discharge following an episode of unstable angina.

[f]Defined as within six days of the onset of myocardial infarction.

Table 3

Comparisons of appropriateness of coronary angiography by
Manitoba and American hospitals

Categories	Manitoba hospital		American hospital number		
	75% positive $(n = 351)^a$	50% positive $(n = 351)^a$	1 $(n = 628)$	2 $(n = 514)$	3 $(n = 535)$
Appropriate	89%	82%	72%	77%	81%
Equivocal	4	8	10	7	4
Inappropriate	6	9	18	17	15
Other	1	1	—	—	—

[a]Assumptions regarding treadmill testing. Overall differences between the Manitoba hospital and the individual American hospitals were statistically at at least the 0.001 level (75% positive assumptions regarding treadmill testing) and at at least the 0.05 level (50% positive assumptions), respectively (by χ^2 tests, $df = 2$, combining "inappropriate" and "other" categories for the Manitoba hospital).

positive treadmill tests, 74 percent of the sample would fall into the appropriate category.

Assuming that at least 50 percent of the exercise tests were positive, the percentage of CA in the Manitoba hospital judged inappropriate was both lower than that in the three comparison hospitals and at the low end of the 8 to 32 percent inappropriate range found in other American data (6, 7) (Table 3). Relatively restrictive criteria for CA imply that fewer patients enter the "funnel" leading to CABS; the criteria for such surgery are also likely to be more stringent.

Coronary Artery Bypass Surgery

Manitoba and American surgical patients differed significantly in clinical presentation. A much larger percentage of Manitoba bypass patients were characterized by unstable angina (Table 4); these differences were larger than those found among patients having angiography (Table 2). In Manitoba, among the most frequent indications for surgery were unstable angina and an ejection fraction of 20 percent or greater with either three-vessel disease or two-vessel disease with left anterior descending coronary artery involvement; these conditions accounted for 20 and 10 percent, respectively, of the bypass operations. Patients with chronic stable angina, left main disease, and an ejection fraction of 20 percent or greater made up 11 percent of the sample, while those having chronic stable angina, three-vessel disease, class III or IV angina, ejection fraction of 50 percent or greater, and undergoing maximal medical therapy accounted for another 12 percent. These figures were all substantially higher than for the American bypass surgery patients.

Table 4

Characteristics of patients undergoing coronary artery bypass surgery by site

	Manitoba hospital (n = 245)	American hospitals (n = 386)
Clinical presentation[a]		
Chronic stable angina	49%	55%
Unstable angina	42	25[b]
Myocardial infarction within past six months	4	13
Asymptomatic or chest pain of unknown origin	5	4
Acute myocardial infarction on hospital admission	<1	2
Intractable ventricular arrhythmias	<1	<1
Vessel disease		
Left main disease	16	12
Three-vessel	51	36
Two-vessel	27	33
One-vessel	6	18
No significant disease	0	1

[a]Differences between the Manitoba hospital and the American hospitals were statistically significant at the 0.001 level ($df = 4$) for clinical presentation and $df = 3$ for vessel disease.
[b]This category includes n = 31 (8%) cases of "following unstable angina."

Sensitivity testing (again primarily involving missing treadmill test results) defined the range of Manitoba appropriateness scores. Table 5 shows the high level of appropriateness of CABS in the Manitoba hospital. When relevant data were missing, all patients assumed to have a positive treadmill test were grouped into the "positive assumptions" category; with "negative assumptions" such tests were assumed to be negative. Making the "negative assumptions," only one of the American hospitals approaches the Manitoba hospital's level of appropriateness.

The presence of a formal waiting list in Manitoba permitted looking at the total length of time from entry on the waiting list to CABS. For patients receiving angiography on an urgent basis (bypassing the waiting list), the time from angiography to surgery was used. Table 6 presents waiting times for the most frequent indications for surgery in Manitoba. Patients with unstable angina moved to surgery considerably more rapidly than those with stable angina. The three- to six-month waiting period for 38 percent of the patients with left main disease and chronic stable angina may represent a problem of some concern.

Patients Not Having Surgery

Thus far, we have focused on the question: Given the patients who have undergone bypass surgery, for what proportion was surgery appropriate? Two

Table 5

Appropriateness of coronary artery bypass surgery in
Manitoba and American hospitals[a]

| Categories | Manitoba hospital | | American hospital number | | |
	Positive assumptions (n = 245)	Negative assumptions (n = 245)	4 (n = 161)	5 (n = 96)	6 (n = 129)
Appropriate	94%	83%	59%	78%	37%
Equivocal	5	14	29	17	40
Inappropriate	1	3	12	6	23

[a]All differences between the Manitoba hospital and the individual American hospitals were statistically significant at at least the 0.001 level, except for the comparison between Manitoba and American hospital number 5 (not significant) based on negative assumptions ($df = 2$).

Table 6

Wait to bypass surgery for the most frequent indications, Manitoba, 1981–83[a]

| Indications | Wait to surgery, % of group | | | |
	≤30 days	1 to 3 months	3 to 6 months	6 to 12 months
Unstable angina (n = 49) Three-vessel disease Ejection fraction ≥20%	55%	33%	12%	0%
Unstable angina (n = 25) Two-vessel disease with LAD involvement Ejection fraction ≥20%	48	36	8	8
Chronic stable angina (n = 26) Left main disease Ejection fraction ≥20%	23	35	38	4
Chronic stable angina (n = 29) Three-vessel disease Class III or IV angina Maximal medical therapy Ejection fraction ≥50%	10	21	52	17

[a]Time was counted from the date wait-listed for angiography to the date of coronary artery bypass surgery. Some patients moved quickly (within a day) to coronary angiography and were not entered on the waiting list. In these cases the time interval was from date of angiography to date of surgery. LAD, left anterior descending coronary artery.

other questions should be asked: What proportion of patients for whom surgery would be appropriate did not have surgery? What are the characteristics of those not receiving surgery? Table 7 summarizes data on the clinical presentation and appropriateness for surgery of patients who did not receive bypass surgery during the 12 months following angiography. These patients' mean age was 57 years, with only 20 percent being over 65 years of age (compared with a mean age of 60 for the Manitoba surgery patients). The information on appropriateness was generally insensitive to the missing data; the negative assumptions on exercise testing were used. Using positive assumptions raised this group's level of appropriateness for bypass surgery to 52 percent from 44 percent.

Those not having bypass surgery were less likely to report either chronic stable angina or unstable angina than were the patients who were operated on. They were more likely to present clinically with a recent myocardial infarction or chest pain of unknown origin. While 51 percent of the bypass patients suffered from three-vessel disease and 16 percent from left main disease, only 6 percent had one-vessel disease. On the other hand, many of those not undergoing surgery had one-vessel disease (41 percent), with only 5 percent suffering from left-main

Table 7

Characteristics of Manitoba patients not undergoing coronary artery bypass surgery

Clinical presentation	Percentage (n = 153)
Chronic stable angina	29%
Unstable angina	23
Myocardial infarction within past six months	13
Asymptomatic or chest pain of unknown origin	20
Acute myocardial infarction on hospital admission	1
Intractable ventricular arrhythmias	1
Other[a]	13
Vessel disease	
Left main disease	5
Three-vessel	22
Two-vessel	18
One-vessel	41
Other[a]	13
Appropriateness of surgery (had it been conducted)	
Appropriate	44
Equivocal	19
Inappropriate	24
Other[a]	13

[a]Insufficient data were available on 20 cases (13%) to determine vessel disease and surgical indication; however, four cases had catheter findings of "normal" and "continued medical management" was indicated on the chart for the remaining 16 cases.

disease and 22 percent from three-vessel disease. At least 68 Manitoba patients met the American appropriateness criteria for surgery; follow-up of the unoperated patients with three-vessel disease would be of particular interest. Such patients meeting appropriateness criteria but not having surgery raise questions as to when an operation is necessary.

Necessary Surgery?

Appropriateness criteria have been derived to give practitioners the benefit of the doubt. Expert panelists are not providing prospective guidelines but rather are asking: "If I'm looking at a patient with these characteristics who has already had a procedure, am I prepared to question whether my colleague was right? Could this be appropriate?" Thus, designating a procedure as "appropriate" does not mean that the surgery is necessary. Failure to proceed in a case that is "appropriate" does not prove that "underprovision" or a denial of care exists. Although the literature is not definitive, Hadorn (17) has suggested that bypass surgery may be "necessary" (compared with "appropriate") under three conditions: First, triple-vessel disease (greater than 70 percent each vessel) with impaired left ventricular function (ejection fraction less than 40 percent); second, high-grade (greater than 70 percent) left-main coronary artery obstruction; and third, unstable or persistent angina unresponsive to maximal medical therapy or with incapacitating side effects.

The Manitoba data permitted looking at 17 patients having the first condition: triple-vessel disease with impaired left ventricular function. Of these 17, 10 had bypass surgery within one year of angiography; three of these surgical patients (30 percent) died by the end of 1987. Of the seven patients who did not have surgery, four (57 percent) died by the end of 1985.

These findings highlight the difficulties of making judgements about necessity of care. Of the medically treated patients, chart reviews indicated that six suffered from either cardiomegaly, congestive heart failure, or both (two patients). The seventh individual was diabetic. Just three of the 10 surgical patients were noted as suffering from cardiomegaly or congestive heart failure; none were diabetic. Surgical patients were more likely to be hypertensive, obese, or smokers.

DISCUSSION

CA and CABS have been identified elsewhere as high priority for medical practice assessment (18) but study results can be difficult to interpret. The lower Manitoba rates of CA and CABS cannot be shown to be more or less "right" than the higher American rate. Lower rates of invasive procedures result in less procedure related mortality, but surgery for some indications leads to better long-term survival and improved quality of life.

More recently, rates of bypass surgery were found to vary markedly among American Standard Metropolitan Areas, but Canadian rates have generally remained lower than those in the United States (19). In comparisons among two American states (New York, California) and three Canadian provinces (British Columbia, Manitoba and Ontario), Manitoba recorded the lowest overall rate of bypass surgery (12) (see Chapter 13). In 1990 one state (New York) with controls on the number of hospitals performing bypass surgery had a lower percentage of inappropriate CA (only 4 percent) and CABS (only 2 percent) than did the American hospitals studied in the early 1980s (20, 21). New York state is probably atypical because of its relatively low rates of coronary bypass surgery and its use of a management registry with screening procedures to help ensure appropriateness of surgery. Such controls may generate a "spillover effect" resulting in better use of related procedures (CA and percutaneous transluminal coronary angioplasty) (22).

As Schoenbaum (23) has noted, appropriateness may be too easy a hurdle to clear. Although Canadians may wait longer for relief from angina than do Americans (24), the lower Canadian bypass surgery rates probably do reflect a lower percentage of inappropriate surgery than in the United States.

By extension, both "appropriateness" and "necessity" reviews would seem desirable for comparing these procedures across countries; such work is ongoing in Canada and the United States. Ideally, studies should not only be cross-sectional (as almost all appropriateness research has been), but should also trace patterns forward in time from angiography. Only through such follow-up can we learn how often patients who might benefit from coronary artery bypass are not having such surgery. Further research into this issue would have to deal with patient preferences, unmeasured comorbidity, conflicting test results, and so on.

The applications of "appropriateness" and "necessity" reviews are not without hazards. Although physician panels provide the best available judgements regarding their specialties, the knowledge base underlying their decisions is not scientifically robust (25). Both the indications for and the efficacy of many treatments are uncertain. At least one set of studies using data banks has found a much greater number of postoperative problems after prostatectomy than those anticipated by expert panels (26, 27).

Practice differences may also affect the applicability of such reviews. A Canadian practice based almost entirely on referrals to a teaching hospital may be organized differently from an American practice with more patient initiated visits. Manitoba cardiologists' reliance on exercise testing seems to reflect an assumption that catheterization is appropriate for referred patients. Canadian physicians, like their British counterparts, are likely to differ from American physicians as to the indications for a particular procedure (7, 8). In 1987, Chassin and colleagues (28) felt it "unlikely that any of the major uses of coronary angiography classified as inappropriate then (1981) would today be considered appropriate." As noted earlier, the high Manitoba levels of appropriateness do not automatically follow from rates generally lower than those in the United States. Low rates in the United Kingdom are not clearly associated with either higher levels of appropriateness or lower levels of inappropriateness, especially if a country is judged by its own (more conservative) criteria (7, 8, 29). Moreover, although Leape and colleagues (6) found that inappropriate use accounted for 28 percent of the variance in American use of CA, the exclusion of just one high-use county made the relationship between rates of appropriateness and angiography rates statistically insignificant. For two other procedures (carotid endarterectomy and upper gastrointestinal tract endoscopy), no significant correlations were found between inappropriateness of use and rate of use.

The Manitoba patients staying on medical management appear to be a combination of relatively well and extremely ill individuals. Better modeling of the outcomes associated with such medical conditions as cardiomegaly and congestive heart failure would make more informed judgements about when surgery is and is not appropriate or necessary (30, 31). That relatively few Manitoba patients with single-vessel disease receive bypass surgery (6%) of the Manitoba surgery patients versus 18 percent of the American sample) suggests more cost-effective medicine in Canada, since "one million US dollars for bypass surgery would produce 134 life-years for middle-aged men with left main disease but only 17 life-years for such men with one-vessel disease" (32, 33). Similar information for two- and three-vessel disease would be useful.

The possibility of modeling at least the mortality outcomes of those who do and do not receive surgery can help deal with the question, "Which rate is right?" (34). Although quality of life issues are important, an improved ability to predict mortality will provide better, more empirically based input for the treatment decision. Such work is one of the tasks of the Medical Effectiveness Treatment Program research on ischemic heart disease. If the links between referral-based practices, lower rates, and better case selection are confirmed by ongoing research, the Canadian approach of regionalized services with restricted growth in surgical caseloads and "rationing by queue" will have obtained important support (35).

APPENDIX:
DIFFERENCES BETWEEN AGE GROUPS

The 55 to 64 and the over 65 year age groups showed only minor differences on a number of relevant clinical characteristics. The groups did not differ significantly in measurements of ejection fraction. The extent of vessel disease among patients in the two groups was almost identical: the largest difference was in the occurrence of left main disease, and even this was only 3 percent (12 percent versus 15 percent for the 55 to 64 and over 65 years age groups, respectively).

Prevalence of vessel disease was also similar between groups, with the over 65 years age group having slightly higher (3 to 5 percent) incidence of aortic and mitral stenosis. The percentage of patients with stable angina differed by 5 percent, while the percentage of patients with unstable angina was virtually identical.

REFERENCES

1. Woolhandler, S. and Himmelstein, D. U. A national health program: Northern light at the end of the tunnel. *JAMA* 262: 2136–2137, 1989.
2. Woolhandler, S. and Himmelstein, D. U. The deteriorating administrative efficiency of the US health care system. *N. Engl. J. Med.* 342: 1253–1258, 1991.
3. Blendon, R. J., et al. Datawatch: Satisfaction with health systems in ten nations. *Health Aff. (Millwood)* 9: 185–192, 1990.
4. Bronow, R. A national health program: Abyss at the end of the tunnel—the position of physicians who care. *JAMA* 263: 2488–2489, 1990.
5. Iglehart, J. K. Canada's health care system faces its problems. *N. Engl. J. Med.* 322: 562–568, 1990.
6. Leape, L. L., et al. Does inappropriate use explain small-area variations in the use of health care services? *JAMA* 263: 669–672, 1990.
7. Brook, R. H., et al. Diagnosis and treatment of coronary disease: Comparison of doctors' attitudes in the USA and the UK. *Lancet* 1: 750–753, 1988.
8. Bernstein, S. J., et al. The appropriateness of the use of cardiovascular procedures: British versus US perspectives. *Intl. J. Tech. Asses. Health Care* 9: 3–10, 1993.
9. Morris, A. L., et al. Managing scarce services: A waiting list approach to cardiac catheterization. *Med. Care* 28: 784–792, 1990.
10. Roos, L. L., et al. Risk adjustment in claims-based research: The search for efficient approaches. *J. Clin. Epidemiol.* 42: 1193–1206, 1989.
11. Anderson, G. M., Newhouse, J. P., and Roos, L. L. Hospital care for elderly patients with diseases of the circulatory system: A comparison of hospital utilization in the United States and Canada. *N. Engl. J. Med.* 321: 1443–1448, 1989.
12. Anderson, G. M., et al. Use of coronary artery bypass surgery in the United States and Canada: Influence of age and income. *JAMA* 269: 1661–1666, 1993.
13. Chassin, M. R., et al. *Indications for Selected Medical and Surgical Procedures— A Literature Review and Ratings of Appropriateness: Coronary Artery Bypass Graft Surgery* (Rand R-3204/2-CWF/HF/HCFA/PMT/RWJ). Rand Corporation, Santa Monica, 1986.
14. Chassin, M. R., et al. Does inappropriate use explain geographic variations in the use of health care services? *JAMA* 258: 2533–2537, 1987.
15. Winslow, C. M., et al. The appropriateness of performing coronary artery bypass surgery. *JAMA* 260: 505–509, 1988.
16. Kosecoff, J., et al. Obtaining clinical data on the appropriateness of medical care in community practice. *JAMA* 258: 2538–2542, 1987.
17. Hadorn, D. C. Setting health care priorities in Oregon: Cost effectiveness meets the rule of rescue. *JAMA* 265: 2218–2225, 1991.

18. Phelps, C. E. and Parente, S. T. Priority setting in medical technology and medical practice assessment. *Med. Care* 28: 703–723, 1990.
19. Health Care Financing Special Report. *Hospital Data by Geographic Area for Aged Medicare Beneficiaries: Selected Procedures, 1986,* Vol. 2. US Department of Health and Human Services, Washington, D.C., 1990.
20. Bernstein, S. J., et al. The appropriateness of use of coronary angiography in New York state. *JAMA* 269: 766–769, 1993.
21. Leape, L. L., et al. The appropriateness of use of coronary artery bypass graft surgery in New York state. *JAMA* 269: 753–760, 1993.
22. Hilborne, L. H., et al. The appropriateness of use of percutaneous transluminal coronary angioplasty in New York. *JAMA* 269: 761–765, 1993.
23. Schoenbaum, S. C. Toward fewer procedures and better outcomes. *JAMA* 269: 794–796, 1993.
24. Rouleau, J. L., et al. A comparison of management patterns after acute myocardial infarction in Canada and the United States. *N. Engl. J. Med.* 328: 779–784, 1993.
25. Chalmers, T. C., et al. Selection and evaluation of empirical research in technology assessment. *Intl. J. Tech. Asses. Health Care* 5: 521–536, 1989.
26. Roos, N. P., et al. Mortality and reoperation after open and transurethral resection of the prostate for benign prostatic hyperplasia. *N. Engl. J. Med.* 320: 1120–1124, 1989.
27. Wennberg, J. E., et al. Use of claims data systems to evaluate health care outcomes: Mortality and reoperation following prostatectomy. *JAMA* 257: 933–936, 1987.
28. Chassin, M. R., et al. How coronary angiography is used: Clinical determinants of appropriateness. *JAMA* 258: 2543–2547, 1987.
29. Gray, D., et al. Audit of coronary and angiography and bypass surgery. *Lancet* 335: 1317–1320, 1990.
30. Pryor, D. B., et al. Trends in the presentation, management, and survival of patients with coronary artery disease: The Duke Data Base for Cardiovascular Disease. In *Trends in Coronary Heart Disease Mortality,* edited by M. W. Higgins and R. Luepker, pp. 76–87. Oxford University Press, New York, 1988.
31. Califf, R. M., et al. The evolution of medical and surgical therapy for coronary artery disease: A 15-year perspective. *JAMA* 261: 2077–2086, 1989.
32. Russell, L. B. Opportunity costs in modern medicine. *Health Aff. (Millwood)* 11: 162–169, 1992.
33. Detsky, A. S. Are clinical trials a cost-effective investment? *JAMA* 262: 1795–1800, 1989.
34. Wennberg, J. E. Which rate is right? *N. Engl. J. Med.* 314: 310–311, 1986.
35. Naylor, C. D. A different view of queues in Ontario. *Health Aff. (Millwood)* 10: 110–128, 1991.

CHAPTER 15

Health and Surgical Outcomes in Canada and the United States

Leslie L. Roos, Elliott S. Fisher, Ruth Brazauskas, Sandra M. Sharp, and Evelyn Shapiro

The ongoing escalation of U.S. health care expenditures threatens both individual incomes and corporate competitiveness. At the same time, an ever-increasing number of Americans are finding adequate health insurance beyond their reach. Two broad policy responses to the crisis are apparent. The first focuses on reform of the financing system. A second major thrust of both government and corporate health policy, however, is to better define value in health care. The critical assumption is that prudent purchasing—whether by consumers or by large organizations—will lead to lower costs and better health.

Many have looked to Canada for insight not only on the organization and financing of the health care system, but also on the value of services provided. For example, U.S. advocates of single-payer systems point to Canada's lower overall costs, administrative efficiency, and higher satisfaction with the health care system (1). At the same time, those concerned with preserving the U.S. health insurance market point to Canada's waiting lists for surgery or, as in George Bush's Comprehensive Health Reform Program, Canada's alleged inability to provide adequate care for certain conditions (2). The latter is a distortion of our previous work comparing short-term surgical outcomes in New England and Manitoba.

This chapter reports findings on three-year mortality rates following common surgical procedures undergone by residents of Manitoba and New England over age 65 (see Chapter 12) (3). We show that for low- and moderate-risk surgical procedures, short-term outcomes differed little, but three-year survival was

Published by *Health Affairs,* Summer 1992, pp. 56–72. Copyright 1992, The People-to-People Health Foundation, Inc., Project HOPE.

substantially better in Manitoba. For certain high-risk procedures, short-term outcomes favored New England, but three-year survival was similar. Overall population mortality among the elderly is lower in Manitoba than in New England. These findings raise important questions for those considering reform of the U.S. health care system, and also for those striving to define value in health care.

Long-term analyses raise questions as to the overall health of the population, which may be reflected both in the longevity of patients coming to surgery and in the longevity of individuals not receiving a given treatment. In the mid-1980s, Canadian life expectancy at age sixty was 23.3 years for females and 18.4 for males, compared with 22.5 years and 17.9 years for American females and males, respectively. Among 33 countries with vital registration systems, Canada ranked considerably better than the United States, both in life expectancy at birth (76.5 versus 75.0 years) and in all-cause, age-adjusted death rate per 100,000 population (4, 5).

Background on Manitoba and New England

The populations of both Manitoba and New England are primarily of European origin. Manitoba's population includes about 5.4 percent Treaty Indians and about 0.5 percent blacks. In the 1986 census, 71.3 percent of Manitobans reported English as the mother tongue and 4.3 percent, French, with 18.6 percent reporting a nonofficial language and 5.8 percent giving a multiple response. As of 1985, about 4.3 percent of New Englanders were black, with smaller numbers of Hispanics and Asians (6–8).

Both the United States and Canada provide universal insurance coverage for the elderly, and Manitoba and New England have similar numbers of physicians and hospital beds per capita, but the health care systems differ in several important ways. Although differences in purchasing power make comparisons only approximate, New England elderly would presumably have benefited from higher regional levels of health care expenditures. In 1987, the United States spent U.S.$2,051 per capita on health care, with Canada at U.S.$1,483 (9). New England's nonfederal hospital expenditures per capita in 1987 were 18 percent higher than the American mean (6, 10). In Manitoba, per capita hospital expenditures are near the Canadian mean (see Chapter 3) (11).

In contrast to Canada's higher proportion of generalist physicians, specialists predominate in the United States. Although Canadians use considerably more physician services overall than Americans, these services primarily involve patient evaluation and management. With a few exceptions (such as cholecystectomy), surgical rates in the United States are generally higher than those in Canada. American programs supporting home care and nursing homes are largely oriented toward short-term recovery, while the Canadian focus is more long-term. Manitoba and other provinces provide home care services without charge, while nursing home care is insured with a room and board charge less than the minimum pension. Canadians use more inpatient days per capita but have roughly similar pharmaceutical expenditures per capita (12, 13).

STUDY METHODS

Data Sources

Both U.S. Medicare and the Manitoba Health Services Commission databases contain computerized information on hospital discharges and patient enrollment in the respective insurance systems. The hospital files include patient and hospital identifiers, admission and discharge dates, and data on diagnoses and procedures. The enrollment files include individual identifiers and specify a date of death, regardless of whether that death occurred inside or outside a hospital.

In Manitoba, all hospital and medical care, with a few minor exceptions (such as private room, cosmetic surgery, and some out-of-province care), is without user fees or limitations on use. The Manitoba health insurance database contains information on all individuals registered in the province. New England Medicare data were based on the hospital claims file (Medicare Part A) and the enrollment file.

Both the Manitoba and New England data sets are population based, containing information on almost all residents age 65 and older, regardless of where their care was received.[1] New England mortality statistics were generated using a 20 percent sample of all Medicare enrollees who were alive, residents of New England, and age 65 or older on December 31, 1984. Population mortality for the Manitoba elderly was taken from life table calculations by Statistics Canada (16).

Procedures Selected

The procedures selected were relatively common, contributed significantly to health care costs, and were well defined using administrative data; some postsurgical mortality is associated with each condition. Except as noted below, the primary procedure on the discharge abstract defined the operations. To minimize potential case-mix differences, we selected relatively homogeneous groups of surgical patients. Patients who received concurrent valve replacement/bypass surgery were analyzed separately. Both diagnostic codes and procedure codes were used to construct the groups for total hip replacement (no hip fracture diagnosis) and for hip fracture repair procedures (hip fracture diagnosis and "surgery for repair" performed). Prostatectomy cases with diagnoses of cancer of

---

[1] Details on the minor exclusions, on the ascertainment of vital status, on the codes used to specify surgical cases, and on statistical power are available elsewhere and from the authors.

the bladder or prostate were excluded (22 percent of the total), as were cholecystectomy cases with cancer of the gallbladder (1.5 percent).

Definition of Variables

We selected covariates for case-mix adjustment based on our previous work. They included age, sex, the absence or presence of high-risk diagnoses that independently predict mortality, and type of operation ("emergency," "scheduled," or "delayed") (3, 17, 18). The high-risk diagnoses were malignant neoplasm, old myocardial infarction, peripheral vascular disease, chronic obstructive pulmonary disease, diabetes, dementia, moderate or severe chronic liver disease, renal failure, and ulcers. Operations were defined according to the number of days between admission and surgery. Emergency operations were those occurring on the date of admission. Scheduled operations were generally performed within two days of admission. Patients hospitalized three or more days prior to surgery were classified as having delayed operations; these may be high-risk cases requiring further diagnostic procedures or sicker patients whose condition must be stabilized before surgery. Length-of-stay before transurethral prostatectomy differed to such an extent between Manitoba and New England that the "type of operation" variable was not included for this procedure.

Statistical Methods

Because of the small numbers of certain procedures performed in Manitoba, we also grouped procedures into three categories according to mortality in the year following surgery: low (mortality rates below 9 percent), moderate (9–18 percent), and high (above 18 percent). To generate adequate numbers of cases, more years of data are used for Manitoba. The main analyses compare mortality after Manitoba surgery performed between 1980 and 1986 with mortality after New England surgery done in 1984 and 1985.

As used here, the odds ratio is an estimate of the probability of death in Manitoba in a given time period, compared with the probability of death in New England in the same time period. Adjusted odds ratios are calculated from logistic regression models.[2] Logistic regression is particularly suitable for calculations using a dichotomous dependent variable (individual dead/alive at 30 days, six months, and so on, after surgery) and generates odds ratios that adjust for case-mix. A ratio greater than 1.0 indicated higher mortality in Manitoba; a ratio lower than 1.0 showed higher mortality in New England.

---

[2] Odds ratios approximate the direct measure of relative risk and are less suitable when mortality rates are relatively high. Where possible, comparisons between the odds ratio and the relative risk measure were made; differences were uniformly small.

RESULTS OF THE COMPARISONS

Our analyses emphasize the importance of considering long-term, postsurgical mortality (Table 1). Considerable mortality within three years of surgery is found for almost all procedures performed on the elderly; for both groups, only patients with hip replacements, simple cholecystectomies, and open prostatectomies show 15 percent mortality or less over these three years.

Figures 1 and 2 show how the Manitoba survival advantage for low- and moderate-risk procedures widens over time. Survival after the two high-risk procedures converges by three years after surgery (Figure 3). Some simple calculations using the unadjusted data highlight the relative number of deaths that might be postponed. If three years after surgery the proportions of New England deaths were the same as those in Manitoba, there would have been 1,102 fewer deaths among New England elderly patients having low-mortality procedures and 223 fewer deaths among those having moderate-mortality procedures. Fifty-four additional deaths would be recorded among the New England elderly undergoing high-mortality procedures.

The case-mix-adjusted odds ratios between Manitoba and New England for 30-day, one-year, and three-year mortality are generally similar to the unadjusted data (Table 2). Both low- and moderate-mortality procedures show significantly better long-term survival for Manitoba elderly than for New England elderly. On the other hand, the New England patients' advantage in 30-day survival for the high-mortality procedures diminishes greatly by the end of a year.

Baseline comorbidity (comorbidity in the population) might better predict patient deaths in long-term follow-up than in the short term. Because the negative results of any single intervention (or illness) tend to occur in close proximity to the event, 30-day mortality will be most affected by events shortly before, during, and shortly after surgery. Later mortality will be more affected by other comorbidity and general health status. A decline in adjusted odds ratios between 30-day and three-year mortality—a pattern consistent both with Manitobans having lower presurgical comorbidity and with better support after surgery—was observed across all conditions: the odds ratio dropped from 0.93 to 0.76 for low-risk procedures, from 0.87 to 0.76 for moderate-risk procedures, and from 1.40 to 0.96 for high-risk procedures. Although adjusted odds ratios for three years after surgery favor Manitoba in nine of the ten comparisons, results for several specific procedures bear close scrutiny.

SPECIFIC COMPARISONS: WHAT CAN WE LEARN?

Hip Fracture

Repair of hip fracture accounts for 97 percent of the high-mortality procedures (with the concurrent valve replacement/bypass operation making up the rest).

Table 1

Risk of death by type of procedure, patients age 65 and older, Manitoba and New England[a]

Procedure	No. of procedures		30-Day mortality		1-Year mortality		3-Year mortality	
	Manitoba	New England	Manitoba[b]	New England[c]	Manitoba[b]	New England[c]	Manitoba[b]	New England[c]
Low mortality								
Total hip replacement	1,568	5,163	1.28	0.97	2.87	3.95	8.35	10.56
Simple cholecystectomy	2,961	9,042	1.52	2.38	4.26	7.66	10.37	16.53
Open prostatectomy	1,004	1,235	1.10	1.05	5.78	4.13	15.64	12.23
Carotid endarterectomy	466	3,802	1.93	2.26	6.44	8.13	15.02	21.73
Transurethral prostatectomy	4,934	15,078	1.26	1.03	8.21	8.79	20.45	22.15
All low-mortality procedures	10,933	34,320	1.34	1.52	6.07	7.52	15.31	18.52
Moderate mortality								
Cholecystectomy with exploration of common bile duct	794	2,346	3.40	4.22	9.07	10.40	19.65	23.19
Coronary artery bypass graft surgery	732	5,152	5.33	5.57	8.47	10.33	12.43	15.99
Heart valve replacement	212	1,231	6.60	7.88	12.74	16.08	19.81	24.94
All moderate-mortality procedures	1,738	8,729	4.60	5.53	9.26	11.16	16.63	19.19
High mortality								
Repair of hip fracture	4,586	16,236	8.05	5.60	24.33	22.39	42.13	41.83
Concurrent valve replacement/bypass surgery	101	435	20.79	12.18	22.77	20.92	27.72	29.43
All high-mortality procedures	4,687	16,671	8.32	5.77	24.30	22.36	41.82	41.50

[a]Sources: For Manitoba data: Manitoba Health Services Commission, admission/discharge abstracts and enrollment file. For New England data: Health Care Financing Administration, Medicare discharge abstracts. *Note:* Mortality rates express risk of death per 100 procedures.
[b]1980–1986.
[c]1984–1985.

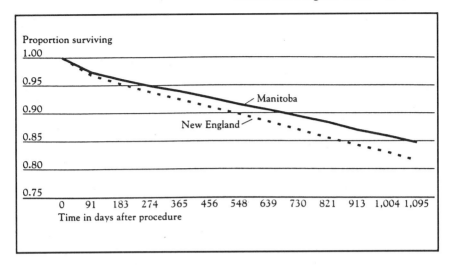

Figure 1. Postsurgical survival for low-mortality procedures, age 65 and older, Manitoba and New England. Sources: For Manitoba data: Manitoba Health Services Commission, admission/discharge abstracts and enrollment file. For New England data: Health Care Financing Administration, Medicare discharge abstracts. *Note:* Manitoba data are for 1980–1986; New England data are for 1984–1985.

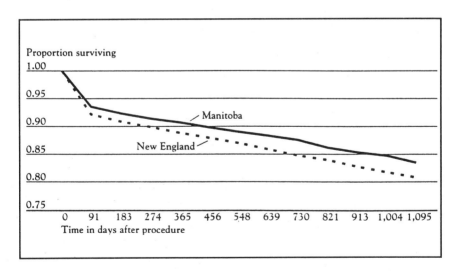

Figure 2. Postsurgical survival for moderate-mortality procedures, age 65 and older, Manitoba and New England. Sources: For Manitoba data: Manitoba Health Services Commission, admission/discharge abstracts and enrollment file. For New England data: Health Care Financing Administration, Medicare discharge abstracts. *Note:* Manitoba data are for 1980–1986; New England data are for 1984–1985.

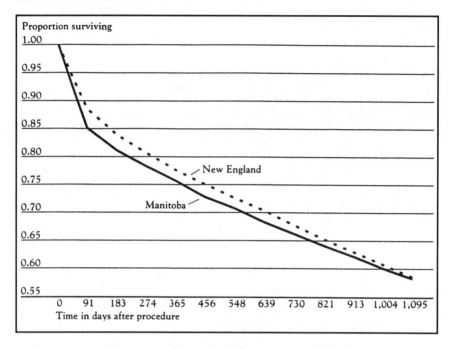

Figure 3. Postsurgical survival for high-mortality procedures, age 65 and older, Manitoba and New England. Sources: For Manitoba data: Manitoba Health Services Commission, admission/discharge abstracts and enrollment file. For New England data: Health Care Financing Administration, Medicare discharge abstracts. *Note:* Manitoba data are for 1980–1986; New England data are for 1984–1985.

Other analyses have shown that increased 30-day mortality following hip fracture in Manitoba holds for all types of repair and all age groups. This short-term mortality appears influenced by the geographic distribution of patients and hospitals in Manitoba: 23 percent of Manitoba patients (and only 5 percent of New England patients) were transferred prior to hip fracture repair.

Manitoba patients first admitted to a smaller hospital and then transferred to a larger hospital for surgery had a higher 30-day mortality rate (8.3 percent) than their counterparts who were not transferred (6.3 percent); hip fracture patients admitted to a hospital from a nursing home had the highest mortality (11.4 percent). Further analyses adjusting for case-mix showed only the latter to have a significantly higher 30-day mortality.

Because most transferred patients incur additional presurgical hospital stays of one or two days, the time lag between fracture and surgery was undoubtedly greater in Manitoba than in New England. Although a delay in surgery to repair hip fracture may increase mortality, the differences in 30-day survival among

Table 2

Unadjusted and adjusted comparisons of mortality (odds ratios) in Manitoba and New England[a]

Procedure	30-Day mortality		1-Year mortality		3-Year mortality	
	Unadjusted	Adjusted	Unadjusted	Adjusted	Unadjusted	Adjusted
Low mortality						
Total hip replacement	1.32	1.19	0.72[b]	0.63[b]	0.77[b]	0.70[b]
Simple cholecystectomy	0.63[b]	0.77	0.54[b]	0.63[b]	0.58[b]	0.67[b]
Open prostatectomy	1.04	1.05	1.42	1.32	1.33[b]	1.32[b]
Carotid endarterectomy	0.85	0.90	0.78	0.81	0.64[b]	0.66[b]
Transurethral prostatectomy	1.22	1.27	0.93	0.98	0.90[b]	0.94
All low-mortality procedures	0.89	0.93	0.79[b]	0.76[b]	0.80[b]	0.76[b]
Moderate mortality						
Cholecystectomy with exploration of common bile duct	0.80	0.83	0.86	0.86	0.81[b]	0.82
Coronary artery bypass graft surgery	0.95	0.87	0.80	0.75[b]	0.75[b]	0.69[b]
Heart valve replacement	0.83	0.87	0.76	0.73	0.74	0.72
All moderate-mortality procedures	0.82	0.87	0.81[b]	0.80[b]	0.84[b]	0.76[b]
High mortality						
Repair of hip fracture	1.48[b]	1.38[b]	1.11[b]	1.05	1.01	0.96
Concurrent valve replacement/bypass surgery	1.89[b]	1.93[b]	1.11	1.13	0.92	0.89
All high-mortality procedures	1.48[b]	1.40[b]	1.11[b]	1.05	1.01	0.96

[a]Sources: For Manitoba data: Manitoba Health Services Commission, admission/discharge abstracts and enrollment file. For New England data: Health Care Financing Administration, Medicare discharge abstracts. Note: Confidence intervals and P values are available from the authors. An odds ratio greater than 1.0 indicates higher mortality in Manitoba: a ratio less than 1.0 indicates higher mortality in New England. Data for Manitoba are for 1980–1986; data for New England are for 1984–1985.

[b]Manitoba/New England differences were significant at $P \leq 0.05$.

263

Manitoba patients labeled as "emergency," "scheduled," and "delayed" were minimal (19).

Analyses of hospital size were only suggestive. Hip fracture patients in low-volume hospitals (39 or fewer repairs annually among the elderly) were only 1.15 times as likely to die in the 30 days after surgery as were their counterparts in higher-volume hospitals. One of five high-volume Manitoba hospitals had relatively high mortality rates.

Cardiovascular Surgery

As stressed in the Bush proposal, 30-day mortality for concurrent valve replacement/bypass surgery was significantly higher in Manitoba than in New England (although the number of Manitoba cases was quite low—101) (2). Because of the "judgment call" made by the surgeon in deciding to perform the concurrent procedure, looking at the three open-heart operations (coronary artery bypass, valve replacement, and the concurrent surgery) is particularly informative. Considering the three procedures together, unadjusted 30-day results favor New England (6.4 percent mortality versus 7.1 percent for Manitoba). While in both regions the number of deaths is greater by one year after cardiovascular surgery (933 deaths in the two regions, versus 511 at 30 days), Manitoba mortality is less than that of New England (10.7 and 12.1 percent, respectively). Manitoba's advantage is even greater after three years—15.4 percent versus 18.5 percent in New England. Adjusted figures show an almost identical trend.

Prostatectomy

Because the results for open prostatectomy were inconsistent with those of the other procedures, we examined the type of procedure (open or transurethral) and the presence of an associated prostate or bladder cancer diagnosis. Two lines of evidence suggest that despite our statistical controls, New England males having open prostatectomies were healthier than their Manitoba counterparts. First, the open procedure is used at a much higher rate in Manitoba (14.9 percent of prostatectomies) than in New England (6.6 percent). Outcomes favored New England only for those having open procedures, with the greatest difference occurring among patients without an associated cancer diagnosis. Long-term survival among males having transurethral procedures favored Manitoba, with the larger difference for those with an associated cancer diagnosis. When all subgroups are combined, the adjusted odds ratios go from 1.08 at 30 days to 0.92 at three years.

Second, international comparisons show 90-day and one-year age-adjusted Manitoba mortality figures close to those reported in Denmark and in Oxford-shire, England (20). Among the four jurisdictions, New Englanders had the highest relative risk when transurethral prostatectomies were compared with the open procedures (an odds ratio of 2.18 for one-year mortality). Such findings are consistent with different selection criteria being applied in New England.

Additional Analyses

Using 1980–1986 Manitoba information and pooling across all procedures, odds ratios for 30-day mortality slightly favor New England. However, the odds ratios for three-year mortality favor Manitoba (0.84 to 0.91, depending on the statistical model); the Manitoba advantage increases even further (0.77 to 0.85) when repair of hip fracture (which has the largest number of cases) is not included.

Although fewer operations are available, Manitoba data from 1983–1986 are closer in time to the New England 1984–1985 data. Comparisons for these sets of years show slightly smaller Manitoba long-term advantages for low- and moderate-mortality procedures. On the other hand, the long-term comparisons suggest a Manitoba advantage following the high-mortality procedures; here, the adjusted odds ratios changed from 1.05 (1980–1986 Manitoba data) to 0.95 (1983–1986 data) for one-year survival and from 0.96 to 0.91 for three-year survival.

Differences in Life Expectancy

Life expectancy in Manitoba for those age 65 and older seems several months longer than the Canadian average, which is in turn slightly greater than the New England mean (16, 21). Manitoba death rates are consistently lower than those in New England for men and women ages 65 to 85 (Table 3). Despite our statistical controls, these differences in the underlying population appear reflected in the surgical outcomes.

Our findings clearly raise more questions than they answer. Nevertheless, they have important implications, not only for those who consider the Canadian system either nirvana or anathema, but also for those trying to define value in health care in the hope that organizational changes or enhanced consumer choice will improve overall health.

WHY DO MANITOBA RESIDENTS LIVE LONGER?

What explains the better Manitoba long-term outcomes and improved population survival, regardless of the type of surgery and relative surgical rates? Population mortality might vary because of differential susceptibility (inherited biologic potential), individual lifestyles (health habits and behavior), physical environment (exposure to physical, chemical, and biological agents), social environment (aspects of social organization, particularly levels of social isolation, deprivation, stress, and powerlessness), and health services (22).

Table 3

Risk of death during the next year for Manitoba and New England elderly[a]

Age	Manitoba[b]		New England[c]		Manitoba/New England ratio	
	Male	Female	Male	Female	Male	Female
65	2.29	1.11	2.61	1.43	.88	.78
70	3.58	1.79	4.15	2.14	.86	.84
75	5.45	2.86	6.86	3.00	.79	.95
80	8.12	4.70	8.75	5.53	.93	.85
85	12.59	9.19	14.43	9.22	.87	1.00

[a]Sources: For Manitoba: reference 16; for New England: Health Care Financing Administration, Medicare enrollment files. *Note:* Risk of death is expressed per 100 procedures.
[b]1985–1987.
[c]1985.

Better health may largely depend on factors beyond the direct control of the health care system. The uniformity of the observed trends across type of surgery, similar causes of death in the two countries, and annual mortality rates favoring Manitoba at each age suggest that disease-specific factors are not responsible (23). Although lifestyle surveys suggest that Canadians smoke more than Americans, Canadians exercise more (24–26). Despite our statistical controls, Canadians' better outcomes may be explained by a lower preoperative risk of death. If an adequately measured Manitoba advantage over New England in presurgical health is real, then in studying postsurgical mortality, the odds ratios should be adjusted in New England's favor. Unfortunately, we know neither the extent of such a statistical adjustment nor whether it should be made.

Health care systems may also contribute to the observed outcomes. The greater accessibility of both primary care and long-term care services in Canada is likely to promote improved health. In the United States, posthospital treatment for the elderly can be provided either at home or in skilled nursing facilities. However, Medicare restricts the duration of such services and requires patient cost sharing. Only the poorest elderly are covered for long-term care without restriction. In Canada, posthospital treatment and care is usually provided either at home or in a geriatric rehabilitation unit, without restrictions as to time or site and at no charge to the patient. These rehabilitation units, generally staffed by certified geriatricians, provide in-facility rehabilitation for as long as required and may continue to provide these services on an outpatient basis. Such services, along with the general freedom from worry about health care costs, no doubt underlie Canadians' greater satisfaction with their health care system (27).

The outcomes of hip fracture in the two countries may be instructive. Since the role of physician discretion in deciding whether to operate is minimized, an important source of variation is essentially eliminated. The health status of patients suffering hip fractures should be similar (after controlling for age) in the two countries. Surgical rates for hip fracture repair were nearly identical in Manitoba (50.0 operations per 10,000 elderly) and New England (50.5). The patients' age (81.6 and 81.9 for Manitoba and New England) and percentage of high-risk diagnoses (22.9 and 25.0, respectively) are quite similar.

To a considerable extent, short-term survival will reflect the timeliness, intensity, and quality of medical care. Thus, the relatively poor 30-day survival of Manitoba hip fracture patients may relate to the difficulty of bringing patients to surgery rapidly. Intensity of treatment may also bring short-term (but not long-term) survival benefits (28).

Both the cause of the higher acute mortality in Manitoba and the improved subsequent survival of Manitoba hip fracture patients bear further scrutiny. Comparisons between jurisdictions highlight areas where quality might be improved; the Manitoba short-term survival rates should not be seen as written in stone. Since the survival curves of New England and Manitoba patients do appear to meet—indicating at least equal long-term survival in Manitoba—the health care system may well contribute to improved longevity.

A robust relationship between socioeconomic status and health has been found in many studies and seems ubiquitous to industrialized countries. Thus, reducing inequalities in economic status may mitigate class differences in health status (29–31). As a percentage of gross domestic product (GDP), public expenditures on health, family benefits, and unemployment insurance are higher in Canada than in the United States. Support for the poor elderly is probably greater in Canada, since American pension benefits are more related to earnings (32, 33). To the extent that Canada's social programs have reduced poverty, they should have improved health status and added to Canadian life expectancy.

On the other hand, factors other than social class also appear important (34, 35). Despite economic, social, and geographic similarities, male and female life expectancies in British Columbia exceed those in the state of Washington by between 1.5 and 2 years. Relatively long life expectancies in rural states such as Iowa point to the importance of lifestyle and physical environment (12). Indeed, the variations in mortality rates across American states are larger than the differences between Manitoba and New England. Controlling for known prognostic factors—variables that measure individual patients' medical conditions—seems unlikely to be able to explain away a large part of these differences (6, 36–38).

The differences in life expectancy noted here are considerably larger in magnitude than the variations associated with many health promotion and medical treatment strategies. Thus, a "best-case" scenario associated with reduction of fat in the American diet leads to an increase in life expectancy of only three to four months (39). From a different perspective, the expected outcomes of watchful waiting versus immediate transurethral resection for benign prostatic hypertrophy varied only 2.94 "quality-adjusted life-months" in an analysis of 70-year-old men (40).

HOW MIGHT WE LEARN MORE?

Competing explanations for our findings and their potential policy importance suggest several lines of inquiry. First, new data collection might provide answers to such questions as: How healthy are Canadian and American patients before and after surgery? How many patients in each jurisdiction are served by home care after surgery? How does the frequency of transfer to a rehabilitation unit for further therapy in Manitoba compare with the frequency of transfer to a skilled nursing facility in New England? Second, adding census data on social class to existing administrative data would help sort out the potential impact of social supports. In Manitoba, recent research has found no statistically significant relationships between several measures of social class and poor health outcomes in the elderly (41). If the Manitoba/New England mortality differences are concentrated in the lowest quintile in income distribution, explanations based on Canada's more generous medical and social programs would become more plausible.

Third, research on long-term treatment outcomes should consider baseline mortality rates across the catchment areas of cooperating hospitals (38). Because the benefits and risks of different treatment alternatives vary with expected life span, the generalizability of findings will be affected by the baseline risks in the population (40). Surgical therapies with short-term risks will generally have higher costs per quality-adjusted life year as mortality (baseline or patient-specific) increases; the average patient will have less time to "recover" the costs and risks of surgery.[3] Recent, well-publicized efforts to better inform patients about the outcomes of various treatment options should take into account local data on both short-term and longer-term mortality (43).

POLICY IMPLICATIONS

Differences in per capita health spending of a magnitude similar to that observed between the United States and Canada are seen across the United States and within states (44, 45). The size of the observed differences in per capita expenditures and the absence of known benefits from higher spending levels suggest that substantial resources may be available within current U.S. health care spending for reallocation to meet currently unmet needs (46, 47). The lower

---

[3] Quality-adjusted life years measure longevity on "a utility scale in which each year of life is weighted by an index (ranging from 0 to 1) that reflects the quality of life in that year (42).

health expenditures and the greater population longevity in Canada suggest that it may even be possible to achieve better population health for fewer dollars.

Our findings indicate that despite talk of a "health care crisis," there is no such crisis in Canada. Up until now, Canada has been relatively successful in controlling costs as a proportion of its wealth while providing universal access. With the Canadian economy in poor shape, the current challenge is to contain costs and further improve quality in a system that, all in all, has outperformed its American counterpart (see Chapter 1) (48–50).

Such goals can be met only if we begin to address the difficult questions of the determinants of population health. When is the appropriate mix of expenditures among ambulatory care, acute hospital care, and long-term care that is associated with the best long-term outcomes? What is the role of social programs in achieving improved survival among the elderly? What is the relationship between short-term outcomes and long-term health status? We recognize that posing trade-offs between health policy and social policy complicates matters greatly. However, the Canadian experience suggests that a comprehensive approach to the problem of health expenditures is warranted. As health care debates in both the United States and Canada continue, our study argues forcefully that we consider the following: Are we asking the right questions as we pursue value in health care?

REFERENCES

1. Woolhandler, S., and Himmelstein, D. U. The deteriorating administrative efficiency of the U.S. health care system. *N. Engl. J. Med.* 324: 1253–1258, 1991.
2. U.S. Government. *The President's Comprehensive Health Reform Program.* Government Printing Office, Washington, D.C., 1992.
3. Roos, L. L., et al. Postsurgical mortality in Manitoba and New England. *JAMA* 263: 2453–2458, 1990.
4. Organization for Economic Cooperation and Development. *Health Care Systems in Transition: The Search for Efficiency.* Paris, 1990.
5. U.S. Centers for Disease Control. Mortality in developed countries. *MMWR* 39: 205–209, 1990.
6. U.S. Bureau of the Census. *Statistical Abstract of the United States, 1990.* Government Printing Office, Washington, D.C., 1990.
7. U.S. Bureau of the Census. *State and Metropolitan Area Data Book, 1986.* Government Printing Office, Washington, D.C., 1986.
8. Statistics Canada. *Profiles: Population and Dwelling Characteristics—Census Divisions and Subdivisions: Manitoba,* Part 1. Catalogue 94-113, 1986. Canadian Government Publishing Centre, Ottawa, 1987.
9. Schieber, G. J., and Poullier, J. P. Overview of international comparisons of health care expenditures. *Health Care Financ. Rev.,* Suppl. 1989, pp. 1-7.
10. Health Care Financing Administration. *Nonfederal Hospital Expenditures, 1969–1987. Special Analyses.* Baltimore, 1990.

11. Newhouse, J. P., Anderson, G., and Roos, L. L. Hospital spending in the United States and Canada: A comparison. *Health Aff.,* Winter 1988, pp. 6–16.
12. Fuchs, V. R., and Hahn, J. S. How does Canada do it? A comparison of expenditures for physicians' services in the United States and Canada. *N. Engl. J. Med.* 323: 884–890, 1990.
13. Organization for Economic Cooperation and Development. *Financing and Delivering Health Care: A Comparative Analysis of OECD Countries.* Paris, 1987.
14. Roos, L. L., et al. Registries and administrative data: Organization and accuracy. 1992.
15. Wentworth, D. N., Neaton, J. D., and Rasmussen, W. L. An evaluation of the Social Security Administration Master Beneficiary Record File and the National Death Index in the ascertainment of vital status. *Am. J. Public Health* 73: 1270–1274, 1983.
16. Statistics Canada. *Life Tables, Canada and Provinces, 1985–1987.* Catalogue 541-044. Ottawa, 1989.
17. Charlson, M. E., et al. A new method of classifying prognostic comorbidity in longitudinal studies: Development and validation. *J. Chronic Dis.* 40: 373–383, 1987.
18. Flood, A. B., and Scott, W. R. *Hospital Structure and Performance.* Johns Hopkins University Press, Baltimore, 1987.
19. Russin, L. A., and Russin, M. A. Hip fracture: A review of 1,116 cases in a community hospital setting. *Orthopedics* 4: 23–34, 1981.
20. Roos, N. P., et al. Mortality and reoperation after open transurethral resection of the prostate for benign prostatic hyperplasia. *N. Engl. J. Med.* 320: 1120–1124, 1988.
21. Wilkins, R., and Adams, O. B. Health expectancy in Canada, late 1970s: Demographic, regional, and social dimensions. *Am. J. Public Health* 73: 1073–1080, 1983.
22. Hertzman, C. Where are the differences which make a difference? Thinking about the determinants of health. *CIAR Population Health Working Paper 8.* Canadian Institute for Advanced Research, Toronto, 1990.
23. Wong, T., and Wilkins, K. How many deaths from major chronic diseases could be prevented? *Chronic Dis. Can.,* September 1990, pp. 73–76.
24. Statistics Canada. *Health and Social Support, 1985,* General Social Survey, Analysis Series, Catalogue 11-612, No. 1. Canadian Government Publishing Centre, Ottawa, 1987.
25. National Center for Health Statistics. *Health, United States, 1988.* DHHS Publication No. (PHS) 89-1232. Government Printing Office, Washington, D.C., 1989.
26. Trivia but not trivial. *Future Health/Perspectives Santé,* Winter 1990, p. 21.
27. Blendon, R. J., et al. Satisfaction with health systems in ten nations. *Health Aff.,* Summer 1990, pp. 185–192.
28. Garber, A. M., Fuchs, V. R., and Silverman, J. F. Case-mix, costs, and outcomes—differences between faculty and community services in a university hospital. *N. Engl. J. Med.* 310: 1231–1237, 1984.
29. Blaxter, M. Health services as a defense against the consequences of poverty in industrialized societies. *Soc. Sci. Med.* 17: 1139–1148, 1983.
30. Bunker, J. P., Gomby, D. S., and Kehrer, B. H. (eds.). *Pathways to Health: The Role of Social Factors.* Henry J. Kaiser Foundation, Menlo Park, Calif., 1989.
31. Haan, M., Kaplan, G. A., and Camacho, T. Poverty and health: Prospective evidence from the Alameda County Study. *Am. J. Epidemiol.* 125: 989–998, 1987.

32. Organization for Economic Cooperation and Development. *Aging Populations: The Social Policy Implications.* Paris, 1988.
33. Organization for Economic Cooperation and Development. *Reforming Public Pensions.* Paris, 1988.
34. Katz, A. and McCarry, M. *A Tale of Two Systems: A Comparative Study of the British Columbia and Washington State Health Care Systems and Their Effects on Access, Costs, and Health.* Washington University Press, Seattle, 1989.
35. Evans, R. G., Barer, M. L., and Hertzman, C. The twenty-year experiment: Accounting for, explaining, and evaluating health care cost containment in Canada and the United States. *Annu. Rev. Public Health* 12: 481–518, 1991.
36. Roos, L. L., Sharp, S. M., and Cohen, M. M. Comparing clinical information with claims data: Some similarities and differences. *J. Clin. Epidemiol.* 44: 881–888, 1991.
37. Daley, J., et al. Predicting hospital-associated mortality for Medicare patients: A method for patients with stroke, pneumonia, acute myocardial infarction, and congestive heart failure. *JAMA* 260: 3617–3624, 1988.
38. Enterline, P. E. Pitfalls in epidemiological research: An examination of the asbestos literature. *J. Occup. Med.* 18: 150–156, 1976.
39. Browner, W. S., Westenhouse, J., and Tice, J. A. What if Americans are less fat? A quantitative estimate of the effect on mortality. *JAMA* 265: 3285–3291, 1991.
40. Barry, M. J., et al. Watchful waiting vs. immediate transurethral resection for symptomatic prostatism: The importance of patients' preferences. *JAMA* 259: 3010–3017, 1988.
41. Roos, N. P., and Havens, B. J. Predictors of successful aging: A twelve-year study of Manitoba elderly. *Am. J. Public Health* 81: 63–68, 1991.
42. Weinstein, M. C., et al. *Clinical Decision Analysis,* p. 216, W. B. Saunders, Philadelphia, 1980.
43. Wennberg, J. E. Outcomes research, cost containment, and the fear of health care rationing. *N. Engl. J. Med.* 323: 1202–1204, 1990.
44. U.S. General Accounting Office. *Health Care Spending: Nonpolicy Factors Account for Most State Differences.* Washington, D.C., 1992.
45. Fisher, E. S., Welch, H. G., and Wennberg, J. E. Prioritizing Oregon's hospital resources: An example based on variations in discretionary medical utilization. *JAMA* 267: 1925–1931, 1992.
46. Wennberg, J. E., Freeman, J. L., and Culp, W. J. Are hospital services rationed in New Haven or over-utilized in Boston? *Lancet,* May 23, 1987, pp. 1185–1189.
47. Wennberg, J. E., et al. Hospital use and mortality among Medicare beneficiaries in Boston and New Haven. *N. Engl. J. Med.* 321: 1168–1173, 1989.
48. Evans, R. G., et al. Controlling health expenditures—the Canadian reality. *N. Engl. J. Med.* 320: 571–577, 1989.
49. Evans, R. G. Tension, compression, and shear: Directions, stresses, and outcomes of health care cost control. *J. Health Polit. Policy Law,* Spring 1990, pp. 101–128.
50. Wilkins, R., Adams, O., and Brancker, A. Highlights from a new study of changes in mortality by income in urban Canada. *Chronic Dis. Can.,* May 1990, pp. 38–40.

PART III. PUBLIC OPINION OF THE CANADIAN AND U.S. HEALTH CARE SYSTEMS

CHAPTER 16

Public Opinion
of Health Care Reform

David U. Himmelstein and Steffie Woolhandler

WOULD AMERICANS PREFER THE CANADIAN
HEALTH CARE SYSTEM?

The Harris polling organization asked a random sample of Americans the question shown below. The responses are displayed in Figure 1.

- In the Canadian system of national health insurance, the government pays most of the cost of health care for everyone out of taxes, and the government sets all fees charged by doctors and hospitals. Under the Canadian system, people can choose their own doctors and hospitals. On balance, would you prefer the Canadian system or the system we have here [in the U.S.]?

WOULD CANADIANS PREFER THE
U.S. HEALTH CARE SYSTEM?

The Harris polling organization asked a random sample of Canadians if they would prefer the U.S. system, using the question shown on page 277. Note that this question provides an overly positive description of the U.S. system. In fact, our government does *not* pay most of the costs of health care for the elderly, the poor, and the disabled. Moreover, most Americans are now covered by insurance policies that limit their choice of doctors and hospitals. The survey responses are shown in Figure 2.

Published in *The National Health Program Chartbook,* 1992, pp. 134–150.

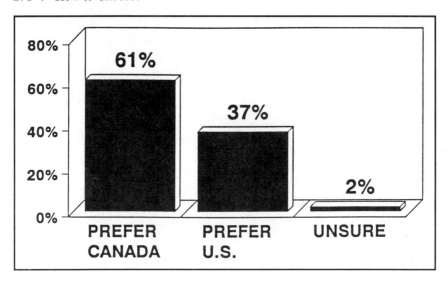

Figure 1. The Harris polling organization surveyed a random sample of Americans, asking them if they would prefer a Canadian-style system: 61 percent replied that they would prefer the Canadian system, 37 percent would prefer the U.S. system, and 2 percent were unsure. Source: Blendon, *Health Manage. Q.* 1: 1, 1989.

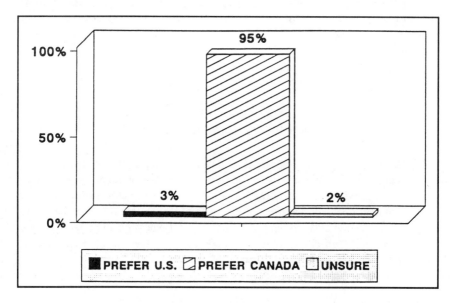

Figure 2. The Harris polling organization asked a random sample of Canadians if they would prefer the U.S. system: 3 percent said yes, 2 percent were unsure, and 95 percent said no. A Canadian colleague pointed out that this 3 percent figure is approximately equal to the illiteracy rate in Canada. Source: Blendon, *Health Manage. Q.* 1: 1, 1989.

• In the U.S. system the government pays most of the cost of health care for the elderly, the poor, and the disabled. Most others either have health insurance paid by their employers or have to buy it from an insurance company. Some have no insurance. Under the U.S. system people can choose their own doctors and hospitals. On balance, would you prefer the U.S. system or the system we have here [in Canada]?

AMERICANS AND CANADIANS:
A SIMILAR SOCIAL ETHIC (Figure 3)

The Harris polling organization surveyed Canadians and Americans about their attitudes toward health care. They expected to find substantial differences between the two nations that would account for the differences in the health care systems. To their surprise, more than 80 percent of the people in both countries favor one-class care, more than 3/4 believe that government should assure access to care, and about 2/3 advocate taxing the rich to pay for care. Fewer than one in five believe that the sick should pay more for care. The pollsters concluded that Americans and Canadians have very similar views of what a health care system should be, but that America's political leadership has not reflected the wishes of the American people.

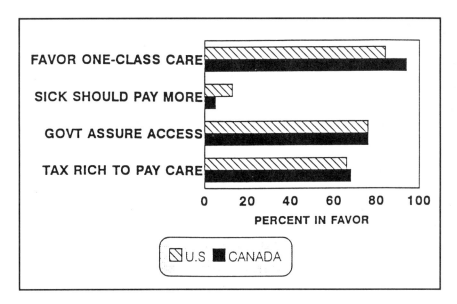

Figure 3. Source: *Health Manage. Q.* 3: 2, 1991.

HOW MANY PREFER
A CANADIAN STYLE SYSTEM? (Figure 4)

Support for a Canadian-style national health program (NHP) is widespread. Majorities of virtually every demographic group support an NHP, in contrast to the more narrow support enjoyed by employer mandate programs. Under an NHP, most Americans' health coverage would improve because copayments and deductibles would be eliminated and long-term care would be covered. Under employer mandate proposals the uninsured might gain coverage, but policies for most Americans would not be improved. As a result, virtually identical proportions of those with coverage and those currently uninsured support an NHP.

WHITES	61%
AFRICAN-AMERICANS	61%
HISPANICS	62%
EXECUTIVES	67%
WHITE COLLAR	59%
BLUE COLLAR	60%
LOW INCOME	58%
MIDDLE INCOME	68%
HIGH INCOME	56%
AMERICANS WHO NOW HAVE HEALTH INSURANCE	**62%**
AMERICANS WITH NO HEALTH INSURANCE	**61%**

Figure 4. Source: *Health Aff.* 8(1): 154, 1989.

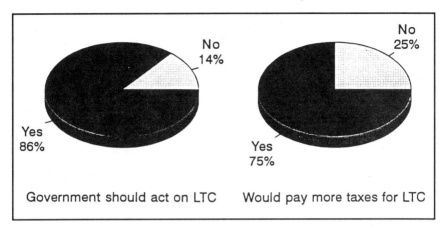

Government should act on LTC   Would pay more taxes for LTC

Figure 5. Sources: R. L. Associates, 1987; L. Harris Associates, 1988.

PUBLIC OPINION
ON LONG-TERM CARE (Figure 5)

Public opinion strongly supports public financing of long-term care: 87 percent of Americans consider the absence of long-term care financing a crisis; a majority prefer public over private funding. Federal administration is favored over private insurance programs by a 3 to 2 margin, and 2/3 believe that private insurance companies would undermine quality of care because of their emphasis on profits. Further, 86 percent of Americans support government action for a universal long-term care program that would finance care for all income groups, and 75 percent would agree to increase taxes to fund it.

Figures 6 through 11 present data on Americans' satisfaction (or lack of) with their health care, their opinions on reform, and their opinions on higher deductibles and copayments.

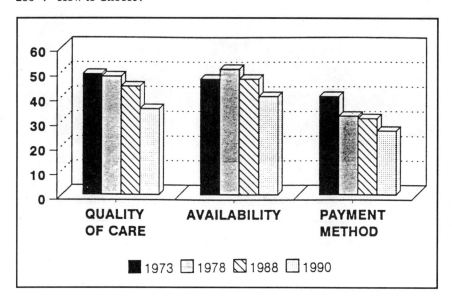

Figure 6. Percent of Americans very satisfied with aspects of their medical care, 1973–1990. The proportion of Americans very satisfied with their care has fallen substantially over the past two decades. Source: Roper, 1991.

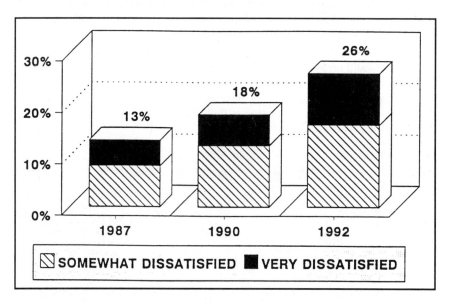

Figure 7. The percent of Americans dissatisfied with their care has doubled in five years. According to polling data, the proportion of Americans who are somewhat dissatisfied or very dissatisfied with their medical care has doubled since 1987. Sources: Harris, 1987, 1990; Commonwealth Foundation, 1992.

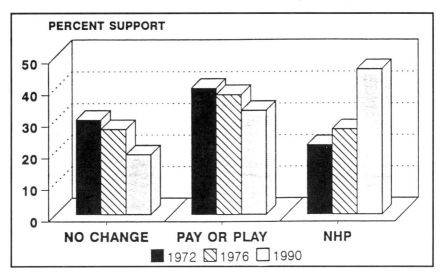

Figure 8. Public support for health reform: 1972, 1976, and 1990. The proportion of Americans wanting to keep the system as it is, or favoring a pay-or-play (employer mandate) approach, has dropped over the past two decades. A national health program is now the preferred approach. Source: Harris, 1990.

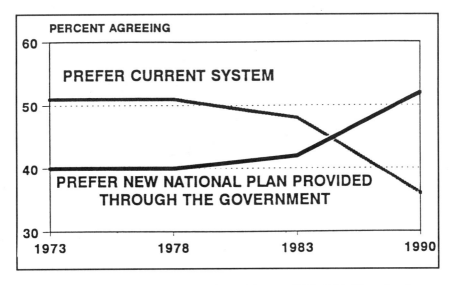

Figure 9. Mandate for radical change in health care, 1973–1990. There has been a dramatic drop in the proportion of Americans who prefer the current system, and a substantial increase in those favoring a government funded national health insurance. The data are derived from repeated surveys by the Roper polling organization. Source: Roper, 1991.

DATE	POLL	PERCENT SUPPORT
1989	NBC (NATIONAL)	67%
1989	LOUISVILLE COURIER J. (KENTUCKY)	62%
1990	LA TIMES (NATIONAL)	72%
1990	ATLANTIC FINANCIAL (WEST VIRGINIA)	62%
1990	CBS/NYT (NATIONAL)	64%
1990	GALLUP FOR BLUE CROSS (NATIONAL)	60%
1990	HARTFORD COURANT (CONNECTICUT)	60%
1990	ROPER (NATIONAL)	69%
1990	ASSOCIATED PRESS (NATIONAL)	62%

Figure 10. Support for a tax-financed NHP: 1989–1990. Recent polls have consistently shown that about 2/3 of the American people support a tax-financed national health insurance program. Source: *Health Aff.* 10(2): 168, 1991.

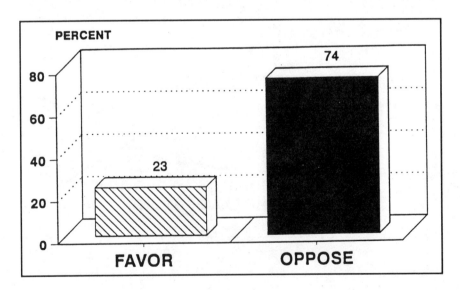

Figure 11. Do Americans favor higher copayments and deductibles to control costs? An overwhelming majority reject cost control strategies based on increasing patients' out-of-pocket costs. While many policy-makers claim that copayments and deductibles will solve the problem, the public thinks copayments and deductibles *are* the problem. Source: *Health Aff.* 8(1): 114, 1989.

PUBLIC OPINION OF HEALTH REFORM

A 1988 survey by the Arthur D. Little Opinion Research Corporation demonstrated that 72 percent of Americans favored national health insurance, including a majority of both Democrats and Republicans. It also found a remarkably egalitarian view of health care: 84 percent of Americans would prohibit paying extra to avoid waiting in a doctor's office, and 56 percent would prohibit paying extra for better care.

* 72 percent favor national health insurance
    90 percent of blacks, 69 percent of whites
    79 percent of low income, 66 percent of high income
    77 percent of Democrats, 61 percent of Republicans
* 56 percent would prohibit paying extra for better care
* 84 percent would prohibit paying extra to avoid waiting in doctor's office
* 30 percent favor expanding Medicaid to cover the poor
* 18 percent favor expanding Medicaid for the unemployed

It is notable that less than 1/3 of Americans favored expanding Medicaid to cover the poor, and only 18 percent favored expanding Medicaid for the unemployed. These patchwork measures would benefit the uninsured, but would fail to address the problems faced by insured Americans. In contrast, a national health program would offer a solution for the insured as well as for the uninsured.

PHYSICIANS' OPINIONS ON HEALTH POLICY

A survey of physicians published by Colombotas and Kirchner ("Physicians and Social Change") in 1986 found that 56 percent favor some form of national health insurance, though about 3/4 of doctors think that most of their colleagues oppose such reform.

* 56 percent favor some form of National Health Insurance (NHI)
* 74 percent think most other doctors oppose NHI
* 64 percent agree: "It is the responsibility of society, through its government, to provide everyone with the best available medical care, whether he can afford it or not."

Figure 12 shows data on physicians' willingness to trade some of their income for less hassle.

Health economists' opinions on health policy, surveyed in 1990, are shown in Figure 13.

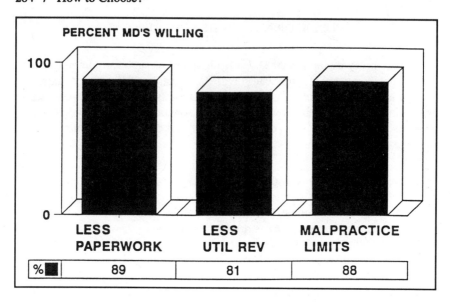

Figure 12. Would physicians accept 10 percent less income for less hassle? The overwhelming majority of physicians would be prepared to trade 10 percent of their income for substantial decreases in paperwork and utilization review, and for tort reform. Source: Metropolitan Life Survey, 1991.

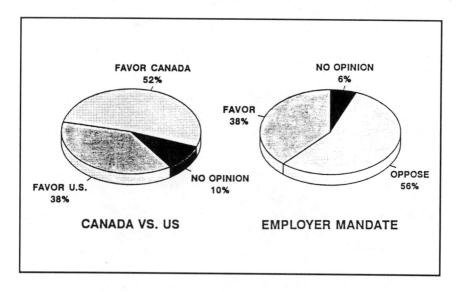

Figure 13. Health economists' opinions on health policy. More than half of all health economists surveyed favor a Canadian-style NHP, whereas only 38 percent support an employer mandate approach. Source: *J. Health Polit. Policy Law* 15: 627, 1990.

CHAPTER 17

Debate on Popular Opinion on Health Care

A

Public Attitudes about Health Care Costs: A Lesson in National Schizophrenia

Robert J. Blendon and Drew E. Altman

Independent forecasts suggest that despite all that is now being done to slow the growth of U.S. health care costs—the enactment of prospective payment for Medicare (diagnosis-related groups (DRGs)); increasing enrollment in health maintenance organizations (HMOs), now 7 percent of the population; hospital rate setting in 12 states; and other changes—the nation's health care expenditures will increase from $322 billion in 1982 to $690 billion in 1990 and to $1.9 trillion by the year 2000 (14 percent of the gross national product) (1, 2). This means an average increase of $50 billion a year and a doubling of the nation's health spending every six years.

The possibility that health care expenditures will rise at this rate is seen by many of the nation's leaders as exacerbating broader problems: a $200 billion federal deficit, the potential bankruptcy of Medicare, the prospect of renewed inflation leading to another recession, and the increasing lack of competitiveness of U.S. goods in world markets. This year, the United States will spend about $1,500 per person for health care, whereas Japan will spend $500, Great Britain $400, France $800, and West Germany $900 (3).

Reprinted by permission of *The New England Journal of Medicine,* from 311(9), pp. 613–616, 1984. Copyright 1984, *Massachusetts Medical Society.*

Why, then, despite the obvious concern about this problem, have we been unable as a nation to agree on a solution? Is it the blocking action of physicians, hospitals, or other interest groups in Washington? Is it the concerns of physicians, which have previously been discussed in the *New England Journal of Medicine* (4)? Is it the change in administration or the honest failure of health professionals or academics to agree on the "right" solution? We believe the answer to all these questions is no. The problem that appears to lie at the heart of the matter is that Americans have much more ambivalent feelings about controlling health care costs than is generally recognized. The public's rather schizophrenic views on this issue have been critical in preventing any single, sweeping solution from being adopted.

What are those views? It seems important to examine them closely, for a resolution of the problem of health care costs will have to be built around the realities of public opinion. Our analysis draws from 15 national public opinion polls conducted between 1981 and 1984 by Gallup, Tarrance and Associates, Yankelovich, Skelly, and White, Research and Forecasts, the Roper Organization, ABC News, and Louis Harris and Associates, as well as from recent surveys by the National Governors' Association and other studies.

Reality 1. Both the public and elected officials see rising costs as the nation's number-one problem in health care. However, neither rank this issue very high on a list of the most important problems now facing the nation.

Surveys show that rising health costs do not appear among the 10 most important problems now facing this country, listed by either the public or elected officials. Unemployment, inflation, social budget cuts, fear of war, excessive government spending, and crime all rank higher (5, 6).

Similarly, when asked to rank the problems believed to be most important at the state level, the nation's governors ranked health number 11. It fell well below more jobs, public safety, and education (7). This was the case despite the fact that outlays for health care are typically the second or third largest state expenditure, the fastest growing, and an issue identified by the National Governors' Association as a critical problem facing state governments (8). Thus, efforts to resolve the complex problem of health care costs take place in an environment in which the public's attention and the energies and political capital of elected officials are largely focused on other national problems.

Realty 2. Americans show great ambivalence about health care costs. They are deeply disturbed by the sharply rising prices of their health care, particularly the increasing cost of a stay in the hospital or a visit to a physician. However, contrary to the views of many national leaders and economists, most Americans are not troubled by the growing share of the nation's economy that is devoted to health care. In fact, most believe that our society currently spends too little rather than too much for these services (9).

In 1983 surveys showed that approximately two out of three Americans saw the high cost of medical care as the major problem facing the nation's health care system (10). Most of those polled (78 percent) recognized that health care costs have been rising at a faster rate than general inflation and believed that this trend has made the costs of their own medical care unreasonable (68 percent) (11, 12). In fact, 25 percent of the public (up from 15 percent in 1974), 51 percent of blacks, and 69 percent of Hispanic Americans reported problems in having enough money to pay for their medical care (5).

Paradoxically, however, Americans are not particularly concerned by the increasing share of the nation's resources that is devoted to health care. Only 14 percent of the public think that our society is spending too much for health care, and 53 percent think we are not spending enough (8). Even with 76 percent of the public seeing our escalating federal deficit as a threat to the economy, two out of three Americans still believe that federal spending for health care should be increased, and 59 percent favor some form of national health insurance, even if coupled with a tax increase to pay for it (13–15).

Although these poll results may seem contradictory, they are consistent with the public's general belief that inflation has made many important family needs, including housing, new automobiles, food, and medical care, prohibitively expensive. Americans believe that their vision of constant material improvement is threatened by the high price of a new home or automobile or a pound of meat, as well as by the cost of a six-day stay in the hospital. It is the unit price that troubles the public most, not the proportion of national resources spent for housing, automobiles, meat, or medical care.

Reality 3. Although most Americans believe that the country's present health care arrangements are not satisfactory, they do not want to change the way in which they currently receive medical care. Surveys show that almost three-quarters of the American public believe that the U.S. health care system requires fundamental change (15). One in four of the general population and one in three of the nation's elderly say that our health care system has so much wrong with it today that "we need to completely rebuild it." Barely one in five Americans think our country's health care arrangements "work pretty well" (16). Sixty-six percent say that doctors are too interested in making money, 68 percent that physician fees are not usually reasonable, and 62 percent that physicians do not spend enough time with their patients (10).

Yet, again, we see extreme ambivalence. In contrast to the public's view of physicians in general, Americans like their own doctors. Seventy-two percent say that their own physician is not too interested in making money, 77 percent that he or she spends enough time with them, and 71 percent that their own physician's fees are usually reasonable (10).

With regard to their own most recent illnesses, 72 percent of those who were hospitalized in the previous year, 78 percent of those who have seen a physician recently, and 63 percent of those who have needed emergency treatment say that they were completely satisfied with the medical care they actually received. The only major complaint (expressed by about 40 percent of those receiving care) was with high out-of-pocket costs that were not paid by an individual's health-insurance plan (17).

This dichotomy between apparent widespread public discontent with the nation's health care system and pervasive satisfaction with personal medical care has important implications for any efforts aimed at slowing the nation's rising health care costs (18).

Reality 4. Because most Americans are reasonably satisfied with the medical care they currently receive and do not see themselves as having created the problem of health care costs, they tend to support only the cost-containment proposals that leave their present personal health care arrangements intact and oppose solutions involving any major reorganization of the nation's health care system.

Surveys show that only about one-quarter of Americans think that they have a great deal of personal responsibility for the nation's rising health care costs. Most believe that the high costs of health care are due to factors other than their own behavior (11). Since this view is coupled with general satisfaction with personal medical care, it is not surprising that the public shows only limited interest in cost-containment proposals that are seen as requiring them to change substantially the ways in which they receive that care. Only 8 percent of Americans give a high priority to enactment of either "socialized" medicine or a national health service (16). Only 33 percent would agree to go to physicians and doctors from a list provided by insurance companies, with no extra charges (10). Only 21 percent wish to limit the use of new, expensive medical equipment and techniques (11). Only 36 percent would be interested in paying a higher health insurance deductible (11). Only 18 percent would be willing to wait longer than usual for an appointment with a physician (10), only 21 percent would be willing to give up the right to sue for malpractice (11), and only 40 percent would like to save money by giving up their personal doctor and being treated by a group of physicians—e.g., at a clinic (10).

The dichotomy between the public's desire for a reorganization of the nation's health care system, on the one hand, and the desire to maintain personal health care arrangements, on the other, can best be seen in the last survey question. The majority of the Americans polled are not in favor of giving up their own personal physicians for care delivered by lower-cost physician groups (10). In fact, studies show that the major reason why many working Americans choose not to join HMOs is their reluctance to break ties with their family physician (19). However, the public is quite enthusiastic (66 percent) about requiring low-income people to use less costly clinics or HMOs (11). The message seems to be: "Reorganize the nation's health care for others, but don't change my own health care arrangements."

The cost-containment approaches strongly favored by most Americans are those that are seen as not disrupting existing individual health care arrangements. In addition, those polled seemed interested in approaches that look as if they might actually improve the quality of their care. For example, over 60 percent of Americans find government price controls on doctor and hospital fees relatively acceptable (16). Likewise, 74 percent of Americans are in favor of regional coordination of expensive hospital services; 58 percent favor a requirement that hospitals budget prospectively; 77 and 84 percent, respectively, favor a requirement that physicians and hospitals publish their fees and charges; and 52 percent would like to see insurance companies reduce premiums for policyholders who do not smoke, do use seat belts, or are not overweight (11).

In terms of saving money through new arrangements that might improve the quality of their health care, Americans see the reduction of unnecessary institutionalization as a positive objective. People are fearful of going to a hospital or nursing home. Thus, 75 percent support the requirement of a second opinion for surgery (11), 56 percent find it acceptable to encourage performance of tests and minor surgery in outpatient clinics and doctors' offices (16), and 46 percent strongly favor home treatment for serious chronic illness (16). Similarly, 70 percent believe that the family of an unconscious, terminally ill patient should be able to have the physician remove life-support systems (11). All these potentially cost-saving measures are seen by the public as improving the quality of life.

Reality 5. With regard to the various proposals that have been advanced for slowing the rise in the nation's health care costs, the views of practicing physicians are often more influential with the public than the opinions of the groups proposing changes—government officials, business, and labor leaders (4).

Surveys show that three out of four people believe physicians bear a major responsibility for the nation's rising health care costs (11), and two out of three say they are beginning to lose faith in doctors (10). In general, however, physicians still maintain a unique credibility with the public.

Survey results indicate that Americans continue to place more confidence in the leadership of American medicine than in almost any other leadership group. Although the public's confidence in medicine has fallen dramatically since the mid-1960s (from 73 to 35 percent), in 1983 it still ranked substantially higher than public confidence in the leadership of the nation's major companies (18 percent), organized labor (10 percent), or the Congress (20 percent) (20, 21).

Likewise, 52 percent of the American people rank physicians high or very high on "honesty and ethical standards," whereas less than 15 percent give similar high marks to the major groups proposing change—government officials (15 percent), business executives (15 percent), and labor-union leaders (12 percent). To bring this home most forcibly, even labor-union families rank physicians higher, in terms of integrity, than labor-union leaders (52 and 14 percent, respectively) (22). All in all, three of four Americans still believe "most doctors are generally dedicated to helping people" (8).

Moreover, the public is more trusting of information from the medical community (79 percent) than from either organized labor (46 percent) or major companies (43 percent) (23). This strong credibility is reflected in public responsiveness to the major concerns of physicians about various cost-containment proposals.

THE IMPORTANCE OF PUBLIC OPINION

It is our belief that public opinion is only one of many factors that influence the nation's health care decision making (4). Health professionals, business and labor leaders, academics, the Congress, government officials, the courts, and special interest groups all have important roles. However, studies show that in areas such as medical care, in which any major national decision will affect the lives of millions of Americans and their families, public opinion is likely to set the practical and political boundaries within which the nation's decision makers can make acceptable changes (24).

As we have seen from the polls, the public is neither sufficiently concerned (relative to other issues) nor sufficiently single-minded about what should be done to make the adoption of a solution to the health cost problem a realistic possibility. Because the bulk of health care is paid for with funds from business, labor, or government (1), most Americans feel no direct pressure to accept a single solution that would dramatically alter their current arrangements for medical care.

This does not mean, however, that nothing can be done. Public opinion polls also suggest that it may be possible to gain acceptance for a cost-containment program that includes elements of different solutions, which if taken together, could have a substantial impact on our mounting health care bill.

THE PUBLIC'S VIEW OF THE
AVAILABLE CHOICES

Generally, the suggested solutions to the problem of rising health care costs can be categorized as either short term or long term. The long-term approaches are of two types: biomedical breakthroughs and major positive changes in life style. Not surprisingly, both are acceptable to the general public. Polls show that the public rates medical research as the highest priority for national research support (25). In addition, more than half of those polled believe we should give more emphasis to the prevention of disease (26). Unfortunately, however, neither of these long-term approaches is likely to have a large impact on health costs in the next decade.

The short-term solutions that have been proposed to slow the increase in health care costs include (a) regulation—reimbursement, utilization, and capital-investment controls (recently, with Medicare DRGs and state hospital rate setting, reimbursement controls have been the most prominent); (b) competition—the restructuring of health insurance benefits and the development of alternative health plans, such as HMOs and preferred-provider organizations; (c) voluntary programs—private initiatives to contain the costs of medical care through voluntary "freezes" and community and "business coalitions," which now number more than 100; (*d*) curtailment of services to the poor—through major reductions in public sector support of health services for low-income citizens and the unemployed; (*e*) rationing of high-cost equipment and procedures; and (*f*) nationalization of the industry—the British and Swedish solution to the problem.

Polls tell us that the last two options are not seen by most Americans as desirable for the United States (1, 2). Although there is support (74 percent) for regionalizing "big ticket" technological equipment, such as nuclear magnetic resonance and CAT scanners, only 21 percent of Americans are in favor of rationing costly new technological approaches (11). In fact, 90 percent of Americans favor the continued development of highly expensive heart, kidney, and other organ transplantations (23). Ninety-two percent of Americans show no strong interest in either "socialized medicine" or a British-style health system (16).

On the other hand, there is support for the first two short-term solutions—regulation and competition—though they are grounded in different premises. Such support is limited, however, and does not suggest a blanket endorsement of either strategy. For example, 58 percent of the public support the idea of paying hospitals a fixed, prospectively set payment for their services (11). However, the majority of Americans are opposed to a comprehensive federal regulatory system to control health care costs (10) or to limitations on the use of expensive medical procedures (11).

Similarly, some Americans will accept higher out-of-pocket payments as part of their insurance coverage (11) or are willing to receive care from less costly groups of physicians (10, 11), but the majority are opposed to or uncomfortable with these alternatives. There is a common theme here, with respect to both the regulatory and competitive approaches: the more a particular solution will alter current medical care arrangements, the less the public will support it. Not surprisingly, since they have only indirect effects on personal health care arrangements, proposals to cut insurance payments to physicians and to introduce prospective reimbursement for hospitals are viewed as acceptable by the American public (11, 16). For similar reasons, most Americans are willing to use less costly physician groups on a voluntary but not on a mandatory basis (10).

Public opinion about the acceptability of the third short-term approach, voluntary freezes or coalitions, is not known. However, surveys show that most corporate benefits officers, insurance executives, hospital administrators, union officials, and physicians are generally supportive of private sector initiatives of this kind (16).

This leaves one final short-term solution: curtailment of public programs supporting health care for the poor—an approach that may prove extraordinarily expensive over the long haul in both human and economic terms. Though polls show public support for the Medicaid program, in practice, eligibility for

Medicaid is closely linked to the nation's welfare programs (9), and in striking contrast to medical care, welfare is an area in which most Americans (71 percent) want no additional spending (14).

CONCLUSION

Health care costs are predicted to rise at a rate of $50 billion a year over the next decade. Unless some major new initiatives are undertaken, we will see the nation's health spending double every six years.

Public opinion surveys show that, more than ever before, Americans want the problem of rising health care costs addressed. However, they are unwilling to support the adoption of any solution that would produce a dramatic change in their own medical care arrangements.

Many people in business, labor, government, academia, and medicine remain deeply committed to one or another proposal as the *only* solution to rising health care costs. This allegiance to single solutions stands in the way of aggressive national efforts to solve the problem. The task ahead for the nation's leaders is to move away from the search for a single solution and to build a consensus around a cost-containment program that realistically reflects public opinion.

REFERENCES

1. Freeland, M. S., and Schendler, C. E. Health spending in the 1980s: Integration of clinical practice patterns with management. *Health Care Financ. Rev.* 5: 1–68, 1984.
2. Tyson, K. W., and Merrill, J. C. Health care institutions: Survival in a changing environment. *J. Med. Educ.,* 1984.
3. Macrae, N. Health care international: Better care at one eighth the cost: *Economist,* April 28, 1984, pp. 17–18.
4. Iglehart, J. Opinion polls on health care. *N. Engl. J. Med.* 310: 1616–1620, 1984.
5. Shriver, J. (ed.). Making ends meet. *Gallup Rep.* 220–221: 25, 1984.
6. Shriver, J. (ed.). The most important problem. *Gallup Rep.* 220–221: 28–29, 1984.
7. National Governors' Association. *Governors' Priorities: 1983,* pp. 3–4. Washington, D.C., 1983.
8. National Governors' Association. *Governors' Guide to Health Care Cost Containment Strategies,* pp. 1–2. Washington, D.C., 1984.
9. Navarro, V. Where is the popular mandate? *N. Engl. J. Med.* 307: 1516–1518, 1982.
10. Lance Tarrance and Associates. *Public Opinion on Health Care Issues: 1983,* pp. 1–25. American Medical Association, Chicago, 1983.
11. Yankelovich, Skelly and White, Inc. *Health and Health Insurance: The Public's View,* pp. 5–29. Health Insurance Association of America, Washington, D.C., 1984.
12. Jeffe, D., and Jeffe, S. B. Losing patience with doctors: Physicians vs. the public on health care costs. *Public Opinion* 7(1): 45–47, 1984.
13. Lipset, M. L., and Wattenberg, B. J. (eds.). Opinion roundup. *Public Opinion* 6(5): 26–27, 1983.

14. Lipset, M. L., and Wattenberg, B. J. (eds.). Opinion roundup. *Public Opinion* 6(2): 26–27, 1983.
15. Shriver, J. (ed.). The economy: Threats to recovery. *Gallup Rep.* 218: 8, 1983.
16. Louis Harris and Associates. *The Equitable Health Care Survey: Options for Controlling Costs*, pp. 6–55. Equitable Life Assurance Society, New York, 1983.
17. Louis Harris and Associates. *Access to Health Care Services in the U.S.: 1982*, pp. 65–91. New York, 1982.
18. Andersen, R., Fleming, G. V., and Champney, T. F. Exploring a paradox: Belief in a crisis and satisfaction with medical care. *Milbank Mem. Fund Q.* 60: 329–354, 1982.
19. United States Department of Health and Human Services. *Employer Attitudes Toward Health Maintenance Organizations*, pp. 60–61. DHHS Publication No. (HRS-M-HM)83-2. Government Printing Office, Washington, D.C., 1983.
20. Lipset, M. L., and Wattenberg, B. J. (eds.). Opinion roundup. *Public Opinion* 2(5): 30–31, 1979.
21. Louis Harris and Associates. Unpublished data.
22. Shriver, J. (ed.). Honesty and ethical standards. *Gallup Rep.* 214: 4–29, 1983.
23. National Science Board. *Science Indicators 1982: An Analysis of the State of U.S. Science, Engineering, and Technology*, pp. 154, 321. National Science Foundation, Washington, D.C., 1983.
24. Wilson, J. Q. *American Government: Institutions and Policies*, Ed. 2. D. C. Heath, Lexington, Mass., 1983.
25. National Science Board. *Science Indicators 1980*, p. 167. National Science Foundation, Washington, D.C., 1981.
26. Louis Harris and Associates. *The Prevention Index: A Report Card on the Nation's Health, Summary Report*, p. 6. New York, 1984.

B

A Response to Conventional Wisdom

Vicente Navarro

Several contributors, the editor, and the publisher of *Health Affairs* have, on several occasions, repeated statements I believe need to be questioned.[1] One is that there has been a *popular mandate since 1980 to cut government health*

---

[1] This, along with Drew E. Altman's response, was originally published as a letter to the editor of *Health Affairs*, Fall 1984.

Parts B, C, and D were published in *International Journal of Health Services*, 15(3), pp. 511–519, 1985.

expenditures, including expenditures for the poor, elderly, and handicapped (1). In those statements it is indicated that while Americans supported those government health programs in the sixties and seventies, they weakened their support at the end of the seventies and beginning of the eighties. All available evidence, however, shows otherwise. A survey of all major polls, including the Harris and Gallup polls, from 1976 to 1983, show that (*a*) American public opinion is not so volatile as it is assumed to be, and (*b*) there has been strong and undiminished support by the majority of the American people throughout this period for federal government health expenditures for the elderly, poor, and handicapped. Moreover, while agreeing that the federal government expenditures may need to be cut to balance the budget, the overwhelming majority of Americans believe (according to George Martin of Yankelovich, Skelly, and White Surveys) that "balancing the budget should be done by cutting down defense and increasing corporate taxes, not by cutting social (including health) expenditures." In brief, any detailed analysis of people's opinion shows that there is not a popular mandate for current federal health policies which include cutting of expenditures for those vulnerable populations.[2] Quite to the contrary. According to pollster Louis Harris (3):

> . . . people all over the country have been profoundly shocked to find that the people running the country seem to want to abandon the poor and the elderly and the minorities . . . and that the American people [think] that America could be systematically stripped of all its compassion for decency and humanity . . . but they are just beginning to get fighting mad about it.

Actually, it is usually forgotten that the majority of the electorate did not vote for Reagan in 1980. They voted for someone else or did not vote. And even among those who voted for him, there is evidence that many did not support his social policies. The current policies of cuts in federal health expenditures do not respond to a popular mandate.

Another position that frequently appears in the pages of *Health Affairs* is that *those cuts in federal health programs were a consequence of the taxpayer's revolt that began in California and spread through the country* (4). It is repeatedly said that Proposition 13 in California was an indicator of a revolt that appeared in the late seventies in this country against increased taxation and that this revolt has forced tax and spending cuts. By definition, however, a revolt assumes a heightening of protest that creates a new situation different from the previous one. An analysis of the popular mood toward taxes, however, does not show evidence of such a revolt. Taxes have been, for the most part, unpopular since they were established. The major changes have been on variations of which of the many

---

[2] For a review of all the polls on federal health programs since 1976 to 1983 see reference 2.

(federal, state income and sales, and property taxes) is the worst. Since 1968, the percentage of those who feel taxes are too high (by type of tax) has not changed much, as shown in Table 1.

In spite of popular awareness of the inequities of the tax structure and its unpopularity, tax reform has not been considered to be a popular top priority. When we look at the open-ended Gallup question (asked since 1939) as to what is the most important issue facing the nation, we find fewer people mentioning taxes in the seventies than in the fifties. In the 1970–1980 period, less than 3 percent named taxes, and these respondents were often more concerned with the relative incidence of taxes than with their level. This confirmed the finding of many polls that the concern with taxes seems to focus not on their level but on equity and incidence questions, with the fairness of the tax system rather than the amount of taxes being the major concern (5).

It was not a heightening of popular discontent about taxes that triggered the passage in California of Proposition 13. The changes in popular mood happened after, not before, Proposition 13. Peretz (5) has convincingly shown how the debate that followed the passage of Proposition 13 (due in large part to the rapid growth of property taxes in a state that had a state budget surplus) raised the level of unpopularity of paying taxes, a level that fell back afterwards to approximately the same level as that of one year earlier. Just two years after the passage of Proposition 13, Proposition 9 (which would have cut state income taxes) failed by a decisive margin of 62 percent to 32 percent.

It is worth stressing that even at the time of highest dissatisfaction with taxes (immediately after Proposition 13), the June 1978 Harris Poll found that the majority of respondents opposed tax cuts if they thought they would lead to cuts in aid to the elderly, disabled, and poor (71 percent opposed), and cuts in services in public hospitals and health care (62 percent).

Another position frequently put forward in *Health Affairs* is that *national health insurance has lost its way because of lack of supporters*. In the

Table 1

Percentages of Harris Poll respondents who felt taxes were too high, by type of tax, 1969–1978

Type of tax	July 1969	Feb. 1973	June 1974	Jan. 1975	Aug. 1976	March 1977	June 1978
Federal income	73	67	73	77	77	73	74
Federal corporate	44	40	25	21	25	45	48
Federal capital gains	55	54	47	48	59	57	—
State income	58	60	52	52	57	56	52
State sales	65	58	62	55	58	53	47
Local property	73	75	67	65	71	73	70

introduction of the Winter issue of 1983 (6), your publisher indicates that "there has been a demise of any real constituency of national health insurance." This position seems to ignore that, since the early seventies, all major polls that have asked people's opinions about a comprehensive universal health program show that either large pluralities or the majority of Americans favor it (2, 7). One would hope that in a democratic society a plurality or majority of people (depending on the year) count as a major constituency after all.

In light of all the already published evidence that contradicts those positions it is clear that the uncritical acceptance of large segments of the medical and academic establishments of the existence of a popular mandate to reduce rather than expand federal health expenditures and related statements cannot be seen as a mere reflection of reality in the United States but, rather, as an advocacy statement rationalizing and justifying those policies.

REFERENCES

1. Iglehart, J. K. An interview with Dr. David E. Rogers. *Health Aff.,* Fall 1983.
2. Navarro, V. Where is the popular mandate. *N. Engl. J. Med.* 307: 1516–1518, 1982.
3. Pollster says opposition to Reagan mounting. *Nation's Health* 12(7): 1–2, 1982.
4. Altman, D. E., and Morgan. The role of state and local government in health. *Health Aff.,* Winter 1983.
5. Peretz, P. There was no tax revolt. *Politics and Society* 11(2): 231, 1982.
6. Walsh, W. B. Letter. *Health Aff.,* Winter 1983.
7. Schneider, W. Public ready for real change in health care. *National Journal* 3(23): 664, 1985.

C

What Do Americans Really Want?

Drew E. Altman

I am happy to comment on Vicente Navarro's "Response to Conventional Wisdom." Since the sad fate of most articles is to go unread, I am even more pleased that the interview with David Rogers (1) and my own article (2) may have helped stimulate him to write.

The crux of Professor Navarro's argument is that Americans want more health spending, not less, particularly for the poor and the elderly. He seems easily upset whenever it is suggested that Americans might want government health spending reduced, and especially bothered whenever anyone mentions Proposition 13, which he regards as an isolated event signifying basically nothing.

It seems fruitless to quibble with Professor Navarro about what was said in the article and interview. Rather, the compelling question is what do Americans really want? It seems important to answer this question, since the views of the public are likely to play a major role in setting the political and practical boundaries around what policymakers can do to affect change.

My colleagues and I have recently had occasion to examine what the public really thinks (see Part A) (3) and the fact is that Professor Navarro is about half right. Americans do favor more spending for health, not less. Public opinion polls tell us that only 14 percent of the public thinks that our society is spending too much for health care, while 53 percent think we are not spending enough. Two out of three Americans still believe that federal spending for health should be increased, and 59 percent still favor some form of national health insurance, even if coupled with a tax increase to pay for it. On the other hand, of course, he is also half wrong. In 1983, approximately two out of three Americans saw the high cost of medical care as the major problem facing the nation's health care system. Seventy-eight percent recognize that health care costs have been rising at a faster rate than inflation. Seventy-six percent of the public see our escalating federal deficit as a threat to the economy. Seventy-one percent want no additional spending on welfare (to which Medicaid is obviously closely tied). Most impressive of all, a recent Roper poll found that controlling health care costs ranked third (tied with inflation and behind crime and drugs and unemployment), as the most important priority for the nation as a whole.

Is there, perhaps, a poll to support virtually any position? Having analyzed all of the recent polls, I think not. They are remarkably consistent. Rather, what appears to be much closer to the truth is that Americans are highly ambivalent about health care costs and health spending and about what to do about the problem. Professor Navarro had decided to tell only one part of the story.

What is the nature of their ambivalence? The polls show that Americans are most concerned about the sharply rising prices of their health care and what they pay out of pocket (68 percent believe the costs of their own medical care are unreasonable). However, in contrast to government officials, many business leaders, and many economists, Americans are not particularly troubled by the increasing share of our nation's resources devoted to health, according to the polls. Perhaps more fundamental, most Americans are reasonably satisfied with their own medical care arrangements (72 percent of those hospitalized last year and 78 percent of those seeing a physician were "completely satisfied") and are unwilling to support cost reduction strategies that would change those arrangements to any significant degree. This fact—the public's reluctance to alter their current medical arrangements—much more than the public's complex and somewhat ambivalent feelings about spending for health, will influence what government and business can accomplish in the coming years to reduce health spending and affect change. The perception in Washington of the need for change in our health system, and the insistence of the proregulation and procompetition "camps" on their favorite solutions, will ultimately have to come to grips with this reality. Otherwise, we will do less than we must to control our mounting expenditures for health. (The views expressed in this letter are those of the author and no official endorsement by The Robert Wood Johnson Foundation is intended or should be inferred.)

REFERENCES

1. Iglehart, J. K. An interview with Dr. David E. Rogers. *Health Aff.*, Fall 1983.
2. Altman, D. E., and Morgan. The role of state and local government in health. *Health Aff.*, Winter 1983.
3. Blendon, R., and Altman, D. Public attitudes about health care costs: A lesson in national schizophrenia. *N. Engl. J. Med.* 311(9): 613–616, 1984.

D

In Defense of American People: Americans Are Not Schizophrenic

Vicente Navarro

In my letter to the editor, published in the Fall 1984 issue of *Health Affairs,* I criticized some key positions put forward in the pages of the journal by its publisher, its editor, and several of its contributors (1). Specifically, I provided evidence questioning the statements that there has been a demise of any real constituency for a national health insurance (W. B. Walsh), and that there has also been a popular mandate for cutting government health expenditures, including expenditures for the poor, elderly, and handicapped (D. E. Rogers and J. K. Iglehart). I also questioned that that "popular mandate" was in response to a taxpayers' revolt that began in California and spread through the country (Altman and Morgan). Altman, in his reply in the same issue, grants that: (*a*) there is indeed a national constituency for a national health program; (*b*) there is not a tax revolt in the health sector (59 percent of Americans are willing to pay higher taxes if those taxes are spent in establishing such a nationwide program); and (*c*) there is not a popular mandate for cutting health expenditures, including those for the poor, elderly, and the handicapped; rather, the majority of people are asking for an expansion (2). I am glad that my letter triggered all those corrections and recognitions. Altman, however, does not stop with these recognitions. He moves on and criticizes me for telling the reader only half of the story. Americans also hold a series of views that, according to him, are in contradiction with the three above-mentioned positions. Americans, for example, are also concerned about (d) the rising costs of health services, (e) the need to reduce the federal deficit, (f) the rising expenditures for "welfare," and (g) changing the personal health care arrangements that they like. Thus, he repeats what he and his colleagues have stated elsewhere: that Americans are schizophrenic in their views on health care and that schizophrenia is the reason for the political inability to make substantial changes in American Medicine (3).

A more detailed and rigorous reading of American popular opinion, however, does not show any contradiction in those views. Quite to the contrary. Those views are logical, reasonable, and consequent with the experience of the majority of Americans. Let me expand on each one of the assumed contradictions by referring both to Altman's letter, as well as to the article that he and Blendon wrote in *The New England Journal of Medicine*, which on popular opinions on health care (see Part A), he refers to extensively.

Blendon and Altman see a contradiction between the public being disturbed by the sharply rising prices of their health care on the one hand, and their apparent lack of concern with the growing share of the nation's economy that is devoted to health care on the other. They lament that most Americans believe that our society spends too little rather than too much on medical care services. They also refer to the apparently contradictory view that, in spite of public concern about health care costs. Americans are still willing to pay even higher taxes for health services (3). A more thorough reading and analysis of these views show, however, that there is nothing contradictory in them. Quite to the contrary—one is a logical extension of the other. Americans are rightly concerned that they still pay a very large percentage of their health care bill directly and out of their own pockets, with major health benefits still uncovered. An international analysis of health expenditures shows that this concern is, indeed, a very legitimate one. No less than 27 percent of all health expenditures in the United States are still covered by direct payment, compared, for example, with only 5 percent in the United Kingdom, 8 percent in Sweden, and 12 percent in West Germany (4). This percentage is even higher among some groups in the population. For example, almost two decades after Medicaid and Medicare, our elderly still pay 40 percent of all their expenditures directly and out of their own pockets (5). The other side of the coin is that the United States is the Western developed country where, for the majority of citizens, health benefits are most limited and large percentages of the population have major problems with insurance coverage (public or private). Here are just a few examples: 32 million Americans do not have public or private insurance coverage (6, 7); 100 million do not have any form of catastrophic insurance coverage (8); and one million American families have been refused medical care because of lack of financial means (9).

Because of these problems of coverage, and because (a) health is perceived by the public as an important condition for enjoying life, and (b) health care is considered to be useful and important for improving the public's health, we find a logical and consequent—rather than contradictory—response from the majority of Americans. They want an expansion rather than a reduction of health expenditures, to the point of being willing to pay even higher taxes if those tax revenues are spent on health care. It is indeed a sign of collective wisdom and solidarity that people are willing to pay less in direct payment (the reason for their concern about costs) and more in taxes (the indication of collective responsibility and solidarity). Actually, it is not only a more equitable way of funding health services, but also a more efficient one. Countries where the majority of health services are paid with public funds have better coverage of benefits and of the population (e.g., United Kingdom, Sweden, Canada) than those, like the United States, which still rely on private funding. And they spend less than we do (4).

The other public demand is for major changes in the medical care system. Here the authors see another major, schizophrenic contradiction between the public's desire to keep their own doctors and their personal health care arrangements, and the need for major changes in the health sector (3, p. 614). Here, again, there is nothing schizophrenic about this set of beliefs. The public can, indeed, be satisfied with many of the elements of the system but still be dissatisfied with how those elements relate together in their structurally defined, institutional settings. The medical profession is more than the aggregate of individual doctors and the medical care system is more than the mere aggregate of its individual components. Thus, there is nothing contradictory between liking one's doctor and disliking elements of the corporativist behavior of the medical profession, nor between liking elements of the medical care system and disliking how those elements are organizationally and financially related.

The polls show that the majority of Americans have supported, for quite a number of years now, (a) the establishment of a tax-based comprehensive and universal health program, and (b) the federal control of doctors' fees, hospital costs, and prescription drugs (10–12). The implementation of these proposals would, indeed, mean major changes in medicine. The fact that the first proposal has never been implemented in the United States, and only very few elements of the second, has nothing to do with a nonexistent public schizophrenia, but rather with the power relations within America and its institutions of medicine, which continuously hinder the expression of the public's will. It is quite remarkable that in spite of the limited number of alternatives that are reasonably presented to the public by a highly conservative lay and professional media, the American public is farther ahead than its leaders in terms of needed changes. Contrary to widely held belief, the American media do not only reflect reality but create and reproduce the dominant vision of reality. And this vision tends to be heavily ideological. The use of certain terms are consistently identified with negative ones aimed at triggering a predetermined public response. When the public is asked whether they would like to see "welfare" expenditures reduced, they answer in the affirmative. It is wrong to conclude, however, as Blendon and Altman seem to do, that Americans are not sensitive toward the poor and that they are tolerant of reductions in programs aimed at them (such as Medicaid), as a way of controlling costs. The term "welfare" has been transformed by the media (with the constant image of the welfare cheater) into a heavily ideological one. But, if instead of "welfare" the question is broken down into the different components of welfare expenditures, the responses are dramatically different. The public supports them by large majorities (10). Indeed, the cutting of social (including health) federal expenditures is one of the areas where Americans are expressing major concern (13). Here, again, there is not a contradiction between the public's concern about the federal deficit and the perceived need to reduce it on the one hand, and public willingness to increase federal spending for health and other major expenditures on the other. The major reason for the high rise of the deficit since 1980 has been the largest economic recession since the Depression, occurring during the current [Reagan] administration, as well as the huge growth in military expenditures and the tax cut that has benefited, for the most part, the top 15 percent of the population (14). Thus, it is quite reasonable that the majority of Americans believe that the way of reducing the deficit is by cutting military defense expenditures and raising the taxes of the corporations and high-income individuals, rather than reducing social expenditures (15). The international experience shows that the United States could indeed afford larger federal health expenditures without necessarily enlarging the federal deficit. For example, the United Kingdom, Sweden, West Germany, and Canada have far larger percentages for health expenditures covered by public funds and all have lower government budget deficits than the United States (16).

In summary, the fact that the United States is the only developed, industrialized society—besides South Africa—that does not guarantee efficient and effective health care to the whole population is not due to the schizophrenia of the American public but, rather, to the unresponsiveness of American institutions to the public wishes, which are consistent, reasonable, and clear. The majority of Americans—although not their leaders—want to see major expansions of federal health expenditures side-by-side with major changes in the organization and funding of health care. The possibility and probability of those changes occurring does not depend on the development of consensus but on changes in the power relations within and outside American institutions—making them more responsive to the wishes of the majority of Americans.

REFERENCES

1. Navarro, V. A response to conventional wisdom. *Health Aff.* 3(3): 137–139, Fall 1984.
2. Altman, D. E. What do Americans really want? *Health Aff.* 3(3): 139–141, Fall 1984.
3. Blendon, R. J., and Altman, D. E. Special Report: Public attitudes about health care costs: A lesson in national schizophrenia. *N. Engl. J. Med.* 311(9): 613–616, 1984.
4. Direct payment for consumers. In *Health and Wealth: An International Study of Health Care Expenditures,* edited by R. J. Maxwell, p. 65, Fig. 4-4. Lexington Books, Lexington, Mass., 1981.
5. Gibson, R. M., Waldo, R., and Lairt, K. R. The national health expenditures 1982. *Health Care Financ. Rev.* 5(2): 1–31, 1983.
6. President's Commission for the Study of Ethical Problems in Medicine and Biomedical and Behavioral Research. *Securing Access to Medical Care,* Vols. 1–3. Government Printing Office, Washington, D. C., 1983.
7. Davis, K., and Rowland, D. Uninsured and underserved: Inequities in health care in the United States. *Health and Society* 61: 149, 1983.
8. Califano, J., Secretary of HEW. Memorandum to the President of the United States on national health insurance, May 22, 1978.
9. Louis Harris Poll. *Updated Report on Access to Health Care for the American People.* Robert Wood Johnson Foundation, Princeton, N.J., 1983.
10. Navarro, V. Where is the popular mandate? *N. Engl. J. Med.* 307: 1516, 1982.
11. Schneider, W. Public ready for real change in health care. *National Journal* 3(23): 664, 1985.
12. Louis Harris. *Equitable Health Care Survey.* May–June, 1983.
13. Shriver, J. (ed.). The most important problem. *Gallup Rep.* 220–221: 28–29, 1984.
14. Ackerman, F. *Reaganomics, Rhetoric and Reality.* South End Press, Boston, 1983.
15. Lipset, S. M. Poll after poll after poll warns President on programs. *New York Times,* January 13, 1982, p. 23.
16. Navarro, V. Selected myths guiding the Reagan Administration's health policies. *J. Public Health Policy* 5(1): 65, 1984.

Conclusion

Robert Chernomas and Ardeshir Sepehri

The most recent data comparing the U.S. and Canadian health care systems suggest that the previous trend of a more rapid growth of U.S. health expenditures as percentage of GDP has begun to accelerate. In 1975 the Canadian figure was 7.1 percent, while the U.S. figure was 8.4 percent; by 1993 the corresponding figures were 10.1 and 14.4 percent. Since 1991 the Canadian growth has flattened out, but the U.S. figure grew by 2 percent between 1991 and 1993. In Canada the percentage was 9.9 percent in 1991 and 10.1 percent in 1993; the U.S. percentage grew from 13.2 percent in 1991 to 14.4 percent in 1993. The rate of increase in Canada declined from 3.9 percent in 1991 to 0.06 percent and 1.1 percent in 1992 and 1993, respectively. Overall real per capita health expenditures in Canada declined in 1992 and stabilized in 1993. Of potential interest is the fact that public health expenditures decreased in 1992 and 1993 as a percentage of overall health expenditures whereas the percentage for the private sector increased in both years. In addition, real per capita health expenditures for both hospitals and physicians declined in 1992 and 1993, but real per capita drug expenditures continued to grow (data from *National Health Expenditures in Canada, 1975–1993*, Policy and Consultation Branch, Health Canada, 1994).

In Canada, the trend by a series of federal governments to reduce their responsibility for direct health care expenditures has been accelerated by design under the current Liberal Government. This trend has resulted in a further reduction of federal transfers and replacement of direct expenditures with a transfer of tax points, giving the provinces increasing control over their health care institutions. Critics of this devolution of federal financial responsibility suggest that the federal government is giving up the financial power to enforce the public administration, portability, comprehensiveness, and accessibility promised by the Canada Health Act. The results could be user fees, extra-billing, increased privatization, and a two-class, more expensive, less accessible system.

In the United States, the recent failure to reform the system from the top leaves the chaotic process of reform from below to its own hodgepodge of devices. In

303

the private sector, business spending on health care continues to grow as a percentage of profit. Health care costs are the fastest growing segment of production costs. The effort to cut costs by profit-maximizing firms has led to pressure on employee-based insurance providers and to labor conflict as firms attempt to reduce their responsibility for employees' health care costs. The public sector's preoccupation with deficits and debts has led to attempts to reform Medicaid and Medicare, resulting in political conflict with voters. Providers are confronted with an increasingly bureaucratic and expensive delivery system, while patients are confronted by a bewildering array of options, all seeming to either raise their out-of-pocket expenses, reduce their services, or limit their choice of practitioner.

In the public sector, concerns about health care costs, and outcomes collide with the need to expand services to a growing uninsured population. The growing costs, poor U.S. health care statistics, and declining access all invite purchasers of public and private services to seek new ways of controlling costs while improving quality of outcomes.

The U.S. system is in crisis in the sense that it is going through qualitative change, its very institutional structure now in transition. The Canadian system is being strained to the breaking point, but as yet it is maintaining its institutional framework. Qualitative transition and institutional strain indicate a need for research.

For economists this means continuing the debates on how to measure and what to measure in terms of health care costs. The debate on what to measure may be the more underdeveloped of the two. Capital costs, research and development, population mix, and the costs of equitable access are all underdeveloped areas for research, important for both the United States and Canada. Failure to implement managed competition from the top and a continued bias toward a market structure for health care in the United States suggest that economists need to continue their investigation of the advantages and disadvantages of competition, marketing, and profit maximizing in the health care sector in contrast to the advantages and disadvantages of a single-payer system.

Of equal importance, researchers should be careful about identifying the sectors of the health system being studied and their relationship to the system as a whole. If the U.S. system of diagnosis-related groups is effective at cost control the question becomes: Is it as effective at providing quality of care? If the answer is yes, what is the impact on costs and quality in the rest of the U.S. system if it is only partially constrained? An analogy in Canada would be to contrast cost and quality in the government-constrained hospital, physician, and administrative sectors with those subsectors left to the market.

For researchers studying the access issue the debate must go beyond waiting lists versus the uninsured and underinsured to a careful accounting of who is actually missing what. Some rationing may always be an issue. The question becomes: What are the mortality, morbidity, functioning, and physical and psychological health consequences of waiting or outright exclusion that exists for consumers in the two systems? And what sort of protocols and financing alternatives might improve the process?

Probably the most underdeveloped research area surveyed in this book is that of medical outcomes in the two countries. In the United States, with greater hospital expenditures per patient stay than in Canada and greater use of technology than anywhere else in the world, the question becomes: What impact does this have on mortality, morbidity, functioning, and discomfort vis-à-vis Canada, which spends less and uses less technology? The authors in the few studies alone thus far, as represented in this book, suggest some answers to this question for a few significant medical procedures. A lot of resources and a great deal of human welfare depend on such studies being extended to a broader range of medical interventions.

And finally, researchers must continue to gather and analyze information on the political viability of and consumer satisfaction with the two systems. This is essential as the two systems continue to change, buffeted about by political and economic forces and by issues internal to the health systems themselves.

Index

California. *See* Coronary artery bypass
surgery (CABS)
California Blue Shield, 25
Canada Health Act, 2, 3, 88, 303
Canada's National Health Program
(NHP). *See* also various subject
headings
cardiac-related diagnoses and interventions, 148-150
criteria for provincial plans eligibility
for federal subsidy, 2
difficulties in getting needed medical
care, 146-147
length of stay in hospitals, 151-152
minimum standards for provincial
programs, 145
physician visits per capita, 148, 151
rating the, Canadians, 147-148
safety valve for Canada, U.S. as a, 91,
93, 97, 158, 165
serious symptoms, 146
shortcomings, 88-90
transplants, 150
*Canadian Health Care: The Implications
of Public Health Insurance*
(Neuschler), 66
Capital costs, 84, 95, 103-104, 111
Cardiac-related diagnoses and interventions, 148-150. *See also*
Coronary artery bypass surgery
(CABS)
Cardiovascular surgery
postsurgical mortality, 264
waiting lists, 164-167, 176-179, 184,
191, 194-199, 201, 207-209
Carotid endarterectomy, 217, 219, 220,
260, 263
Case-mix differences, 45, 47, 48, 215,
257-259
Cash collections, fee-for-service, 25
Catastrophic illness, 135-136, 156, 300
Centralization of the cost-control process,
19-20
Cholecystectomy, 217, 219, 220, 260, 263
Clinical outcomes and cost sharing
groups, 139-140. *See also* Post-
surgical mortality

Coalitions, community/business, 291
Coinsurance, 33, 136-137, 139
Community coalitions, 291
Comorbidity in the population, 259
Comprehensiveness and Canadian Health
care system, 2
Computed tomographic (CT) scans,
174
Copayments. *See* Out-of-pocket payments
Coronary angiography and appropriateness standards, 241-246, 250-253
Coronary artery bypass surgery
(CABS)
age distributions, 230-232, 236-237,
238
appropriateness ratings, 241-244,
246-253
control over resources, 228, 237
financial barriers, 237-238
income, 233-235
limitations of the data, 235-236
methods for studying, 228-230
percutaneous transluminal coronary
angioplasty, 236
postsurgical mortality, 217, 219, 220,
222, 260, 263
quality and access to care, differences
in, 227
rates per number of adults, 230, 231
Cost-control process
ambivalent feelings about, publics',
286-288
appropriateness standards, 241
centralization of, 19-20
cost sharing on health outcomes, effect
of, 139-140
effectiveness of, 78-80
HIAA's analysis, 67-71
hospitals, 14-16
personal health care arrangements,
concerns over, 288
public's view of available choices,
290-292
shortcomings of Canadian system,
88-90
uninsured/underinsured population
colliding with, 4, 304